D1256194

EMERGENCY NURSING

EMERGENCY NURSING

Edited by JEANIE BARRY, R.N., M.S.

CRITICAL CARE NURSING INSTRUCTOR
EMERGENCY MEDICAL SERVICES PROGRAM OF HAWAII

McGRAW-HILL BOOK COMPANY
A BLAKISTON PUBLICATION
NEW YORK   ST. LOUIS   SAN FRANCISCO
AUCKLAND   BOGOTÁ   DÜSSELDORF   JOHANNESBURG
LONDON   MADRID   MEXICO   MONTREAL
NEW DELHI   PANAMA   PARIS
SÃO PAULO   SINGAPORE
SYDNEY   TOKYO
TORONTO

NOTICE   Nursing is an ever-changing science. As new research and clinical experience broaden our knowledge, changes in treatment and drug therapy are required. The editors and the publisher of this work have made every effort to ensure that the drug dosage schedules herein are accurate and in accord with the standards accepted at the time of publication. Readers are advised, however, to check the product information sheet included in the package of each drug they plan to administer to be certain that changes have not been made in the recommended dose or in the contraindications for administration. This recommendation is of particular importance in regard to new or infrequently used drugs.

EMERGENCY NURSING

Copyright © 1978 by McGraw-Hill, Inc. All rights reserved. Printed in the United States of America. No part of this publication may be reproduced, stored in a retrieval system, or transmitted, in any form or by any means, electronic, mechanical, photocopying, recording, or otherwise, without the prior written permission of the publisher.

1 2 3 4 5 6 7 8 9 0   DODO   7 8 3 2 1 0 9 8 7

This book was set in Souvenir Light by Monotype Composition Company, Inc. The editors were Orville W. Haberman, Jr., James W. Bradley, and Henry C. De Leo; the designer was Ben Kann; the production supervisor was Robert C. Pedersen. The drawings were done by Russ Peterson. R. R. Donnelley & Sons Company was printer and binder.

Library of Congress Cataloging in Publication Data

Main entry under title:

Emergency nursing.
      "A Blakiston publication."
      Bibliography: p.
      Includes index.
      1. Emergency nursing.   I.   Barry, Jeanie.
[DNLM: 1.   Emergencies.   2.   Nursing care.   WY156
E52]
RT120.E4E47   610.73'6   77-1436
ISBN 0-07-003839-2

to DAVID

CONTENTS

LIST OF
CONTRIBUTORS

Jeanie Barry, R.N., M.S., Critical Care Nursing Instructor, Emergency Medical Services Program of Hawaii, Honolulu, Hawaii

Dorothy A. Bicks, R.N., Nursing Education, Queen's Medical Center, Honolulu, Hawaii

Geralee Bumbaugh, R.N., Mobile Intensive Care Nurse, Los Angeles, California

Pamela K. Burkhalter, R.N., M.S.N., M.A., Nursing Consultant, Honolulu, Hawaii

Percival H. Y. Chee, M.D., F.A.C.S., Clinical Assistant Professor of Surgery (Ophthalmology), University of Hawaii School of Medicine, Consultant in Ophthalmology, Tripler Army Medical Center, Honolulu, Hawaii

Gwendolyn R. Costello, R.N., M.P.H., Nursing Consultant—Research Coordinator, Child Protective Services Center, Kauikeolani Children's Hospital, Honolulu, Hawaii

Virginia R. Dods, R.N., Emergency Medical Technician Instructor, Emergency Medical Services Program of Hawaii, Honolulu, Hawaii

Gene W. Doo, B.A., M.D., Assistant Professor: Otolaryngology, University of Hawaii School of Medicine, Honolulu, Hawaii

J. B. Greenwell, Jr., B.A., M.D., Surgeon—Honolulu Medical Group, Clinical Associate Professor of Surgery, University of Hawaii School of Medicine, Honolulu, Hawaii

Samuel C. Gresham, M.D., Cardiologist, Member of Hawaii's CPR Faculty and Queen's Medical Center CPR Committee, Honolulu, Hawaii

Sandra Gresham, R.N., M.Ed., Executive Director, Hawaii Nurses' Association, Honolulu, Hawaii

Jean T. Grippin, R.N., M.S., Clinical Specialist—Psychiatry, Queen's Medical Center, Honolulu, Hawaii

Robert C. Hinman, B.S., M.D., Associate Professor of Medicine, University of Hawaii School of Medicine, Honolulu, Hawaii

Carl P. Hollenborg, M.D., Chief Medical Resident, University of Hawaii Integrated Medical Residency Program, Honolulu, Hawaii

Jill D. Holmes, R.N., M.S., Cardiovascular Clinical Nursing Specialist, Los Altos, California

Carol Ann Isaac, Capt., A.N.C., R.N., M.Ed., Clinical Nurse—Surgical Intensive Care and Trauma Unit, Tripler Army Medical Center, Honolulu, Hawaii

Christine N. Langworthy, M.S.W., A.C.S.W., Psychiatric Social Worker, Lanai, Hawaii

Marlene Moniz, R.N., C.R.T.T., Clinical Coordinator—Respiratory Therapy, Kauikeolani Children's Hospital, Honolulu, Hawaii

Eileen Mulqueeney, R.N., M.S.N., Assistant Specialist, University of Hawaii, Honolulu, Hawaii

Maurice W. Nicholson, M.D., Attending Neurosurgeon and Clinical Instructor, Department of Neurosurgery, Queen's Medical Center, Honolulu, Hawaii

James Penoff, M.D. F.A.C.S., Department of Plastic and Reconstructive Surgery, Straub Clinic and Hospital, Honolulu, Hawaii

Reta M. H. Pozzi, R.N., Mobile Intensive Care Technician Instructor, Emergency Medical Services Program of Hawaii, Honolulu, Hawaii

Richard K. Quinn, Esq., Medical Malpractice Defense Attorney, Anthony, Hoddick, Reinwald and O'Connor, Honolulu, Hawaii

Judith Ramseyer, M.D., Assistant Professor, Department of Medicine, University of Hawaii School of Medicine, Honolulu, Hawaii

Laurence A. Reich, M.D., Assistant Professor, Department of Obstetrics and Gynecology, University of Hawaii School of Medicine, Honolulu, Hawaii

Lizabeth Love Ryan, R.N., Emergency Nurse, Lawrence and Memorial Hospitals, New London, Connecticut

J. K. Sims, M.D., Training Coordinator, Emergency Medical Services Program of Hawaii, President-Elect, American College of Emergency Physicians, Hawaii Chapter, Honolulu, Hawaii

Mary Wieland, R.N., M.S., Critical Care Clinical Nursing Instructor, Emergency Medical Services Program of Hawaii, Honolulu, Hawaii

FOREWORD

EMERGENCY medical service (EMS) systems are a new and much needed development in the national health-care delivery system. A systems approach to field casualty care has been progressively improved during each successive military conflict since the Civil War. These improvements were initiated after the medical-care and evacuation disaster experienced by the Union Army of the Potomac at Bull Run on July 21, 1861. From this chaotic awakening, a series of reorganizations of the army surgeons, medical corps, ambulances and hospitals was undertaken. During the Civil War, major changes in administration, professional personnel, transportation, hospitals, sanitation, and medical records established patterns that have been continually refined and improved and have been largely responsible for the modern improvements in military field-casualty survival.

Stimulated by pressing demands of war surgery, and coupled with parallel advances in medical care over the last century, an almost unbelievable level of performance was realized in the Vietnam war. Advances in field resuscitation, efficiency of transportation, and energetic treatment of military casualties have proved to be major factors in the decrease in death rates of battle casualties reaching medical facilities: from 8 percent in World War I to 4.5 percent in World War II to 2.5 percent in Korea and to less than 2 percent in Vietnam. As has been repeatedly demonstrated in previous military conflicts, the rapid evacuation of the critically injured to adequately staffed and equipped advanced-treatment units has shown that a highly perfected and well-operated EMS system can also save lives in the civilian peacetime community. While there are considerable differences between the civilian peactime community and a battlefield, many principles for an areawide trauma-system design for accident-patient care are transferable and can be successfully implemented into statewide and regional programs for the comprehensive care of the injured.

It is of some bewilderment and much concern as to why the lessons learned so dearly in the military conflicts over the last half century have not been more effectively incorporated in the peacetime civilian environment. The need for such a system is, of course, as great and even exceeds the need for such a system in the military sphere. Seventy million citizens in this country receive emergency department care each year. Within this massive group of emergency patient responses there are several types of critically ill and injured who require for their survival a competent EMS system response as outlined below:

• Trauma, the third largest killer in the United States, claims 115,000 lives annually and permanently disables an additional 400,000.

• Two million burn accidents occur annually, and less than 10 percent of the 75,000 major burn victims currently receive organized burn care.

• Ten thousand spinal cord injuries occur each year. Only a relatively few (less than 10 percent) of these patients reach special care centers within 4 to 6 hours from injury and are then adequately treated and able to return to active employment.

• It is estimated that 1.0 to 1.5 million people experience acute myocardial infarction each year; one-half of these usually die within 2 hours of the onset of symptoms without any prehospital or hospital emergency care.

• It is known that 2.5 to 3.0 percent of all children born each year have congenital abnormalities and/or difficulty because of size and prematurity which may be lethal or have long-term effects on physiological or mental development. Improved neonatal and perinatal care of these children can reduce major complications by 50 percent if proper recognition, transportation, and special care are provided.

• Each year there are approximately 5 million poisonings. Of these cases, 90 percent involve children; poisoning remains the fourth largest cause of death for children.

• With the recognition of alcoholism as a health problem in this country, the EMS system will be the entry point into health care for an enormous increase of patients with these chemical-physio-logical-psychological problems.

• It is appreciated that psychiatric disturbances may result in suicides. Suicide ranks second as a cause of death for adolescents and college students. Emergency mental health programs must be established and integrated into the existing EMS system, with humane care and major improvements in triage for these and other behavioral emergencies.

The EMS system must be comprehensive and totally operative because of the very nature and needs of these acute and critically injured patients. The EMS system requires purposeful planning. This involves improved reporting and access; better response systems; improved field stabilization and care enroute; optimal resuscitation at the initial care facility; and well-executed, progressive, intensive, critical care from the interhospital phase to the advanced, critical-care treatment and rehabilitation phases.

While there is considerable, justifiable interest in emergency facilities, communications, transportation and treatment techniques, it must be understood that it is really the trained technical and professional EMS personnel working as a team who make the difference in saving the lives of emergency patients. Each EMS professional from the field, hospital emergency departments, and critical-care elements must be adequately prepared to provide a level of clinical judgment and skills appropriate to the demands of each emergency patient.

The EMS team includes all of those professionals involved with the planning, coordination, and provision of emergency care through the entire system. As these new and established team members are identified [nurses, physicians, emergency medical technicians (EMT), systems coordinators, and directors] new roles and interrelationships will need to be identified and refined. Considerable attention and progress has been made in upgrading prehospital emergency personnel: emergency medical technicians—ambulance (EMT-A), and emergency medical technicians—paramedics (EMT-P). Emphasis is currently being placed on cardiopulmonary resuscitation (CPR) training for citizens and other non-EMS personnel (e.g., public safety personnel such as fire fighters, police officers, and lifeguards). Unfortunately, too little attention has been given to an essential element of the EMS team—the emergency department nurse. Nurses working in emergency departments and in critical-care units have not been given the proper attention, educational opportunities, funds, or materials to maintain and upgrade their knowledge and skills so they can perform at their highest potential. Nurses employed in critical-care centers have enjoyed more intensive educational opportunities because of the high demand for their skills and their close association with physicians interested in developing a true team concept in the critical-care specialties.

Emergency department nurses and their educational needs have only very recently come into focus as an essential part of the EMS team. With this long overdue recognition, the emergency department nurses must assert their obvious need for continued education, expanded educational opportunities, and special educational tools.

Emergency nurses play a key role in a changing delivery system and are part of a very flexible and interdependent EMS team. The acute demands of emergency patients require competent nursing personnel with the essential skills, background, and judgment to anticipate and treat occult injuries and illness in order to prevent complications and further deterioration of the critically ill and injured patients. The emergency department nurse must be a clinical specialist who is able to function independently in the busy emergency department even when physicians are readily available. This is true and even more important in the rural hospital where the physician is often unavailable and where the emergency nurses must function independently in order to serve the needs of those seriously ill patients in their charge.

As EMS systems further develop, a select number of emergency department nurses will find their skills and responsibilities extending beyond the emergency department walls via radio and telephonic linkages (telemetry) to paramedics in the prehospital phase. This group of nurses should readily accept this new challenge and take a leadership position in the training of these prehospital EMT-A and paramedics. These nurses should also assume positions of responsibility in on-line supervision of these new team members as they perform life saving techniques beyond and during transport to the hospital.

Another select group of emergency department and critical-care nurses will be called upon to occasionally leave their hospital environment to assist in resuscitation care at an accident scene and also to travel from regional advanced-care centers to outlying hospital facilities to assist nurses and physicians in maintaining and furthering life support during intrahospital transportation.

In order to attain some of the goals outlined above, *Emergency*

Nursing is a major contribution to this important, national effort and one that will greatly assist the currently developing educational programs for emergency department nurses. The text is clear, concise, and represents the most modern techniques that should be used by all emergency personnel. The text of this book is comprehensive in all areas with which the emergency department nurse should be familiar. The sections on biological basics and pathophysiology are well written. I am pleased to see that a major section of this book deals with the emotional aspects of communicating with patients' friends and family under very stressful conditions. The emergency department nurse has traditionally been called upon to assist the grieving family, who usually are not prepared to receive the catastrophic news of an emergent illness or death. The instruction of this text will assist in further developing the emergency nurse's competence in communication skills and will add an essential, humane aspect to emergency care.

This textbook is written primarily by nurses for nurses. It meets most of the needs of emergency department educational programs, and it is a welcome addition to the rapidly expanding literature for emergency personnel. The Emergency Department Nurses Association (EDNA) has recently developed a core curriculum for emergency nurse education and *Emergency Nursing* should serve as an excellent text for this educational program. *Emergency Nursing* is an important addition to the library of every educational program for emergency department nurses. In this rapidly developing field, even this comprehensive text will need periodic revision, and I trust that the editor and authors will respond to this obligation with the same vigor and clarity as they have incorporated into this initial edition.

The authors and, most importantly, the editor of this text are to be congratulated for this excellent addition to the literature of emergency health care.

DAVID R. BOYD, M.D.C.M.
Director,
Division of Emergency Medical Services,
U.S. Department of Health, Education, and Welfare

PREFACE

IN the past, the greatest advances in emergency medical care have been in wartime. War, with its multiple-trauma patients, has been a testing ground for the improvement of emergency medical care. However, with the increase in high-speed transportation accidents and other emergencies associated with highly populated urban areas, emergency medical care has gained more and more importance.

The concept of an emergency medical services system has been devised by Dr. David Boyd and propagated by the United States Department of Health, Education, and Welfare. The delivery of prehospital emergency care has been stressed by the emphasis on training of emergency medical technicians and paramedics and the development of sophisticated portable equipment. Too little has been written regarding the role of emergency department nurses and the knowledge necessary for them to render high-quality emergency nursing care.

Jeanie Barry, R.N., M.S., the editor and major contributing author of this book, is the Emergency and Intensive Care Nursing Instructor for the Emergency Medical Services (EMS) Program of Hawaii. The other contributing authors have lectured for this same program. The authors and editor have developed a very comprehensive textbook for emergency department nursing. The textbook is clear and concise; it presents the most modern techniques for various emergency situations.

This text has a great potential and should be widely used by emergency personnel. The authors and editor are reminded of the necessity to update this text from time to time in order to present the most current modes of therapy in emergency department treatment.

The EMS Program of Hawaii is federally funded through the Department of Health, Education, and Welfare to the City and County of Honolulu. Mayor Frank F. Fasi of Honolulu, Hawaii, has subcontracted the program to the Hawaii Medical Association. It is with these federal funds that *Emergency Nursing* has been written.

LIVINGSTON M. F. WONG, M.D.
Project Director
Emergency Medical Services
Honolulu, Hawaii

ONE

THE
BIOLOGIC BASIS
OF
EMERGENCY NURSING

CHAPTER 1
THE INTERNAL ENVIRONMENT OF THE BODY

EILEEN MULQUEENY, R.N., M.S.

T HE evaluation of the acutely ill or injured patient, by necessity, begins with a brief pertinent history and physical inspection. The initial neurological, cardiovascular, and respiratory assessments include observation of the level of consciousness, skin color and warmth, degree of movements, and respiratory and cardiac rate and rhythm. In performing these observations, the members of the health team must familiarize themselves with the internal status of the emergency patient. For them to accomplish this, knowledge of cell physiology, normal fluid and electrolyte theory, and the aberrations of specific pathologies must be part of their basic and continuing education.

Life is dependent on the integrity of cellular functioning. This functioning, in turn, is very much dependent on precise ranges of normal concentrations of fluids and electrolytes, both intracellular and extracellular. This chapter discusses the cell, its membrane, intracellular organelles, and cellular physiology. It also explores some of the major concepts concerning fluid and electrolyte theory.

THE CELL

As illustrated in Fig. 1-1, the cell is a complex "factory" of subcellular structures, called *organelles.* The major structures include the nucleus, nucleolus, cytoplasm, endoplasmic reticulum and ribosomes, Golgi complex, mitochondria, lysosomes, and the cell membrane.

Figure 1-1 Sketch of a generalized cell, with the organelles emphasized. *(Taken from Langley, L., Telford, I., and Christensen, J., Dynamic Anatomy and Physiology, 4th ed., McGraw-Hill, New York, 1974, p. 29.)*

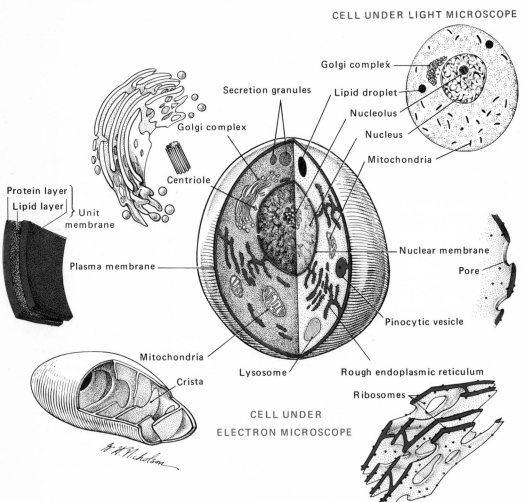

CELL UNDER LIGHT MICROSCOPE

Golgi complex

Lipid droplet

Nucleolus

Nucleus

Mitochondria

Secretion granules

Golgi complex

Centriole

Protein layer
Lipid layer
Unit membrane

Plasma membrane

Nuclear membrane

Pore

Pinocytic vesicle

Mitochondria

Crista

Lysosome

Rough endoplasmic reticulum

Ribosomes

CELL UNDER
ELECTRON MICROSCOPE

The *nucleus* is present in all cells that divide and consists largely of chromosomes. The basic unit of the chromosome is the gene which is responsible for regulating the hereditary characteristics of each person or animal. Deoxyribonucleic acid (DNA) is the building block of the gene.

A *nucleolus* is present in the nucleus of most cells, especially in growing cells, and is the probable site of synthesis of messenger ribonucleic acid (RNA). Messenger RNA is responsible for providing a template (i.e., model) for the synthesis of protein by the cell.

Cytoplasm is the viscid substance outside the nucleus (but inside the plasma membrane) which contains a variety of organelles. *Endoplasmic reticulum* is a series of tube-like passageways which provide a communication channel between the nucleus and the cytoplasm and the cytoplasm and the cell membrane. Granular endoplasmic reticulum is encrusted with dense particles called *ribosomes*. Ribosomes, containing 65 percent RNA and 35 percent protein, are sites of protein synthesis. Agranular or smooth endoplasmic reticulum (i.e., with no ribosomes) may be the site of steroid synthesis in some cells, while in others it is the site of detoxification of unnecessary cell substances.

The *Golgi complex* is a collection of tubules and vesicles near the nucleus. It is said to be an area where proteins, such as hormones and enzymes, are collected and wrapped in membranes so they can be stored as granules or enclosed particles for later secretion of the granule contents.

Mitochondria are centers of cellular respiration and energy production. Adenosine triphosphate (ATP), the principal energy source of the body, is synthesized within this organelle. Mitochondria are more abundant in areas of the cell where more energy is needed for biochemical processes. They are also seen in higher concentrations in cells requiring more energy output such as cardiac cells.

Lysosomes are organelles which contain enzymes capable of destroying most cellular components. Alien substances such as bacteria or necrotic cellular structures are engulfed into the lysosomes, destroyed, and then dumped into the cytoplasm for excretion.

The intracellular contents are completely enclosed by the *cell* or *plasma membrane*. This semipermeable structure allows *selective passive* movement of substances between the intra- and extracellular compartments. The membrane also actively *pumps* specific electrolytes to their appropriate compartment against natural concentration gradients. In addition, molecules and particles, such as glucose and hormones, are carried to the inside of the cell through this membrane.

FLUID AND ELECTROLYTES

The general and brief description of the cell and its structures given above can only allude to the complexities of the cellular activities needed to support the life processes. The continuation of these activities is dependent on appropriate nutrients and energy sources, as well as proper fluid and electrolyte concentrations. Cellular functions appear to have a narrow tolerance for change before toxic effects are manifested.

FLUID DISTRIBUTION

Approximately 60 percent of the body is composed of *water*. This amount may range from 45 to 75 percent depending on age and body composition. As illustrated in Fig. 1-2, the infant and baby, up to 1 year of age, have a high percentage of body water in comparison with body solids, whereas in the child and adult approximately 60 percent of the body consists of water. *Fat content* in the body also influences water content. Since fat is water-resistant, the higher the body fat content, the lower the percentage of body water.

Figure 1-2 Distribution of body water and solids in children and adults. *(Adapted from Talbot, R., and Crawford, J. D., Metabolic Homeostasis, Harvard University Press, Cambridge, Mass., 1959.)*

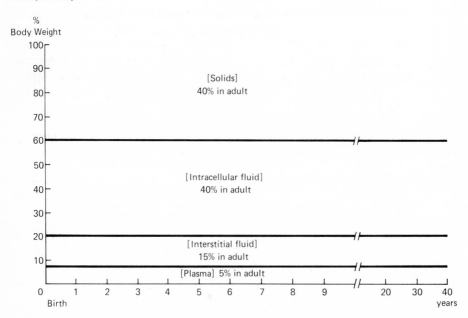

Water is distributed in two major compartments of the body, the *intracellular* and the *extracellular*. The extracellular compartment is subdivided into two areas—the *interstitial space* and the *plasma*. Intracellular fluid constitutes 40 percent of body weight, interstitial fluid 15 percent, and plasma (intravascular fluid) only 5 percent. A variety of pathologies and traumas can influence these normal distributions. Dehydration and overhydration can affect the fluid and electrolyte concentrations in the plasma. Edema or hemorrhage into the interstitial space can be a hidden area of fluid concentration and must be considered in the nursing assessment. Cellular dehydration and overhydration also influence fluid and electrolyte concentration in the intracellular compartment.

ELECTROLYTES AND NONELECTROLYTES

Aqueous solutions (or pure water) do not exist in the body. The fluid distributed in all the compartments has a variety of particles or solutes dissolved in it at all times. Some of these particles are electrolytes and others are nonelectrolytes. An *electrolyte* is a compound which dissociates into ions when dissolved in water. *Ions* may be defined as electrically charged particles. A positively charged ion is called a *cation*, and a negatively charged particle is referred to as an *anion*.

The ionic charge is dependent on an imbalance between the number of orbiting electrons (negative charge) and protons (positive charge) found in the nucleus of the atom (see Fig. 1-3). Since an anion needs a positive charge to be balanced electrically and the cation needs a negative charge, a physical attraction exists between them. When united, they form a stable electrolyte. The term "electrolyte" is commonly misused in references to singular ions such as potassium, but this need not be a stumbling block. Pure ions are not given therapeutically, but rather are given in an electrolyte form.

Figure 1-3 Schematic representation of (*a*) an atom possessing no electric charge; (*b*) an atom representing an anion; and (*c*) an atom representing a cation. (+ is a proton; N is a neutron, which has no electric charge; − is an electron.)

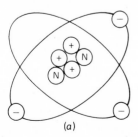
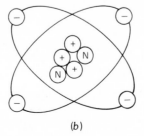
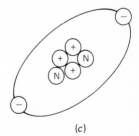

(*a*)   (*b*)   (*c*)

Examples of these electrolytes are sodium chloride, sodium bicarbonate, potassium chloride, and magnesium sulfate.

MILLIEQUIVALENCY

All ions exert an electric force which is dependent on their electric charge. An ion may have more than one electric charge, which implies that there is an imbalance of more than one electron in comparison with the protons. The number of unbalanced electric charges a particle has, either positive or negative, is referred to as its *valence*. Potassium (K^+) and sodium (Na^+) are monovalent cations. Magnesium (Mg^{++}), a bivalent cation, has two free positive electric charges. It is one ion, but it has two electric equivalents or charges which must be balanced by two negative electric charges. Electrolytes, or ions, are most commonly reported in *milliequivalents*. Milliequivalency refers to the number of electric charges available rather than to the number of molecules present. If, for example, 10 ions of magnesium were in solution, this would be reported as 20 equivalents because there are two charges per atom. Ten ions of sodium, a monovalent ion, would be reported as 10 equivalents. (A milliequivalent is 1/1000 of an equivalent.)

Electrolytes are extremely important in the maintenance of the cellular functions, and their distribution in the body compartments is quite specific. Figure 1-4 depicts the normal concentrations of the major body electrolytes in the plasma, the interstitial compartment, and the cell. Later in this chapter, a more specific explanation of the actions of the major electrolytes in the cell is provided. At present, though, it is important to recall that the concentrations of electrolyte vary greatly in the two major compartments of the body. Since practitioners must rely on plasma values as a determinant of electrolyte levels, they must constantly remember that these values only indirectly reflect the electrolyte values of the intracellular compartment.

Figure 1-4 also depicts the level of nonelectrolyte solids in these compartments. Nonelectrolytes carry no electric charge, but they serve a very important role in the regulation of fluid distribution in the body as well as function in a nutritional or metabolic role. Both electrolytes and nonelectrolytes participate in the dynamic movement of fluid and electrolytes by diffusion and osmosis.

PRESSURE GRADIENTS

As described above, the cell membrane is a selective semipermeable membrane. In addition, it is the site of an active transport mechanism which pumps many electrolytes against their natural concentration level. Due to these concentration differences, pressure gradients are created.

DIFFUSION Since nature is constantly attempting to remove imbalances, there tends to be a movement of molecules from an area of *higher* concentration to an area of *lower* concentration. This movement is called *diffusion*. It occurs in gases, liquids, and solids and does not require an active energy transport system. Diffusion ceases once equilibrium is reached. Since the cell's ability to respond to an electric stimulus is dependent on the maintenance of a concentration difference, the cell membrane must work to prevent this equilibrium. This takes a large amount of energy which is supplied to the cell membrane from the subcellular structures, especially from the mitochondria.

OSMOSIS Since the cell membrane prevents diffusion of the electrolytes and nonelectrolytes from achieving total equilibrium, *water* moves through this semipermeable membrane from areas of *lower* particle concentration to areas of *higher* concentration. This movement helps to

Figure 1-4 Electrolyte and nonelectrolyte distribution in the capillary, the interstitial space, and the cell.

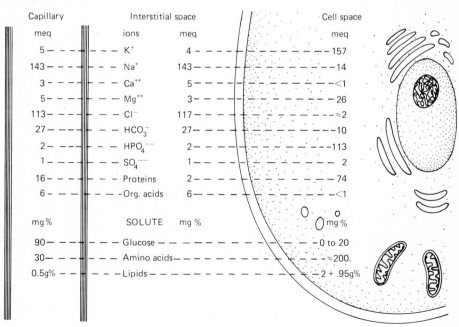

Capillary	Interstitial space		Cell space
meq	ions	meq	meq
5	K⁺	4	157
143	Na⁺	143	14
3	Ca⁺⁺	5	<1
5	Mg⁺⁺	3	26
113	Cl⁻	117	≈2
27	HCO₃⁻	27	10
2	HPO₄⁻⁻	2	113
1	SO₄⁻⁻	1	2
16	Proteins	2	74
6	Org. acids	6	<1
mg %	SOLUTE mg %		mg %
90	Glucose		0 to 20
30	Amino acids		≈200.
0.5g%	Lipids		2 + .95g%

dilute the highly concentrated areas, thus reducing the pressure gradient. Because of the increased flow of water, total weight or volume on the concentrated side of the membrane increases. This movement of water is called *osmosis;* it is a physical process which requires no outside energy source and ends when concentration differences disappear. Since water passes freely through most membranes, all fluids in the body are in osmotic equilibrium.

OSMOLARITY   Osmotic pressure is the drawing force that is exerted by particles to attract water to them. The particles, regardless of their electric charge or their weight, exert a force to draw water from another area. The *osmolarity,* or the measurement of the osmotic pressure of the molecules or particles in solution, can give information about the concentration status of the circulating blood volume and can help the nurse to anticipate the consequences of abnormal concentrations. Normal plasma osmolarity is about 270 to 290 milliosmoles per kilogram (mosmol/kg).

If the osmolarity of the blood volume is increased over the normal value by loss of intravascular water, hemoconcentration occurs. This means that the percentage of fluid (i.e., plasma) in the blood would be lower and the number of dissolved particles would be higher. Such *hyperosmolarity* could be caused by fluid loss from vomiting, diarrhea, or hemorrhage. An abnormally high solute content, as seen in polycythemia vera or with excessive parenteral infusion of salt, dextrose, or other solutes, can also cause an increase in serum osmolarity.

Hypoosmolarity, or an abnormally lowered number of particles in solution in the blood, could indicate overhydration from excessive parenteral administration or excessive solute loss (especially plasma proteins) as in malnutrition. Renal or hormonal disease resulting in abnormally high urinary loss of electrolytes can also cause hypoosmolarity.

Any state of abnormal osmolarity can alter drug action. Overdose effects in hyperosmolar states and lack of desired therapeutic effects in hypoosmolarity must be anticipated. Symptoms of cellular malfunction throughout the body must be also anticipated. With hyperosmolarity, fluid moves from the cell to help dilute plasma concentration, resulting in cell shrinkage; with hypoosmolarity, water moves from the extracellular compartment into the cell, causing cellular swelling. In either state, cell irritability and malfunction can result, especially in the nerves and muscles of a seriously injured or ill patient. Initial manifestations are observed in an abnormal mental response ranging from apprehension, confusion, listlessness, or drowsiness to coma. Gastrointestinal symptoms such as nausea, vomiting and diarrhea, and muscular cramping or weakness are not unusual. Cardiac arrhythmias vary from occasional premature beats to serious arrhythmias such as ventricular tachycardias or ventricular fibrillation. Congestive heart failure may also occur if fluid overload is the cause of the hypoosmolarity. Many of the above symptoms are due to electrolyte imbalances resulting from a change in osmolarity.

FLUID MOVEMENT AT THE CAPILLARY LEVEL *Hydrostatic pressure:* As blood moves through the cardiovascular system from the heart toward the microcirculation, blood pressure progressively decreases from its highest pressure area in the left ventricle to the capillaries (see Fig. 3-13). The pressure created by the flow of blood through and against the constantly narrowing vascular tree is called the *hydrostatic pressure.* Once the blood reaches the capillary level, the hydrostatic pressure is no longer resisted by thick impermeable arterial walls. Rather, the capillary walls are thin membranes which have many semipermeable pores. The walls are impermeable only to large particles such as proteins, red blood cells, and large sugar molecules. Thus, even though the hydrostatic pressure is greatly decreased in the capillaries, the vascular walls offer minimal resistance to this pressure, and outward filtration is enhanced. Fluid in the interstitial space also creates a small amount of hydrostatic pressure resulting from the constant movement of fluid within this space. A portion of this fluid movement is directed toward the vascular tree and resists the hydrostatic pressure generated inside the capillary wall.

Colloidal pressures: A specific type of osmotic pressure due solely to plasma colloids, especially *plasma proteins,* is called *colloidal osmotic pressure* or the *oncotic pressure.* Due to their large size, plasma protein molecules are relatively nondiffusable into the interstitial space and create an osmotic pressure. The osmotic pull or pressure is a very strong force keeping fluid in the vascular compartment. Protein in the interstitial space exerts the same water-drawing force.

Figure 1-5 illustrates and explains the joint effect of hydrostatic and colloidal pressure at the capillary level.

ACTIVE TRANSPORT Movement of fluid and solutes at the capillary level occurs from diffusion and osmosis; this does not require an active energy transport system. Tissues receive necessary nutrients, oxygen, fluid, and electrolytes and eliminate unneeded substances by a constant flux between the capillaries and tissues.

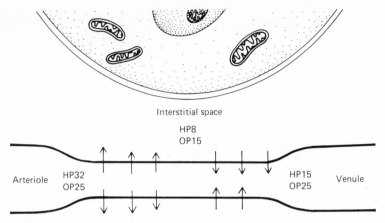

Interstitial space

HP8
OP15

Arteriole   HP32
OP25   HP15   Venule
                                        OP25

Figure 1-5 Schematic representation of pressure gradients and filtration at the capillary level: the arrow indicates direction of filtration flow; HP is hydrostatic pressure; OP is oncotic pressure. At the arteriolar end an HP of 32 mmHg is forcing outward filtration while an OP of 25 mmHg resists this flow. The result is a 7-mmHg filtration gradient. The tissue resists this capillary flow with an HP of 8 mmHG but enhances the filtration with 15 mmHg OP, resulting in a 7-mmHg drawing force. The net arteriolar filtration gardient is 14 mmHg. At the venule end, HP decreases to 15 mmHg, but the OP remains the same, and so there is an inward capillary pull of 10 mmHg. The tissue pressures remain the same with 7 mmHg resistance. Therefore, fluid is reabsorbed into the capillary pressure gradient of 3 mmHg.

At the cellular level, an *active transport* mechanism is needed to pump electrolytes into and out of the cell. This cellular active transport system is often called the "sodium pump" and works *against* normal pressure gradients (see Fig. 1-6). The energy to run this pump is supplied by the intracellular breakdown of glucose (see Fig. 5-6). The main task of this pump is to actively contribute to the dynamic equilibrium of intracellular sodium and potassium.

As Fig. 1-4 shows, all the electrolytes and nonelectrolytes exhibit concentration differences across membranes. The cell's ability to remain in a living, responsive state depends on the cell membrane's ability to maintain fairly exact differences in intracellular and extracellular concentrations. These differences create a *resting potential,* which implies that a concentration difference is being actively created by the sodium pump. When this active transport ceases, ionic fluxes occur in an effort to reestablish a homeostatic or equilibrium state. Movement of these particles can generate an electric current which is spread throughout the cell and to all adjacent cells. These cells also have a potential and are therefore capable of being stimulated. The major ions responsible for the creation of the resting potential are potassium, sodium, chloride, and anionic intracellular protein.

ELECTRICAL GRADIENT   In the resting cell, there exist not only concentration differences across the plasma membrane but also total electric charge differences. At the cell membrane, there tends to be a faster movement of potassium to the outside of the cell in comparison with the slower movement of sodium to the inside of the cell. This contributes to an *electronegative* charge which exists *intracellularly*. There is also a large number of anionic intracellular proteins which are relatively nondiffusable. These anions, along with the high intracellular concentration of the anionic phosphates, contribute to a strong intracellular negative electric charge of approximately -90 mV for nerve, skeletal muscle, and cardiac cells. (The exact electronegativity measurements vary above and below -90 mV, depending on the cell type.)

Thus, the cell membrane creates many differences in concentration and electric charges. Without differences, there would be no resting potential; the cell would not be capable of performing certain types of work and would not respond to stimuli. A "live" cell is dependent on its ability to maintain these differences within a very specific range, if the important life processes of the organism are to be carried out.

Figure 1-6 The sodium pump: As potassium diffuses out of the cell and sodium diffuses into the cell, an active transport system, supplied with energy produced in the cell by glucose metabolism, delivers sodium back to the extracellular compartment and potassium to the intracellular compartment.

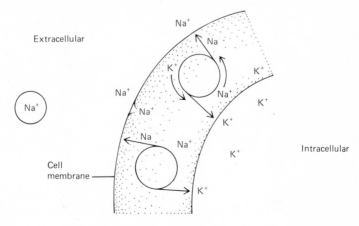

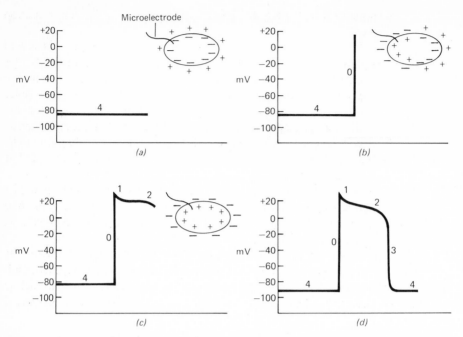

Figure 1-7 The different phases of the action potential for a ventricular muscle cell. (*a*) Polarized cell; (*b*) depolarization; (*c*) slow repolarization; (*d*) rapid repolarization.

ELECTRICAL PHASES OF THE CELL

Much information can be gained about the cell through the experimental technique of inserting a microelectrode into an individual cell to measure and record the electrical differences at various phases of rest and action. Figure 1-7*a* depicts a *polarized cell* at rest. When recorded, this phase is referred to as *phase 4* and has an electric charge of −90 mV (intracellular negative relative to extracellular).

The cell remains in this resting state until it receives a *threshold* stimulus. This stimulus represents the electric force capable of evoking *depolarization* or excitation of a cell. Stimuli can be received from the nervous system, or external mechanical sources (e.g., trauma, parenteral injection), or from fluid and electrolyte imbalances, hypoxia, and many other sources. Unless a threshold level is reached, the cell does not respond. Once this level is reached, the cell responds totally. An increase in the stimulus above the threshold level does not make the cell respond to any greater extent than it did at the minimal threshold level. This is often referred to as the "all or nothing law."

When the cell is stimulated to its threshold level, rapid diffusion of sodium occurs. Due to the electronegativity of the polarized cell, the initiating event of depolarization is marked by the rapid movement of the most abundant extracellular cation, *sodium,* into the intracellular compartment. This results in the cell becoming slightly electropositive and is labeled phase O, which represents depolarization or excitation (Fig. 1-7*b*). The cell at this point does not have a resting potential, but rather it has an action potential. An *action potential* is defined as the change in electrical potential which occurs when a cell is depolarized. A period of slow *repolarization* then occurs, labeled phases 1 and 2 (Fig. 1-7*c*). The length of this period varies from cell to cell and is influenced by pathology such as injury, ischemia, or infarction, as well as by specific drugs.

When the active transport of sodium and potassium is restarted by the Na-K-ATP pump in the cell membrane, rapid repolarization occurs. This specific repolarization is called phase 3 of the action potential. This phase ends when the polarized state is reestablished at −90 mV, or phase 4 (Fig. 1-7*d*).

CARDIAC CELLS

All cardiac cells have a threshold level and respond to all the various stimuli mentioned previously. The major difference between some cardiac cells and the other cells of the body is that certain cardiac cell membranes possess *automaticity.* This is the ability of the cardiac cell membrane to gradually begin its own slow depolarization until it reaches its own "threshold" level, whereupon rapid depolarization (phase 0) results. In Fig. 1-8 one can see a gradual incline of the phase 4 period until depolarization occurs.

Figure 1-8 Action potential of a cardiac cell possessing automaticity. The sloping phase 4 represents automaticity.

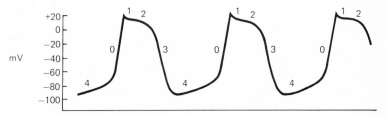

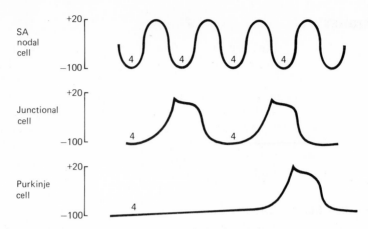

Figure 1-9 Representation of action potentials of an SA nodal cell, a junctional cell, and a Purkinje cell.

While most cardiac cells possess automaticity, each type of cardiac cell possesses a different automaticity rate (Fig. 1-9). The sinoatrial (SA) node normally has the fastest automaticity rate of approximately 80 cycles per minute. Atrioventricular (AV) junctional cells are capable of demonstrating an automaticity rate of approximately 60 cycles per minute. Purkinje cells usually possess an automaticity rate of 20 to 40 cycles per minute. The cell which reaches threshold first and depolarizes spreads the depolarization wave to the other areas of the heart.

The cardiac cells, as well as the other cells of the body, are quite susceptible to changes in interstitial fluid and electrolyte concentrations. The fluid and electrolyte values in this space approximate the serum fluid and electrolyte values. One can assume that the fluid and electrolyte status in the circulating blood volume represents the fluid and electrolyte bath surrounding each cardiac cell. It must also be remembered that the maintenance of this "bath" within normal limits is essential for life.

REGULATORY MECHANISMS

In the normal occurrences of daily living, the body is able to regulate its constantly changing fluid and electrolyte concentrations through the regulatory mechanisms of the kidney, lungs, blood, gastrointestinal tract, and skin.

KIDNEY

The kidney performs many major functions in controlling the internal environment of the body. First, the kidney is able to regulate pH through the elimination or retention of excess hydrogen ions and the maintenance of an appropriate bicarbonate level. Second, it helps control the fluid level by either increasing or decreasing urinary output by responding to the hormonal control of antidiuretic hormone (ADH) and aldosterone. Third, the kidney eliminates or retains specific electrolytes and is specifically able to regulate sodium through the hormonal regulation of aldosterone.

ANTIDIURETIC HORMONE   When the osmolarity of the blood increases, sensitive osmoreceptor cells located in the hypothalamus react by losing intracellular fluid and shrinking in size. A message is sent to the pituitary neurohypophysis and ADH is released. ADH acts mainly on the renal collecting tubules to produce an increase in water reabsorption from urine. When hypoosmolarity occurs, the osmoreceptor cells take in water and swell; the pituitary produces less ADH, and a more dilute urine is excreted.

ALDOSTERONE   *Aldosterone,* which is secreted from the adrenal cortex, produces an expansion of the fluid in the vascular system by initiating interactions that eventually stimulate the Na+ pump of renal tubule cells. Sodium and water are retained; the excretion of the potassium or hydrogen ion is promoted.

LUNGS AND BLOOD BUFFERS

The lungs help maintain a proper pH by eliminating or retaining carbon dioxide. The blood buffer systems also respond in the control of the acid-base balance. This is important to electrolyte balance because high levels of extracellular hydrogen ions tend to be taken up by all the cells of the body. Because the intracellular compartment must maintain an equal ratio of anions to cations, when hydrogen, a cation, enters the cell, a cation must leave. Since potassium is the most abundant intracellular cation, it tends to be lost from the cell and eventually lost from the body through the kidney. If this loss is severe, serious arrhythmias and even lethal cardiac problems can occur.

Various regulating mechanisms help to maintain the intracellular and extracellular fluid and electrolyte balances in a functional state. Trauma and/or acute physiological disorders can disrupt this homeostatic state. When extreme and continuous stress cannot be compensated for by the regulating mechanisms, serious fluid and electrolyte imbalances develop. Basic knowledge of the normal laboratory values of fluid and electrolytes is not enough to allow safe and appropriate care. The nurse practitioner must be familiar with the internal process causing the current electrolyte status as well as the various possible changes which could occur as the therapy is instituted. Physical assessment skills, ECG monitoring, and laboratory results must be utilized in an integrated, comprehensive, problem-solving approach to achieve the highest quality of care.

BIBLIOGRAPHY

Ganong, W., *Review of Medical Physiology,* Lange, Los Altos, Calif., 1974.

Guyton, A. C., *Textbook of Medical Physiology,* Saunders, Philadelphia, 1976.

Metheny, N. M., and Snively, W. D., *Nurses' Handbook of Fluid Balance,* 2d ed., Lippincott, Philadelphia, 1974.

Reed, G. N., and Sheppard, V. F., *Regulation of Fluid and Electrolyte Balance: A Programmed Instruction in Physiology for Nurses,* Saunders, Philadelphia, 1971.

CHAPTER 2
THE NERVOUS SYSTEM
RETA M. H. POZZI, R.N.

TO begin, the reader is urged to clear away all past misconceptions that say that neurology is difficult. Basic neurology is not difficult unless one has already decided that it is.

A simple definition of the nervous system to make its function obvious is to call it a system within the body which enables one to be aware of and react to his or her internal and external environment. The external manifestations of those responses are analogous to the signs and symptoms exhibited by the patient during a neurological emergency. To better understand these manifestations, a basic knowledge of the anatomy and physiology of the nervous system is essential.

OVERVIEW OF NEUROANATOMY

THE NEURON

The nervous system is made up of cells known as *neurons*. Each neuron is composed of a dendrite, a cell body, and an axon (see Fig. 2-1). Usually the cell body of the neuron does not have a centrosome, indicating that nerve cells are incapable of mitosis; once a cell

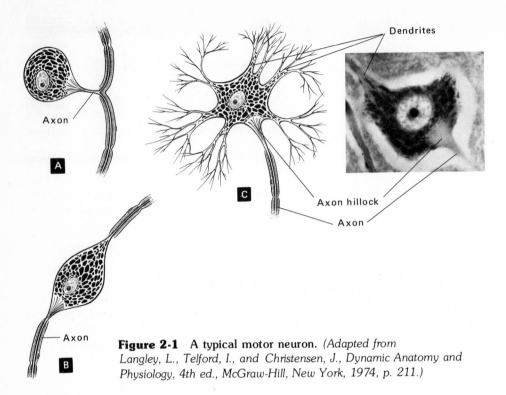

Figure 2-1 A typical motor neuron. *(Adapted from Langley, L., Telford, I., and Christensen, J., Dynamic Anatomy and Physiology, 4th ed., McGraw-Hill, New York, 1974, p. 211.)*

body is destroyed, there is no regeneration. The *dendrite* transmits the nerve impulse to the cell body, and the *axon* transmits the impulse away from the cell body to the next neuron, to an end organ, or a muscle. The physical gap between the axon of one neuron and the cell body or dendrite of the next neuron is called a *synapse*. The synaptic vesicles of the terminal axon store the chemical neurotransmitter which facilitates the transmission of the impulse across the synapse.

The peripheral endings of afferent neurons have *receptors*, which respond to and translate chemical and physical environmental changes (mechanical energy) into action potentials (electric energy) which are propagated along the peripheral neuron. *Afferent* or *sensory neurons* conduct impulses from the receptor sites to the central nervous system, and *efferent* or *motor neurons* conduct the impulse from the central nervous system to the effector organ. Most peripheral nerves are composed of both afferent and efferent neurons. Within the central nervous system, *internuncial neurons* connect or act as bridges between the afferent and efferent neurons. For example, pain sensation is picked up at receptor sites in the fingertip; afferent or sensory neurons carry the impulse to the central nervous system, and internuncial neurons relay the impulse to higher centers where the sensation is interpreted as pain. Efferent or motor neurons then carry the impulse from the central nervous system to the muscle or effector organ, and by muscular contractions in the shoulder, forearm, hand, and fingers, the finger is probably removed from the pain source. This afferent-efferent pathway on a given spinal level constitutes a *simple reflex arc* (see Fig. 2-2).

The nervous system is divided into two parts: (1) the *central nervous system,* consisting of the brain and spinal cord, and (2) the *peripheral nervous system,* consisting of the cranial and spinal nerves and the portions of them which compose the *autonomic nervous system.*

CENTRAL NERVOUS SYSTEM: THE BRAIN

PROTECTIVE COVERINGS OF THE BRAIN   The *scalp* is the thick, highly vascular covering of the skull. The scalp's blood supply is derived primarily from the external carotid artery. This rich blood supply is the source of profuse bleeding when minor scalp lacerations occur, but there is

Figure 2-2   Components of a simple reflex: a sensory, an internuncial, and a motor neuron. *(Taken from Langley, L. Telford, I., and Christensen, J., Dynamic Anatomy and Physiology, 4th ed., McGraw-Hill, New York, 1974, p. 280.)*

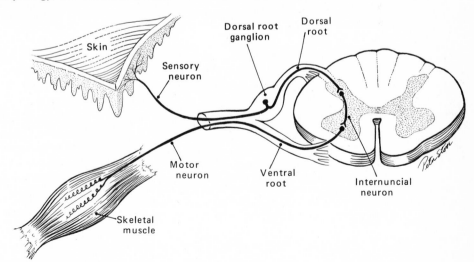

little subsequent infection of the site, even when it is quite contaminated. The scalp is primarily the only pain-sensitive structure that covers the brain, which is itself insensitive to pain. (There are nerve endings in the dura which are activated by painful stimuli.) In fact, neurosurgery can be performed with only local anaesthesia to the scalp.

The *skull* is a bony, nonexpandable vault which encloses the brain (see Fig. 2-3). This lack of expansibility is the reason for the most life-threatening of all neurosurgical emergencies—increased intracranial pressure. If the pressure within the skull is increased, most commonly by hemorrhage and edema, extrusion of the brainstem through the

Figure 2-3 **Lateral view of the skull.** *(Taken with permission from Chusid, J., Correlative Neuroanatomy and Functional Neurology, 15th ed., Lange, Los Altos, Calif., 1973, p. 61.)*

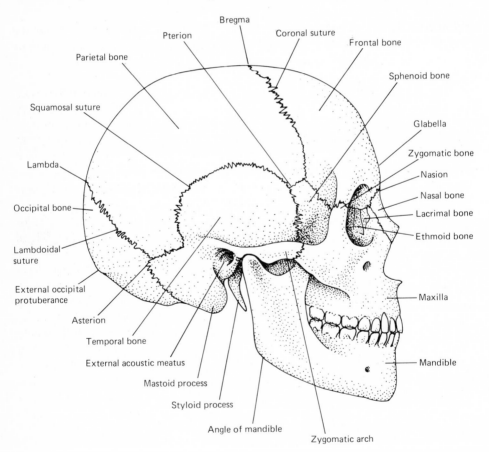

foramen magnum may occur. Herniation of the vital centers of the medulla (respiratory, vasomotor, cardiac) is almost invariably fatal.

Within the skull the brain is covered by three protective membranes, the *meninges:* the outer membrane, dura mater, or "dura" (this is the inner periosteum of the skull), the middle membrane or arachnoid, and the inner membrane, pia mater, or "pia." The largest artery of the dura is the middle meningeal which lies primarily within grooves in the temporal bone of the skull. It often gives rise to serious epidural hemorrhage if it is torn by overlying fractures of this portion of the skull. The meninges extend down from the brain and enclose the spinal cord in one continuous covering. An important concept to bear in mind, even at this early point, is that the brain and spinal cord are continuous. The spinal cord is an anatomical extension of the brain—both are composed of neurons, and in some instances the same neurons—as illustrated in Fig. 2-4.

DIVISIONS OF THE BRAIN   The brain cells which are formed during the prenatal period and the first few months of the postnatal period form the four major divisions of the brain (see Fig. 2-4).

Cerebrum: The *cerebrum,* anatomically the largest area of the brain, occupies the biggest part of the cranial cavity (see Fig. 2-5). It is made up of a surface layer of grey matter (neuron cell bodies) which is called the *cerebral cortex.* The cerebral cortex is the most sophisticated part of the brain. Beneath the cortex is the white matter which consists of nerve fibers arranged in tracts. The cerebral cortex is folded into convolutions or *gyri* (the hills). Between the convolutions lie the fissures or *sulci* (the valleys) of the cortex. Each sulcus is named and has importance according to its anatomical reference for the lobes of the cerebrum. The cerebrum consists of two lateral hemispheres, right and left, resembling a neatly opened walnut. The *falx cerebri,* an extension of the dura, lies along the longitudinal fissure to separate these two hemispheres. The *corpus collosum,* a thick band of communicating nerve fibers, links corresponding regions of the two hemispheres. Each hemisphere controls the activity of the opposite half of the body because the nerve tracts decussate (cross) in the medulla, thus causing contralateral control of function (see Fig. 2-6). In every person one hemisphere of the cerebrum is more intensively trained in association processes. If the left hemisphere is dominant, the person is right-handed, and vice versa. Each hemisphere is divided into four lobes which are named according to their locations under the skull.

Pressure on or interruption of the blood supply to any of the

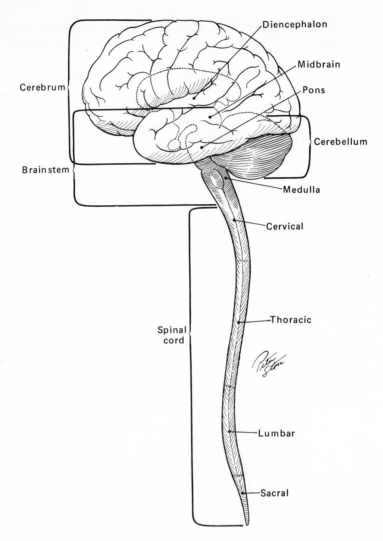

Figure 2-4 Lateral view of the central nervous system. *(Taken from Langley, L., Telford, I., and Christensen, J., Dynamic Anatomy and Physiology, 4th ed., McGraw-Hill, New York, 1974, p. 228.)*

specific areas of the cerebrum may produce a disturbance in the functional activity appropriate to that area of the brain. For example, occipital tumors may cause visual disturbance, such as diplopia or blindness. Trauma to the right frontal lobe with hemorrhage anterior to the central sulcus may result in motor weakness or paralysis of the left leg. In general, hemiplegia indicates brain damage, while para-plegia and quadriplegia are indicative of spinal cord injury.

Diencephalon: The *diencephalon* is located deep in the central part of the brain between the cerebrum and the midbrain. The *thalamus* and *hypothalamus* are important structures located in this area. The *pituitary gland,* a part of the hypothalamus, is located in the sella turcica.

Brainstem: The *brainstem* is located between the cerebrum and the spinal cord. It consists of the midbrain, pons, and medulla oblongata. The *midbrain* is the area located between the two cerebral hemi-spheres. The *pons* (meaning "bridge") and *medulla* form a pathway of nerve tracts which connect the cortex and spinal cord. The pyrami-dal nerve tracts decussate near the junction of the medulla and the spinal cord and become the lateral corticospinal tracts of the spinal cord. The medulla is continuous with the spinal cord at the foramen magnum.

Figure 2-5 (A) Lateral view of the cerebrum. Note the shaded line that demarcates the parietal and temporal lobes. The insula is deep in the temporal lobe. (B) A portion of the cortex in cross section. *(Taken from Langley, L., Telford, I., and Christensen, D., Dynamic Anatomy and Physiology, 4th ed., McGraw-Hill, New York, 1974, p. 229.)*

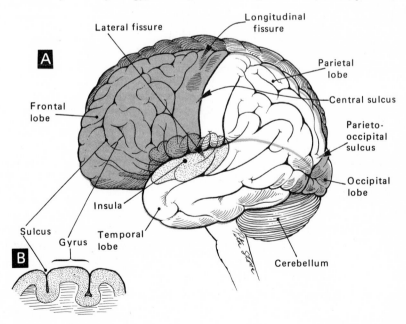

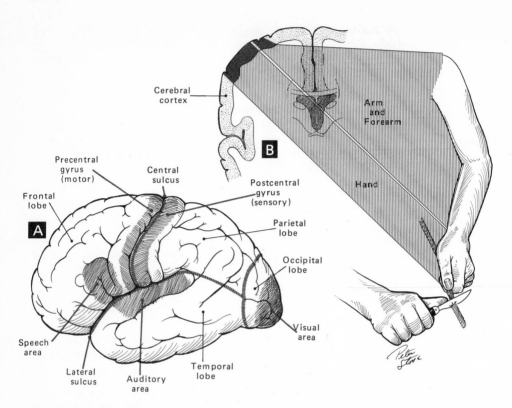

Figure 2-6 Lateral view of the cerebrum. (*a*) Functional areas of the cortex. (*b*) Representation of the left upper extremity on the primary motor (or sensory) areas of the cortex. *(Taken from Langley, L., Telford, I., and Christensen, J., Dynamic Anatomy and Physiology, 4th ed., McGraw-Hill, New York, 1974, p. 230.)*

    Cerebellum: The *cerebellum* lies in the posterior fossa of the cranial cavity at the base of the brain and is located posterior and superior to the brainstem. It is separated from the cerebrum by the *tentorium,* an extension of the dura.

    The functions of the various areas of the brain are briefly outlined in Table 2-1.

VASCULAR SYSTEM OF THE BRAIN The arterial blood supply to the brain is derived from the *internal carotid arteries* and the *vertebral arteries* (see Fig. 2-7*a*). The latter join to form the *basilar artery.* Communicating arteries between the internal carotid and basilar artery make up the arterial *circle of Willis* at the base of the brain (see Fig. 2-7*b*).

    The *cerebral veins* pierce the arachnoid space and the subdural space, then empty into the *dural venus sinuses.* Subdural hemorrhage results from the rupture of these veins as they cross the subdural space. The venus sinuses eventually drain into the *internal jugular vein* (see Fig. 2-8).

Figure 2-7a Arteries of the face and neck. *(Taken from Langley, L., Telford, I., and Christensen, J., Dynamic Anatomy and Physiology, 4th ed., McGraw-Hill, New York, 1974, p. 442.)*

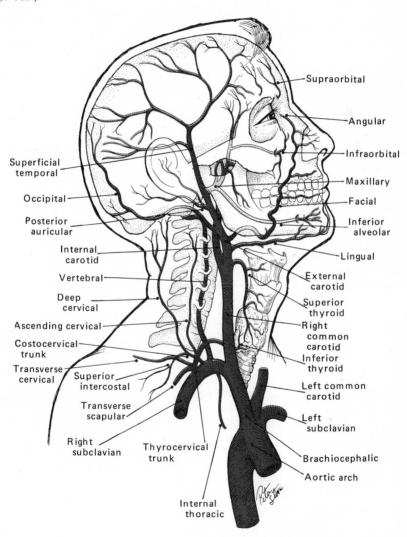

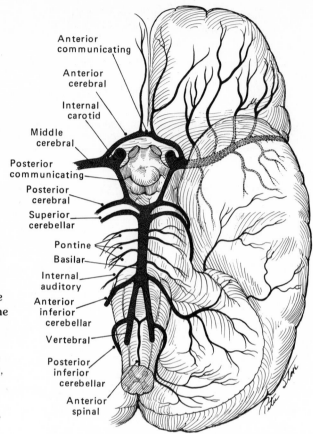

Figure 2-7b Arteries of the brain. The circle of Willis, at the center, joins branches of the basilar and internal carotid arteries. *(Taken from Langley, L., Telford, I., and Christensen, J., Dynamic Anatomy and Physiology, 4th ed., McGraw-Hill, New York, 1974, p. 443.)*

Table 2-1 Functions of areas of the brain

Area	Functions
I. Cerebrum	
A. Frontal lobe	1. Responsible for abstract reasoning and mature judgment which formulate behavior and socialization skills.
	2. Contains the center for voluntary motor function. Massive chaotic discharges from the motor strip result in the tonic and clonic movements of an epileptic seizure. Expressive or motor aphasia occurs due to lesions of Brocca's speech area. The patient is unable to speak intelligently, even though he understands what he wishes to say and recognizes his errors.
B. Parietal lobe	1. Contains the sensory area where incoming impulses reach consciousness.

           2. Responsible for body image awareness. Lesions of this area result in parts of the body not being recognized or confusion as to left and right sides of the body.

C. Temporal lobe

1. Controls comprehension of the spoken and written word. Language is usually controlled by the hemisphere of motor dominance. Lesions in this area of the dominant hemisphere result in receptive aphasia. Auditory receptive aphasia occurs due to lesions of Wernicke's area. The patient cannot comprehend spoken language. He can speak but his speech is meaningless because of lack of comprehension.
2. Auditory impulses are deciphered here.

D. Occipital lobe

1. Contains centers responsible for vision and for formulating sensory stimuli into visual images and comprehending their meaning.

II. Diencephalon

A. Thalamus

1. Relay station for sensory impulses transmitted to the cortex.
2. Registers the awareness of stimuli (perception) and determines the emotional response to stimuli (feelings of pleasure or unpleasantness).

B. Hypothalamus

1. Controls the body's internal environment through integration of endocrine and autonomic nervous system functions.
2. Maintains normal body temperature by integrating autonomic centers with the mechanisms of vasodilation, sweating, vasoconstriction, and shivering.
3. Controls appetite.
4. Regulates water balance through control of the production of antidiuretic hormone from the posterior lobe of the pituitary gland.

III. Brainstem

A. Midbrain

1. Contains nerve tracts which connect the two cerebral hemispheres.
2. Contains visual pathways which relay impulses from the retina to the occipital lobe.

B. Pons

1. Contains nerve tracts which link the cerebellum with the midbrain and the medulla.

C. Medulla

1. Contains control centers for the most vital of the body functions—respiratory, cardiac, vasomotor centers.
2. Also controls vomiting, coughing, sneezing, swallowing, salivation, and sleep.

IV. Cerebellum

1. Contains centers responsible for the coordination of muscle groups and for the timing of their contractions, allowing for smooth and accurate movements. As such, it is important in maintaining equilibrium. Ataxia or gait disturbances occur as the result of damage to the cerebellum.

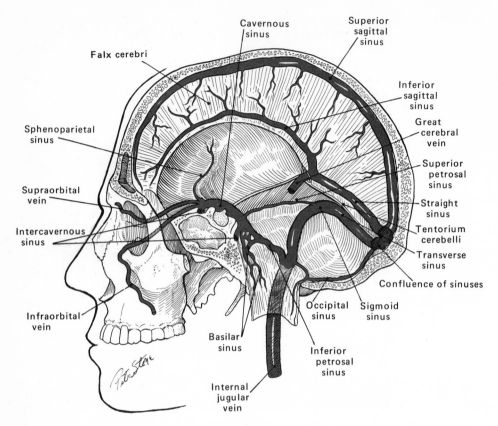

Figure 2-8 Dural sinuses. Superficial veins of the face empty into the cavernous sinus. *(Taken from Langley, L., Telford, I., and Christensen, J., Dynamic Anatomy and Physiology, 4th ed., McGraw-Hill, New York, 1974, p. 455.)*

Glucose is the primary substance which can be metabolized rapidly enough to supply the brain with its high energy requirements. Glucose storage in the brain is minute; therefore the brain depends upon a continuous supply of blood to deliver glucose and oxygen to its cells. During rest the brain receives 15 to 20 percent of the body's total blood supply. When brain cells are deprived of blood supply, they cease to function and they die. Lack of oxygen for 4 to 6 minutes initiates the process of brain death. Lack of glucose causes brain damage within 10 to 15 minutes. Therefore, cerebral circulation is essential to brain function.

Control of the cerebral vascular circulation by the nervous system is very poor. Cerebral vessels are also generally insensitive to the circulating and administered catecholamines. Primarily, variation in the size of cerebral vessels occurs in response to pH, $PaCO_2$, and PaO_2. Elevations in $PaCO_2$, lowered pH, and lowered PaO_2 cause vasodilation. The reverse of this situation causes vasoconstriction. Hyperventilation of patients with intracranial hemorrhage has been advocated since respiratory alkalosis causes vasoconstriction and allows for a decrease in intracranial pressure.

CEREBROSPINAL FLUID   The brain and spinal cord float in a protective buffer of clear watery *cerebrospinal fluid*. This fluid is formed in the ventricles and circulates within the subarachnoid space surrounding the brain and spinal cord (see Fig. 2-9). It is produced by selective blood ultra-filtration and active secretion within the vascular *choroid plexuses* which may be thought of as "the kidney of the brain." These choroid plexuses are found in the ventricles which are communicating cavities or spaces within the brain. In the adult there is about 125 cc CSF. It is constantly produced, circulated, and reabsorbed into the cerebral venous system through the arachnoid villi in the walls of the superior sagittal sinus. In the normal individual, intracranial pressure is main-tained relatively constant by variation in cerebrospinal fluid volume. When the brain swells due to trauma, homeostatic mechanisms decrease the production of CSF in an attempt to maintain normal intracranial pressures.

Because some substances do not pass from the blood to the cere-brospinal fluid, it is believed that a mechanism known as the *blood-brain barrier* exists as a protective barrier between the blood and sensitive brain tissue. It prevents some substances, including penicil-lin, steroids (except Decadron), and catecholamines, from crossing to the brain tissue, except in small quantities. However, it carefully maintains the ionic concentration of fluid bathing the brain cells. Water, glucose, and respiratory gases move freely across the barrier. This blood-brain barrier also exists at the capillary–nerve cell level.

CENTRAL NERVOUS SYSTEM: SPINAL CORD

The *spinal cord* lies within a bony protective spinal column consisting of 33 *vertebrae:* 7 cervical, 12 thoracic, 5 lumbar, 5 sacral, and 4 fused coccygeal vertebrae (see Fig. 2-10). Between every two verte-brae is a tough fibrocartilagenous cushion or *intervertebral disk*. The vertebrae are held together by multiple ligaments and muscles. Motion of the spine occurs at the articular facets of the vertebrae and through the intervertebral disks (Fig. 2-10).

The first cervical vertebra, or *atlas,* serves as a support of the skull. (Remember this by associating it with the mythological Atlas who

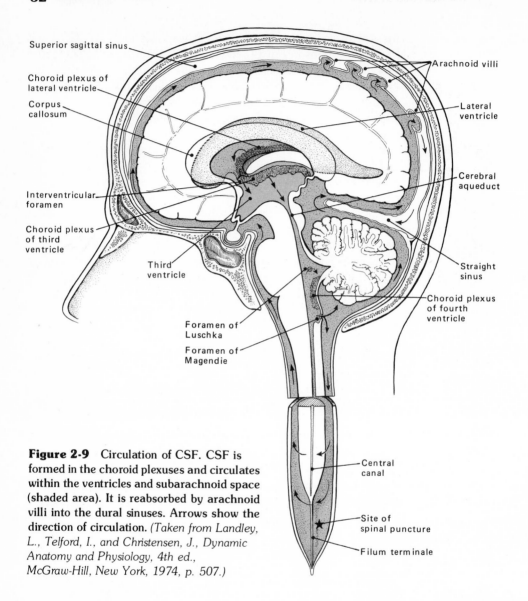

Superior sagittal sinus

Arachnoid villi

Choroid plexus of lateral ventricle

Corpus callosum

Lateral ventricle

Interventricular foramen

Cerebral aqueduct

Choroid plexus of third ventricle

Third ventricle

Straight sinus

Choroid plexus of fourth ventricle

Foramen of Luschka

Foramen of Magendie

Central canal

Site of spinal puncture

Filum terminale

Figure 2-9 Circulation of CSF. CSF is formed in the choroid plexuses and circulates within the ventricles and subarachnoid space (shaded area). It is reabsorbed by arachnoid villi into the dural sinuses. Arrows show the direction of circulation. *(Taken from Landley, L., Telford, I., and Christensen, J., Dynamic Anatomy and Physiology, 4th ed., McGraw-Hill, New York, 1974, p. 507.)*

Figure 2-10 The vertebral column. The primary (convex) curvature in the thoracic and sacral regions is present at birth. Secondary (concave) curvatures develop in the cervical region when the baby begins to move his head, in the lumbar region when he begins to stand and walk. *(Taken from Langley, L., Telford, I., and Christensen, J., Dynamic Anatomy and Physiology, 4th ed., McGraw-Hill, New York, 1974, p. 96.)*

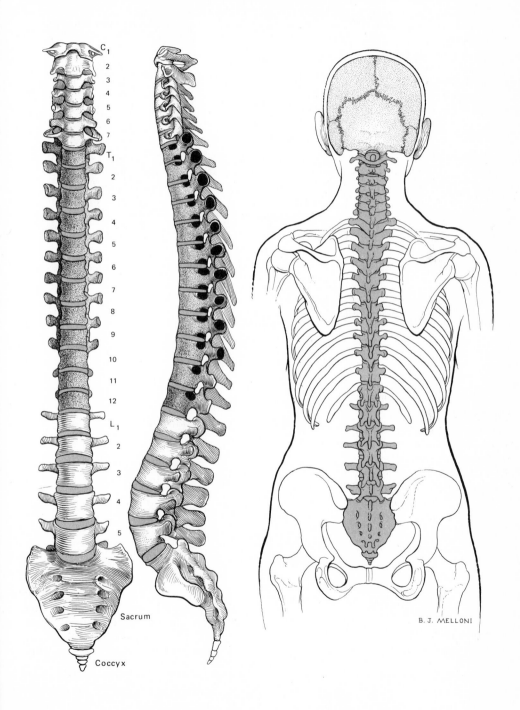

C1
2
3
4
5
6
7
T1
2
3
4
5
6
7
8
9
10
11
12
L1
2
3
4
5

Sacrum

Coccyx

B. J. MELLONI

held up the world.) It is distinguished by the absence of a body and a spinous process. The second cervical vertebra, or *axis,* is notable for its *odontoid process,* a vertical projection extending into the spinal canal of the atlas like a stick in a hoop. Strong ligaments hold the two together but allow for considerable rotational movement. When these ligaments are torn or the odontoid is fractured by trauma, such as a diving accident, the atlas may slip on the axis and crush the cord, resulting in immediate death (see Fig. 2-11).

The spinal cord extends from the foramen magnum at the base of the skull to the lower border of the first lumbar vertebra (see Fig. 2-12). Spinal taps are always done below the first lumbar vertebra to eliminate the danger of trauma to the spinal cord. The cord is surrounded by the pia mater, cerebrospinal fluid, arachnoid, dura, and a cushion of epidural fat within the neural cavity of the bony vertebrae. The *filum terminale* is a thread of fibrous tissue which is continuous with the pia mater and is attached to the first portion of the coccyx.

The spinal cord itself is composed of *white matter* surrounding an H-shaped internal mass of *gray matter* (see Fig. 2-13). A *central canal* extends the length of the spinal cord. It is filled with cerebrospinal fluid and communicates with an opening in the fourth ventricle of the brain.

The spinal cord serves as a two-way path to conduct sensory and

Figure 2-11 Odontoid process (viewed from behind and above).

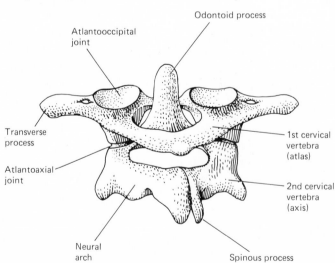

motor impulses between the brain and peripheral nerves. Ascending tracts contained within the *posterior (dorsal) gray column* conduct sensory impulses up the cord to the brain. Descending tracts contained within the *anterior (ventral) gray column* conduct motor impulses down the cord from the brain. The preganglionic cells of the autonomic nervous system are contained within the lateral gray column. The white matter of the spinal cord consists of nerve fibers which link the various segments of the spinal cord and connect the spinal cord to the brain.

Injuries to the spinal cord are of serious consequences, since no regeneration of destroyed or divided nerve tracts occurs. Some degree of recovery may take place from lesser injuries, such as contusion or compression.

PERIPHERAL NERVOUS SYSTEM

The nerve processes which connect the brain and spinal cord to the periphery of the body and its various organs constitute the *peripheral nervous system*. It consists of the spinal and cranial nerves and the portions of them which compose the autonomic nervous system.

SPINAL NERVES Thirty-one pairs of *spinal nerves* originate from the spinal cord: 8 cervical, 12 thoracic, 5 lumbar, 5 sacral, and 1 coccygeal pair. All arise from the spinal cord and emerge through the appropriate foramen located between every two vertebrae, except the lumbar, sacral, and coccygeal which descend from the lower end of the spinal cord to form the *cauda equina* (horse's tail) before emerging from their respective foramen. The cauda equina fills the spinal canal below the termination of the spinal cord.

Each spinal nerve attaches to the spinal cord by means of two roots—one *anterior* and one *posterior*. (See Fig. 2-12.) Each root contains bundles of nerve fibers. Spinal nerves contain both sensory and motor fibers and serve as two-way conduction pathways between the periphery and the spinal cord, making possible both sensations and movements. Motor fibers which originate in the gray column of the spinal cord form the *ventral roots* and communicate with skeletal muscle. Sensory fibers convey impulses to the CNS from visceral and somatic structures through *dorsal roots* to the posterior gray column. *Rami communicantes* are branches of motor fibers which join the spinal nerves to the sympathetic ganglion.

CRANIAL NERVES Twelve pairs of *cranial nerves* arise directly from the under surface of the brain, except for the cerebellum. They emerge from

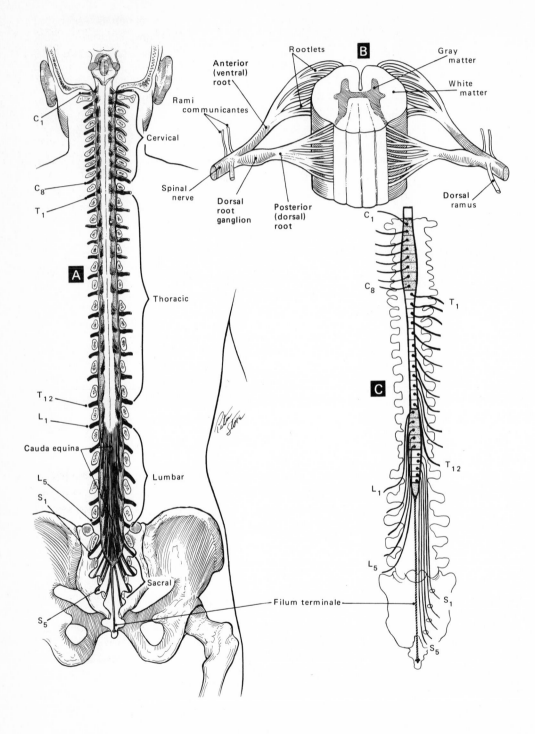

the skull through the *foramen magnum.* Some consist of both afferent and efferent fibers; others consist of only afferent or only efferent
fibers. The names of the cranial nerves identify their distribution or
function, and the numbers indicate the order in which they emerge
from the brain, proceeding from front to back (see Fig. 2-12).

Severe head injuries often damage one or more of the cranial
nerves, producing symptoms analogous to the functions of the nerve
affected. For example, injury to the 6th cranial nerve causes the eye
to turn inward owing to paralysis of the abducting muscle. A bulging
aneurysm of one of the middle cerebral arteries with resultant pressure on the nearby oculomotor nerve causes the pupil on the same
side to become dilated and nonreactive to light. The specific functions of the cranial nerves are summarized in Fig. 2-14.

DIVISIONS OF PERIPHERAL NERVOUS SYSTEM   The peripheral nervous system
may be subdivided according to function. The following is a brief
summary of some of the pertinent anatomical features of each
division.

Afferent division: This division, consisting of afferent fibers, carries
impulses from the *peripheral receptors* to the *central nervous system.*
The afferent neurons have multiple branches which innervate various
receptors. Each afferent neuron has one long axon extending to the
cell body which lies outside but close to the brain or spinal cord. A
second axon extends into the central nervous system where it
synapses with other neurons. These are sometimes called sensory
neurons.

Somatic division: The somatic division, consisting of efferent fibers,
innervates *skeletal muscle.* The somatic division is made up of all the
nerve fibers which carry impulses from the *central nervous system* to
skeletal muscle. The cell bodies of these neurons are located within
the brain or spinal cord, often in groups called *nuclei.* Axons extend

Figure 2-12   (A) The vertebral column with the surface of the spinal cord exposed.
Samples of CSF are usually taken in the lumbar region, where the meninges extend
below the cord. (B) A spinal cord segment. (C) Schematic view of the spinal cord. Note
that, beginning in the thoracic region, spinal nerves emerge from the vertebral column
at points progressively lower than their origin. The spinal nerves below the spinal
cord are collectively termed the cauda equina. *(Taken from Langley, L. Telford, I., and
Christensen, J., Dynamic Anatomy and Physiology, 4th ed., McGraw-Hill, New York, 1974,
p. 240.)*

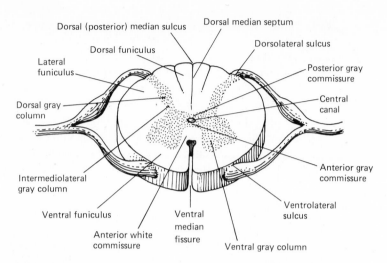

Figure 2-13   Anatomy of the spinal cord. *(Taken from Chusid, J., Correlative Neuro-anatomy and Functional Neurology, 15th ed., Lange, Los Altos, Calif., 1973, p. 243.)*

directly, without synapse, to the skeletal muscle cells. It is a one-neuron chain. Stimulation of somatic efferent neurons results in skeletal muscle contraction.

Autonomic division: The autonomic or involuntary division, consisting of efferent fibers, innervates the smooth muscle of *viscera, cardiac muscle,* and *glandular organs.* The autonomic nervous system is further subdivided into the parasympathetic and the sympathetic divisions. The *parasympathetic* division arises from the *cranial* and *sacral* spinal nerves. The parasympathetic division generally transmits impulses which are concerned with the *slowing* of body functions.

The *sympathetic* division arises from the *thoracic* and *lumbar* spinal nerves. The sympathetic division generally transmits impulses which are concerned with *speeding up* body functions to effect emergency protective mechanisms which help one to cope with stressful conditions. Most organs innervated by the autonomic nervous system have dual parasympathetic and sympathetic innervation (see Fig. 2-15). For example, parasympathetic innervation slows the heart rate while sympathetic innervation speeds up heart rate. A balance between these two divisions maintains the body in homeostasis.

Autonomic ganglia: A *ganglion* is a collection of nerve cell bodies. The efferent fibers of the autonomic nervous system synapse outside

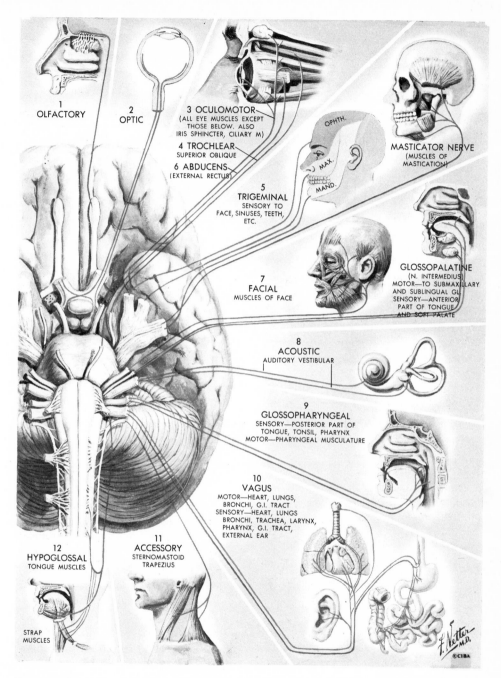

Figure 2-14 The cranial nerves. *(Taken from Netter, F., The Nervous System, vol. I, Ciba Pharmaceutical, Summit, N.J., 1972.)*

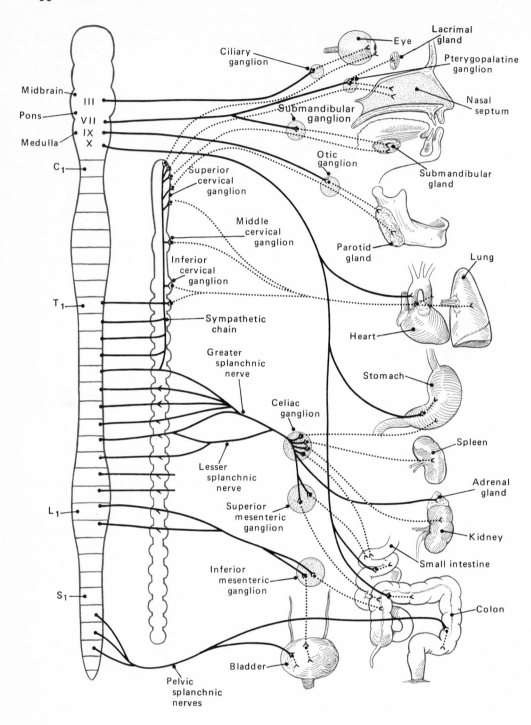

the central nervous system at ganglia and again at neuroeffector junctions. The efferent fibers passing from the central nervous system to ganglia are called *preganglionic autonomic fibers,* and those fibers connecting the ganglia to the effector organ are called *postganglionic autonomic fibers.* Therefore, impulses transmitted from the central nervous system to viscera must traverse a two-neuron pathway. The preganglionic nerve cell body is located in the brainstem or spinal cord, while postganglionic nerve cell bodies lie within the ganglia outside the central nervous system. Most sympathetic ganglia lie close to and along both sides of the spinal cord in chains. The ganglia extend from the base of the skull to the coccyx; the preganglionic fiber is short and the postganglionic fiber, extending from ganglia to effector organ, is long. This sympathetic ganglionic chain allows for the transmission of sympathetic impulses to the organs of the head and pelvis. Most parasympathetic ganglia lie near or within the walls of the effector organ; the preganglionic fiber is long, and the post-ganglionic fiber is short.

OVERVIEW OF NEUROPHYSIOLOGY

The functions of neurons include the transmission of nerve impulses as well as integration and storage of information. The generation and propagation of the *action potential,* which is a neuron function, originates by activation of receptors, by synaptic input from other neurons, or by spontaneous neuron activity. Mechanical stimulation, such as pressure, to the receptor site causes an increase in the membrane permeability of the peripheral endings of the afferent neuron. This allows for an increase in the movement of ions between the intracellular and extracellular fluid. The *resting potential* of the nerve cell membrane is about -70 mV with the greatest concentration of potassium ions being inside the cell. With increased cell membrane permeability there is a dramatic shift of *sodium ions* to the inside of the cell and a relatively lesser shift of potassium ions out of the cell.

Figure 2-15 Schematic diagram of the autonomic nervous system. Parasympathetic (craniosacral) fibers are shown in black. Sympathetic (thoracolumbar) fibers are shown shaded. Preganglionic fibers are depicted as solid lines, postganglionic fibers as dotted lines. *(Taken from Langley, L., Telford, I., and Christensen, J., Dynamic Anatomy and Physiology, 4th ed., McGraw-Hill, New York, 1974, p. 290.)*

This *ionic shift* results in the inside of the cell becoming positively charged and a decreased membrane potential or depolarization. Thus, an action potential is generated and propagated in the same manner until it traverses the length of the axon. This constitutes *a nerve impulse.*

The activity of the neuron depends upon ionic imbalance at the cellular membrane. The creation, maintenance, and reestablishment of these imbalances require work. The source of *energy* for this work is *adenosine triphosphate* (ATP) which is primarily derived from the intracellular catabolism of *glucose* (see Fig. 5-6).

SOMATIC PERIPHERAL NERVOUS SYSTEM

As previously mentioned, it has been hypothesized that the axon secretes a *neurotransmitter* which bridges the synapse to accomplish the transmission of the impulse from one neuron to another. In the *somatic* portion of the peripheral nervous system, this neurotransmitter which functions at the neuromuscular junction, or synapse, is *acetylcholine.* At the nerve ending, acetylcholine transmits the impulse to the muscle. Acetylcholine pours out of the vesicles and diffuses across the synaptic gap to combine with muscle receptor sites (see Fig. 2-16). It is believed that calcium ions facilitate the release of acetylcholine from the vesicles. The combination of acetylcholine with the receptor site causes changes in the permeability and potential of the membrane of the muscle cell.

Figure 2-16 The end of the presynaptic fiber of the axon of one neuron is enlarged to form a synaptic bulb or terminal button. The synaptic vesicles contain the neurotransmitter responsible for synaptic transmission of the nerve impulse to the dendrite of another neuron.

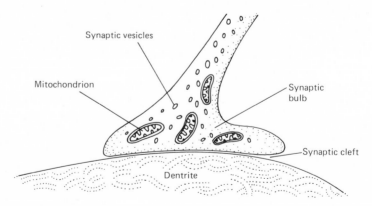

At the excitatory synapse of muscle cells the combination of neuro-transmitter and receptor site increases the permeability of the cell membrane to positively charged ions. As previously stated, some potassium ions move out of the cell and a large number of sodium ions move into the cell, creating a net movement of positive ions into the cell. The negative resting potential of the cell is brought to thresh-old level and an action potential is created. The combined effect of many synapses results in *depolarization* of the muscle cell. This depolarization stimulates *contraction* of the muscle cell. Synaptic activity is terminated when acetylcholine is chemically transformed into an inactive substance by an enzyme known as *acetylcholines-terase* which is produced by the muscle.

It should be noted that many drugs and toxins affect the synapse by modifying the synthesis, storage, release, inactivation, or uptake of the chemical mediator, or by blocking the receptor sites on the muscle cell to prevent combination with the chemical mediator. In myasthenia gravis there is a deficiency in the amount of acetylcholine released at the neuromuscular synapse. Treatment consists of the administration of drugs, such as neostigmine, which block cholines-terase, allowing for more prolonged action of acetylcholine and less muscle weakness.

AUTONOMIC NERVOUS SYSTEM

As previously mentioned, most involuntary organs have both sym-pathetic and parasympathetic innervation. These divisions produce opposing reactions: i.e., stimulation of the fibers of one division produces effects antagonistic to those produced by stimulation of the fibers of the other division (see Table 2-2).

AUTONOMIC NEUROTRANSMITTERS One reason for the opposing functions within the autonomic nervous system is the neurotransmitter pro-duced at the postganglionic fibers. In the *parasympathetic* division, *acetylcholine* is the neurotransmitter between the postganglionic nerve ending and the visceral organ. Nerve fibers which liberate acetylcholine are called *cholinergic fibers*. In the *sympathetic* divi-sion, the neurotransmitter which mediates transmission of the im-pulse from the postganglionic nerve ending to the visceral organ is *norepinephrine.** Nerve fibers which liberate norepinephrine are

* The two exceptions to these characteristics within the sympathetic nervous system are the sweat glands and some blood vessels within skeletal muscles which are inner-vated by sympathetic nerves whose impulse transmission is facilitated by acetylcholine at the postganglionic synapses.

Table 2-2   Autonomic function. *(From Langley, L., Telford, I., and Christensen, J.: Dynamic Anatomy and Physiology, 4th ed., McGraw-Hill, New York, 1974, p. 296.)*

Organ	Effect of sympathetic stimulation	Effect of parasympathetic stimulation
Heart	Increased rate	Slowed rate
Muscle	Increased force of beat	Decreased force of atrial beat
Arterioles	Dilation (?)	Constriction (?)
Systemic blood vessels		
Abdominal	Constriction	
Muscle	Constriction (adrenergic) Dilation (cholinergic)	Dilation
Skin	Constriction (adrenergic) Dilation (cholinergic)	
Blood		
Coagulation	Increased	
Glucose	Increased	
Lungs		
Bronchi	Dilation	Constriction
Blood vessels	Mild constriction	
Intestine		
Lumen	Decreased peristalsis and tone	Increased peristalsis and tone
Sphincter	Increased tone	Decreased tone
Eye		
Pupil	Dilation	Contraction
Ciliary muscle		Contraction
Glands		
Nasal	Vasoconstriction	Stimulation of secretion
Lacrimal	Vasoconstriction	Stimulation of secretion
Parotid	Vasoconstriction	Stimulation of secretion
Submaxillary	Vasoconstriction	Stimulation of secretion
Gastric	Vasoconstriction	Stimulation of secretion
Pancreatic	Vasoconstriction	Stimulation of secretion
Sweat	Copious secretion (cholinergic)	
Liver	Glucose released	
Kidney	Decreased output	
Ureter	Inhibition	Excitation
Bladder muscle	Relaxation	Contraction
Penis	Ejaculation	Erection
Basal metabolism	Increased	

called *adrenergic fibers*. In both the parasympathetic and sympathetic divisions the preganglionic neurotransmitter is acetylcholine (see Fig. 2-17). Both acetylcholine and norepinephrine are synthesized in the vesicles of the postganglionic nerve endings. Figure 2-18 summarizes the process of synthesis for both of these autonomic neurotransmitters.

To review the process of neurotransmission, the nerve impulse reaches the synapse, initiates the influx of calcium ions, which in turn initiates events resulting in an outpouring of acetylcholine from the vesicles. It is thought by some authorities that norepinephrine is also released by a similar mechanism. Acetylcholine is immediately

Figure 2-17 Efferent divisions of the peripheral nervous system. *(Taken from Vander, A., Sherman, J., and Luciano, D., Human Physiology: The Mechanisms of Body Function, 2d ed., McGraw-Hill, New York, 1975, p. 165.)*

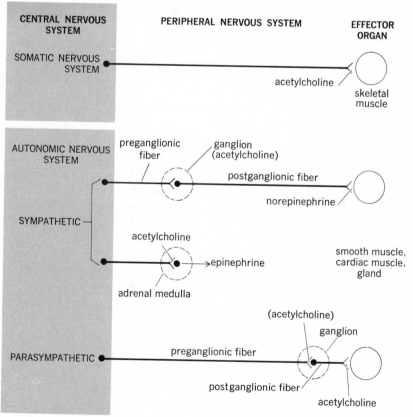

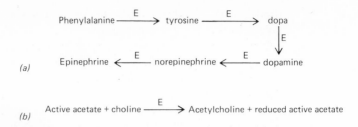

(a)

(b)

Figure 2-18 (*a*) The biosynthesis of catelcholamines. The amino acid phenylalanine is converted to tyrosine in the liver. Tyrosine is then transported to the sympathetic nerve endings where the necessary enzymes for the biosynthesis of norepinephrine are found. Note that dopamine, a drug currently used in the treatment of shock, is formed in this biosynthesis. The additional enzyme for the synthesis of epinephrine is found in the adrenal medulla. (E stands for enzyme.) (*b*) The biosynthesis of acetylcholine. The necessary enzyme for this reaction is found in high concentrations in cholinergic nerve endings. In fact, its presence in high concentrations in any neural area indicates that the synapses are cholinergic.

inactivated by acetylcholinesterase. Norepinephrine, after being secreted, is taken back into the nerve ending or is inactivated by enzymes present at the adrenergic nerve ending. Both acetylcholine and norepinephrine are active for a very short period of time.

Many drugs stimulate or inhibit the synaptic transmission within the autonomic nervous system. Those which stimulate synaptic transmission of norepinephrine and so mimic the effects of the sympathetic nervous system are called *sympathomimetic drugs*. An example of this type of drug is *phenylephrine*. Drugs which inhibit synaptic transmission and block the effects of norepinephrine are called *sympatholytic drugs*. An example of this type of drug is *propanolol*. Drugs, such as *prostigmine,* which stimulate synaptic transmission of acetylcholine and so mimic the effects of the parasympathetic division are called *parasympathomimetic drugs*. Those, such as *atropine,* which inhibit synaptic transmission and block the effects of acetylcholine are called *parasympatholytic drugs*.

ALPHA AND BETA RECEPTORS The actions of the autonomic nervous system depend not only on the postganglionic neurotransmitter but also on the type of receptor at the cell membrane of the effector organ. Through analysis of function it has been hypothesized that two types of receptors exist within the sympathetic division. These are *alpha-adrenergic* and *beta-adrenergic receptors*. The concept of specific binding sites or receptors on postsynaptic cell membranes has been used to explain the sometimes opposite effects of epinephrine and norepinephrine.

Norepinephrine acts predominately at alpha receptor sites while epinephrine acts at both alpha- and beta-receptor sites. *Alpha receptors* are principally located in the *blood vessels,* and their stimulation by norepinephrine causes *vasoconstriction. Beta receptors* are located primarily in the *heart* and the *bronchi.* A few are found in the blood vessels. Stimulation causes increased *strength* of myocardial contraction, increased *heart rate, bronchial dilation,* and minimal *vasodilation.* So-called *beta-mimetic drugs,* such as *isoproterenol,* stimulate beta receptors in the heart, blood vessels, and bronchi, producing the above responses. Through the same mechanism, drugs which are *beta-blocking agents,* such as *propranolol,* bind the beta-receptor sites in the heart, blood vessels, and bronchi. The results are directly opposite to those produced by stimulation of beta receptors, i.e., decreased strength of myocardial contraction, decreased heart rate, bronchoconstriction, and minimal vasoconstriction.

The autonomic nervous system, in conjunction with the endocrine activity, has a vast influence on the functions of the body's internal organs and its internal environment. Blood pressure, heart rate, gastrointestinal activity, glandular secretion, and body temperature are precisely controlled through the integrated activity of these two systems.

Knowledge of nervous system anatomy and physiology is essential for the emergency nurse. With this knowledge, she or he may provide optimal care of the patient with neurological insult and develop increased awareness of the pharmacological action of drugs which affect or mimic the autonomic nervous system.

BIBLIOGRAPHY

Alexander, E., Burley, W., Ellison, D., and Valleri, R., *Care of the Patient in Surgery,* 5th ed., Mosby, St. Louis, 1972.

Anthony, C. P., and Kolthoff, N. J., *Textbook of Anatomy and Physiology,* 9th ed., Mosby Co., St. Louis, 1975.

Chusid, J., *Correlative Neuroanatomy and Functional Neurology,* 15th ed., Lange Medical Publications, Los Altos, Calif., 1973.

Ganong, W., *Review of Medical Physiology,* Lange, Los Altos, Calif., 1974.

Gatz, A., *Clinical Neuroanatomy and Neurophysiology,* 4th ed., Davis, Philadelphia, 1970.

Langley, L., Telford, I., and Christensen, J., *Dynamic Anatomy and Physiology,* 4th ed., McGraw-Hill, New York, 1974.

Plum, F., and Posner, J., *Stupor and Coma,* 2d ed., Davis, Philadelphia, 1972.

Vander, A., Sherman, J., and Luciano, D.: *Human Physiology: The Mechanisms of Body Function,* McGraw-Hill, New York, 1975.

CHAPTER 3
THE CARDIOVASCULAR SYSTEM
JEANIE BARRY, R.N., M.S.

THE HEART

THE heart is a four-chambered muscular organ located within the mediastinum of the thoracic cavity (see Fig. 3-1). It is composed of three layers of tissue: a glistening *endocardium,* a thick muscular *myocardium,* and a serous *epicardium.* The innermost layer of the ventricular myocardium is covered with numerous fibromuscular bands called *trabeculae carnae.* A tough fibrous sac called the *pericardium* surrounds the epicardial surface of the heart and lends support to the organ. A few milliliters of pericardial fluid is found between these two layers and permit frictionless beating of the heart.

The heart initiates blood flow in two separate circuits (see Fig. 3-2). A septal wall prevents admixture of arterial and venous blood while the cardiac valves prevent regurgitation. Since the left side of the heart must generate a higher pressure to deliver blood to systemic circulation, the walls of its chambers are three times thicker than those of the right side. Figure 3-3 provides a diagrammatic summary of cardiopulmonary flow; the cardiac valves are shown in Fig. 3-4.

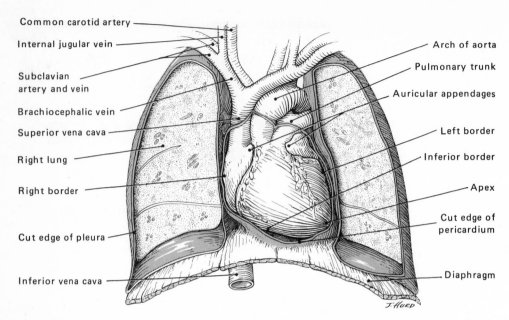

Common carotid artery

Internal jugular vein

Subclavian
artery and vein

Brachiocephalic vein

Superior vena cava

Right lung

Right border

Cut edge of pleura

Inferior vena cava

Arch of aorta

Pulmonary trunk

Auricular appendages

Left border

Inferior border

Apex

Cut edge of
pericardium

Diaphragm

J. HURD

Figure 3-1 Longitudinal section through the thoracic cavity. The mediastinum is the
area between the two lungs. *(Taken from Langley, L., Telford, I., and Christensen, J.,
Dynamic Anatomy and Physiology, 4th ed., McGraw-Hill, New York, 1974, p. 400.)*

Extending from both ventricular walls are the *papillary muscles*.
By means of a number of slender strands of fibrous tissue called
chordae tendineae the papillary muscles attach to the leaflets of the
atrioventricular valves (see Fig. 3-5). When the ventricular muscle
contracts, so also do the papillary muscles, thus preventing the
valvular leaflets from bulging into the atria with consequent regurgitation of blood. Rupture of the chordae tendineae or papillary
muscles from a myocardial infarction can produce severe valvular
insufficiency with consequent congestive heart failure.

CORONARY BLOOD FLOW

The blood flow to the heart is supplied by two main coronary arteries
which originate from the root of the aorta (see Fig. 3-6). The *right*
coronary artery normally supplies the posterior surface of the heart.
The *left main* coronary artery is very short (5 to 20 mm) and rapidly

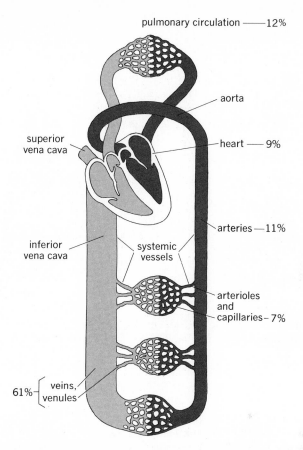

Figure 3-2 Distribution of blood in the different portions of the cardiovascular system. *(Taken from Vander, A., Sherman, J., and Luciano, D., Human Physiology: The Mechanisms of Body Function, 2d ed., McGraw-Hill, New York, 1975, p. 261.)*

bifurcates into the *left anterior descending* branch and the *left circumflex* branch. The left anterior descending branch supplies blood to the anterior surface of the heart, and the left circumflex branch provides blood to the lateral wall of the left ventricle. Estimates hold that 60 percent of all coronary occlusions occur in branches of the left coronary artery. The coronary veins follow roughly the same pathways as the coronary arteries and return venous blood from coronary circulation to the right atrium via the coronary sinus.

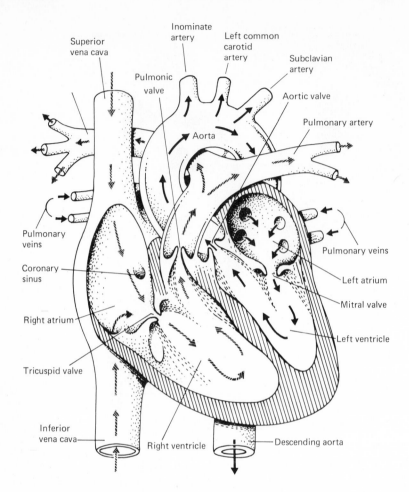

Figure 3-3 Cardiopulmonary circulation.

CARDIAC MUSCLE FIBERS

Cardiac muscle consists of two distinct types of fibers: those which initiate and conduct electric impulses and those which contract the heart. This means that the heart performs two separate kinds of work: *electrical work* (conduction) and *mechanical work* (contraction). It is critically important to realize that electric current must flow through the heart before contraction can occur.

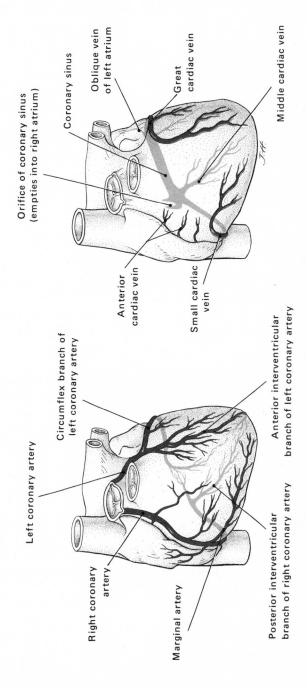

Figure 3-6 Coronary blood vessels. Arteries are at the left, veins at the right. *Taken from Langley, L., Telford, I., and Christensen, J., Dynamic Anatomy and Physiology, 4th ed., McGraw-Hill, New York, 1974, p. 404.*

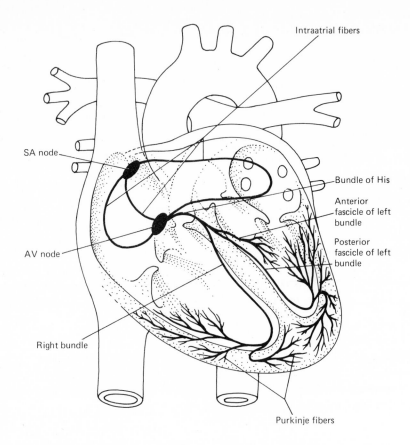

SA node

AV node

Right bundle

Intraatrial fibers

Bundle of His

Anterior fascicle of left bundle

Posterior fascicle of left bundle

Purkinje fibers

Figure 3-7 The electrical conduction system of the heart. The term "junction" is used to refer collectively to the AV node and bundle of His. *(Adapted from Bilitch, M., A Manual of Cardiac Arrhythmias, Little, Brown, Boston, 1971, p. 4.)*

the potassium ion is believed to be the cause of this spontaneous discharge of electricity. In the healthy heart, the SA node tends to reach electrical threshold 60 to 80 times per minute. This rate of spontaneous discharge is faster than the discharge rate of the cells of the junction or the ventricular Purkinje fibers. Thus, the SA node is called the *normal pacemaker* of the heart. In abnormal circumstances, other areas of the ECS may become irritable and develop a more rapid rate of automatic discharge. In these situations, the irritable area of the heart may become an ectopic pacemaker.

CONTRACTILE UNIT OF CARDIAC MUSCLE The atria and ventricles are tightly bound by muscle fibers which combine properties of both skeletal and smooth muscle. Following the flow of electricity via the electrical conduction system, the muscle fibers contract.

Skeletal muscle properties: The cardiac fiber is comprised of striated cylindrical elements known as *myofibrils*. These myofibrils contain delicate myofilaments which form the *sarcomere*. Physiologists believe that the sarcomere is the basic contractile unit of muscle (see Fig. 3-8). Surrounding each myofibril is a sleeve-like structure known as the sarcoplasmic recticulum. The *calcium ion,* which is essential for contraction, is stored within this structure and released following electrical depolarization of the muscle fiber. The positive inotropic action of calcium explains its frequent use during situations of cardiac arrest.

Smooth muscle properties: Cardiac muscle fibers are joined by branching extensions. The points of union between these extensions

Figure 3-8 Representation of the sarcomere, the contractile unit of skeletal muscle. Note the sliding movement of the actin and myosin myofilaments during muscular contraction. *(Adapted from Vander, A., Sherman, J., and Luciano, D., Human Physiology: The Mechanisms of Body Function, 2d ed., McGraw-Hill, New York, 1975, p. 195.)*

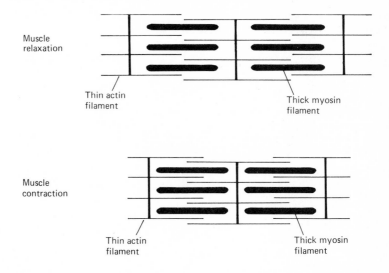

are known as *intercalated disks.* A firm cellular union is provided by these disks so that one muscle fiber rapidly activates the adjoining fibers. Within these disks are points of cellular membrane fusion, known as *tight junctions.* These junctions provide a low-resistance bridge between muscle fibers, and electric impulses can rapidly flow from fiber to fiber. Following the rapid depolarization of the muscle membranes, coordinated cardiac contraction occurs. Efficient pumping of the cardiac muscle is facilitated by the specialized electrical conduction pathway and the low-resistance bridges between muscle fibers.

AUTONOMIC INNERVATION OF THE HEART

The heart is innervated by the autonomic nervous system (see Fig. 3-9). In times of stress, the *sympathetic* division predominates, accelerates the rate of automatic discharge in the SA node, and enhances contractility. When the need for increased cardiac activity ceases, the *parasympathetic* division predominates. Both responses are brought about by the release of a chemical mediator from nerve

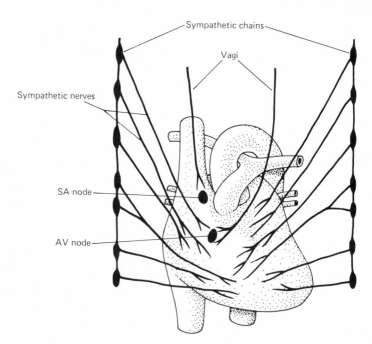

Figure 3-9 Distribution of autonomic nervous fibers to the human heart. *(Taken from Hudak, C., Gallo, B., and Lohr, T., Critical Care Nursing, Lippincott, Philadelphia, 1973, p. 36.)*

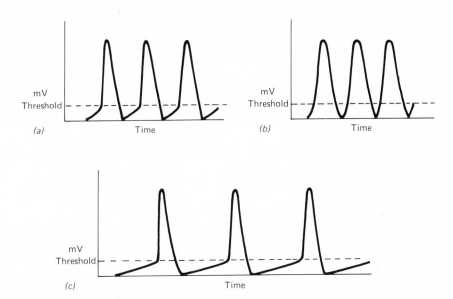

Figure 3-10 (*a*) Intrinsic rate of SA node discharge. (*b*) Effect of norepinephrine on intrinsic rate of SA node discharge. (*c*) Effect of aceylcholine on intrinsic rate of SA node discharge.

endings of each autonomic division. These mediators alter cellular permeability to the potassium ion and thus alter the rate of automatic discharge. The parasympathetic mediator is *acetylcholine,* and the sympathetic mediator is *norepinephrine* (see Fig. 3-10).

BLOOD VESSELS

The blood vessels are a closed system of conducting tubes which transport blood within the cardiovascular system. Arteries and arterioles carry blood away from the heart while venules and veins return it. These vessels are not arranged as a simple one-channel system connecting the left ventricle with the right atrium. There are numerous routes which blood may take as it circulates through the arterial tree, capillaries, and venous vessels (see Fig. 3-11).

ARTERIES

The arteries are essentially elastic tubes which serve a dual function: (1) as transportation pathways of blood away from the heart; and (2) as pressure reservoirs to drive blood through the arterioles and

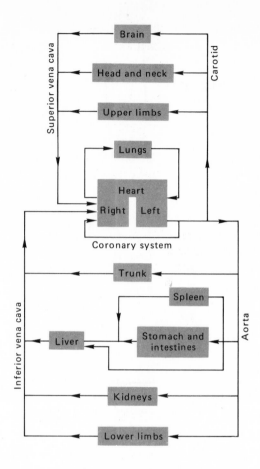

Figure 3-11 Diagrammatic representation of the circulation of the blood. Note the many parallel routes. *(Taken from Langley, L., Telford, I., and Christensen, H., Dynamic Anatomy and Physiology, 4th ed., McGraw-Hill, New York, 1974, p. 467.)*

capillaries. Arterial walls are composed of three layers: (1) inner tunica intima consisting of an endothelium and an elastic membrane; (2) middle tunica media containing numerous elastic and muscular fibers to enhance distensibility; and (3) tunica adventitia consisting of loose collagenous fibers. The walls of the arteries have their own blood supply provided by minute vessels called the *vasa vasorum.*

ARTERIOLES

The arterioles are the primary *resistance* vessels in the body. The smooth muscle lining the arterioles is richly innervated by *sympathetic* nerves and has the ability to constrict and dilate. The pattern of blood flow distribution is primarily determined by the degree of arteriolar constriction or dilatation within the various organs and tissues of the body. The diameter of the arterioles and consequently the resistance to blood flow is closely regulated by a number of factors which are discussed later.

CAPILLARIES

The smallest vessels within the circulatory system are the capillaries, having thin semipermeable walls only one cell layer thick and a surprisingly complex anatomical structure (see Fig. 3-12). At any one time, only 5 percent of the circulating blood volume flows through the capillaries. Yet this 5 percent of blood is the most important part of the entire blood volume since the exchange of oxygen, carbon dioxide, and other metabolites occurs within the capillary network. The oxygen demands of the tissues served by the capillary bed appear to control capillary blood flow. As tissue hypoxia develops, the precapillary sphincter relaxes and blood flows into the capillary. Once the oxygen demand is satisfied, the sphincter constricts, flow stops, and hypoxia again develops. This intermittent flow is often referred to as *rhythmic vasomotion*.

VENULES AND VEINS

After passing through the capillaries, the blood enters the venous vessels to be returned to the heart. Venules are only slightly larger than the capillaries and consist of an endothelial lining and a few smooth muscle fibers.

Figure 3-12 Diagrammatic representation of a capillary network. All the vessels except the true capillary (site of actual metabolic exchange) are enclosed in smooth muscle capable of contraction. Current shock research indicates inadequate cellular perfusion may be caused by precapillary sphincter constriction with microarteriovenous shunting of blood resulting *(Taken from Langley, L., Telford, I., and Christensen, J., Dynamic Anatomy and Physiology, 4th ed., McGraw-Hill, New York, 1974, p. 481.)*

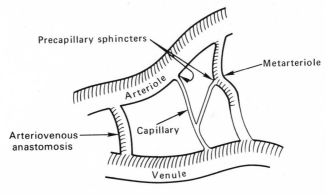

The veins, like the arteries, are composed of three layers. However, their walls are thinner and easily distended. Those veins which return blood to the heart against the force of gravity contain valves which permit unidirectional blood flow. Veins act as both conducting tubes and reservoirs for blood (see Fig. 3-2). In times of stress, the stored blood is pumped into circulation, and venous return is augmented.

PRINCIPLES OF HEMODYNAMICS

Maintenance of adequate blood flow to the tissues and organs of the body is the vital function of the cardiovascular system. This system is precisely regulated by a number of circulatory control mechanisms. It is beyond the scope of this book to present a comprehensive analysis of all hemodynamic factors. However, the major principles can be stated and briefly explained.

Blood flows because of differences or *gradients* in pressure between the arterial and venous sides of circulation. It always flows from areas of *higher* pressure to areas of *lower* pressure (Fig. 3-13).

ARTERIAL PRESSURE AND FLOW

The two primary determinants of arterial pressure are *cardiac output* and *peripheral resistance*. The relationship between pressure, flow (cardiac output), and peripheral resistance can be expressed as follows:

$$Pressure = flow \times resistance$$

CARDIAC OUTPUT   The volume of blood ejected by each ventricle per minute is called the cardiac output. It is determined by multiplying the *heart rate* per minute and the *stroke volume* (amount of blood pumped from the ventricle per beat). Normal resting cardiac output can range from 4 to 6 liters. During periods of stress, it can reach values of 20 to 25 liters. Obviously, both heart rate and stroke volume must increase. For the nurse to accurately determine cardiac output in liters per minutes, fairly elaborate invasive techniques must be utilized. Two commonly used techniques are computation via the Fick principle and the thermodilution indicator method. An indirect, non-invasive method based on knowledge of the factors influencing arterial pressure and the signs and symptoms of decreased cardiac output can also be utilized. With this method, the nurse can rapidly

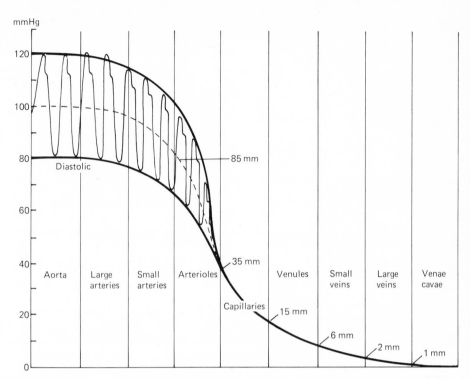

Figure 3-13 Blood pressure gradient. Dotted line indicates the average or mean systolic pressure in arteries. *(Taken from Anthony, C., and Kolthoff, W., Textbook of Anatomy and Physiology, 9th ed., Mosby, St. Louis, 1975, p. 355.)*

assess the patient and intervene appropriately. Nursing assessment of cardiac output is explained in detail in Chap. 14.

Stroke volume: Cardiac muscle, like other muscle, increases its strength of contraction when stretched. The length of the cardiac fiber is determined by the amount of blood which flows into the ventricle during diastolic filling (*preload*) and the end-systolic or residual volume (*afterload*). The greater the volume of blood, the greater the muscle fiber is stretched, and the more forceful the contraction which results. However, marked overstretching of the cardiac muscle can cause a decrease in the force of ventricular contraction. Stroke volume is diminished, and cardiac output may be adversely affected. This intrinsic mechanism by which the heart adjusts to changing end-diastolic volumes is known as *Starling's law of the heart.*

Stroke volume may also be altered via the sympathetic nervous system, circulating catecholamines, and plasma electrolytes. Norepinephrine increases cardiac contractility in addition to enhancing SA nodal automaticity. Circulating catecholamines (epinephrine and norepinephrine) which are released from the adrenal medulla have a profound effect on the heart by enhancing heart rate and contractility. Extracellular concentrations of potassium, calcium, and sodium affect cardiac function in the following ways:

1. Increases in serum potassium decrease the rate and force of cardiac contractility. A decreased potassium gradient between the inside and outside of the myocardial cells may be the cause of this cardiac depression.

2. Elevation of calcium levels stimulates the heart. The positive inotropic effect of this ion has already been noted.

3. Elevations in sodium also depress the heart. Authorities believe that the additional sodium ions compete with calcium ions. This competition inhibits the stimulatory effect of calcium.

Heart rate: Both tachycardias and bradycardias can adversely affect cardiac output. With tachyrrhythmias, diastolic filling time and end-diastolic volume are diminished and stroke volume and cardiac output decrease. While the healthy heart can tolerate rates up to approximately 200 beats per minute, the diseased myocardium has little reserve, and even minor elevations in heart rate can reduce cardiac output. Causes of tachyrrhythmias include hypoxia, electrolyte imbalance, increased sympathetic stimulation, excessive catecholamine release, and drugs such as isoproterenol, amphetamines, and aminophylline. Causes of bradyrrhythmias include a conditioned myocardium, excessive parasympathetic discharge, heart blocks, hypothyroidism, electrolyte imbalances, ischemia to the SA node, and drugs such as digitalis and propranolol.

PERIPHERAL RESISTANCE   The second determinant of arterial pressure is peripheral resistance. Very simply, this is the amount of friction that blood encounters as it travels through the vascular tree. Both the *viscosity* (thickness) of the blood and the *diameter* of the *arterioles* affect peripheral resistance. The numbers of red blood cells and plasma proteins in circulation are the most important factors affecting blood viscosity. As blood viscosity increases, so does peripheral resistance. If the hematocrit of the blood exceeds 60, the blood becomes too viscid for the heart to pump effectively and the cardiac output may decrease.

As the arterioles constrict, peripheral resistance to blood flow also increases and arterial pressure increases. Conversely, arteriolar vasodilation causes a decrease in peripheral resistance. As previously mentioned, arteriolar diameter is precisely regulated by both systemic and local controls.

Systemic controls: The smooth muscle lining the walls of the arterioles is richly supplied by sympathetic nerve fibers. These fibers control the degree of arteriolar constriction by adjusting the amount of *tonic neuron discharge* released at the arteriolar smooth muscle. Increased discharge causes vasoconstriction while decreased sympathetic activity results in vasodilation.

The activity of these sympathetic fibers is coordinated at various levels of the nervous system. The most highly developed center of control is the *vasomotor center,* located in the medulla. It is composed of a cluster of neurons which control arteriolar diameter by varying the degree of constrictor discharge. Peripheral *pressoreceptors* and *chemoreceptors* located in the carotid sinus and aortic arch, the *hypothalamus,* and the *cerebral cortex* are other areas of the nervous system which help to regulate arterial blood pressure.

Humoral agents can also evoke systemic alterations in arterial pressure. Circulating norepinephrine, epinephrine, and angiotensin II elevate blood pressure through arteriolar vasoconstriction. (Epinephrine can also cause arteriolar vasodilation in certain vascular beds, particularly the skeletal muscle.)

In addition to vasoconstricting agents, the body produces certain vasodilating chemicals. Bradykinin causes vigorous vasodilatation. Histamine which is released in response to injury also causes arteriolar dilation.

Local control: Specific organs and tissues, especially the heart and skeletal muscles, can drastically increase their blood flow following an increase in metabolic demands. Decreases in oxygen tension, increases in carbon dioxide tension and hydrogen ion concentration, and local release of histamine and bradykinin following vessel injury have all been demonstrated to cause local vasodilatation. In addition, it has been shown that following vessel injury, epinephrine and serotonin are released from platelets, causing a local vasoconstriction.

Figure 3-14 summarizes the multiple factors influencing cardiac output and peripheral resistance.

ARTERIAL BLOOD PRESSURE MEASUREMENT During left ventricular contraction blood is ejected into the aorta, and the elastic walls of the arteries distend with additional blood (*systole*). During ventricular relaxation (*diastole*) the arterial walls recoil. This elastic recoil drives the blood

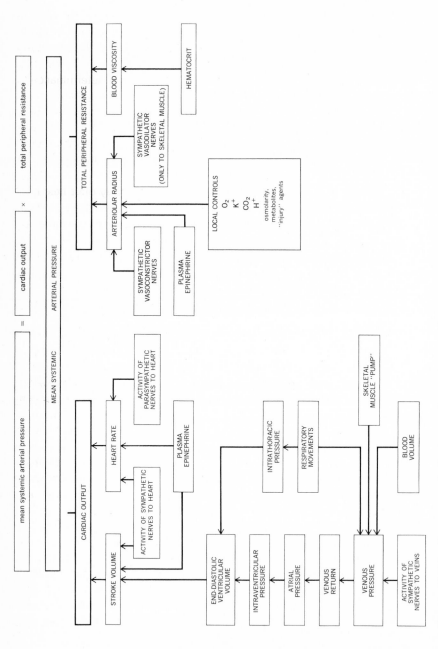

Figure 3-14 **Summary of effector mechanisms and efferent pathways which regulate systemic arterial pressure.** (*Taken from Vander, A., Sherman, J., and Luciano, D., Human Physiology: The Mechanisms of Body Function, 2d ed., McGraw-Hill, New York, 1975, p. 268.*)

through the arterioles. The arterial pulse is due to the gradient or difference between systolic and diastolic pressure. This gradient is called the *pulse pressure,* which is the difference between systolic and diastolic pressures.

Mean arterial pressure: One of the most important arterial pressure measurements is the *mean arterial pressure.* Very simply, this is the average pressure driving the arterial blood through all the organs and tissues during the entire cardiac cycle. Diastole lasts longer than systole and thus has a greater influence on the determination of average or mean arterial pressure. In other words, the mean arterial pressure is not simply the value halfway between those two pressures, but rather a value closer to diastolic pressure. The actual mean pressure can be computed only by highly complex methods, but a rough approximation can be obtained by adding one-third of the pulse pressure to the diastolic pressure.

Because the arteries have a large diameter, they offer little resistance to blood flow, and the pressures are remarkably similar throughout the arterial tree. Thus, measurement of brachial artery pressure gives important information regarding aortic pressure. This knowledge is valuable since aortic pressure influences coronary blood flow.

VENOUS PRESSURE AND FLOW

One of the most significant factors affecting cardiac output is the *venous return* to the heart. The force driving the venous blood back to the right atrium is the venous pressure. The pressure within the veins depends upon the interactions of three factors: (1) the degree of venoconstriction; (2) the blood volume; (3) and the pumping action of the heart.

Central venous pressure (CVP) can be measured to assess the relationship of these three factors. Since venous valves and local venoconstriction can impede flow, peripheral veins do not accurately reflect the above factors. Therefore, the central venous system, which consists of the inferior and the superior venae cavae and the right atrium, must be used (see Fig. 3-3). This system reflects the filling pressures of the *right ventricle.* CVP cannot be relied upon for information regarding left ventricular end-diastolic filling pressures. This has been noted numerous times in the management of patients with acute myocardial infarction. In these patients, CVP can be within normal limits (3 to 15 cmH$_2$O), yet left ventricular pressures are elevated. The recent development of flow-directed catheters (*Swan-Ganz catheters*), which can be threaded via the venous system into a branch of the *pulmonary artery*, has assisted in the measurement of left ventricular pressures. The pulmonary artery diastolic pressure (8 to 10 mmHg), which can be continuously monitored, correlates well with the filling pressures in the left ventricle.

Three important factors assist in returning blood to the right side of the heart. These are: (1) the process of breathing; (2) skeletal muscle contraction; (3) venous valves.

PROCESS OF BREATHING   During inspiration the diaphragm contracts and the pressure within the thorax decreases. Pressure within the intrathoracic veins drops; an increase in the pressure gradient between the central and the peripheral veins occurs, and venous return is temporarily facilitated. The diaphragm also pushes on the abdominal contents, and abdominal pressure increases. This increased abdominal pressure compresses the large veins of the belly, and blood is pushed toward the right side of the heart. Deep breathing intensifies these effects.

SKELETAL MUSCLE CONTRACTION AND VENOUS VALVES   These contractions serve as "booster pumps" for the blood. With each contraction, venous blood is pumped against gravity toward the right atrium. The venous valves prevent the column of blood from regurgitating as the muscle relaxes.

This chapter has provided an overview of the normal anatomy and physiology of the cardiovascular system. Comprehension of the succeeding chapters on cardiovascular pathology is dependent on this knowledge.

BIBLIOGRAPHY

Anthony, C. P., and Kolthoff, N. J., *Textbook of Anatomy and Physiology*, 9th ed., Mosby, St. Louis, 1975.

Ganong, W., *Review of Medical Physiology*, Lange, Los Altos, Calif., 1974.

Guyton, A. C., *Textbook of Medical Physiology*, Saunders, Philadelphia, 1976.

Hudak, C., Gallo, M., and Lohr, S., *Critical Care Nursing*, Mosby, St. Louis, 1973.

Langley, L., Teflord, I., and Christensen, J. B., *Dynamic Anatomy and Physiology*, 4th ed., McGraw-Hill, New York, 1974.

Vander, A., Sherman, J., and Luciano, D., *Human Physiology: The Mechanisms of Body Function*, 2d ed., McGraw-Hill, New York, 1975.

CHAPTER 4
BASIC TWELVE-LEAD ELECTRO-CARDIOGRAPHY

SANDRA GRESHAM, R.N., M.Ed.

THE heart does two types of work, electrical work which includes stimulation and conduction of electric impulses, and mechanical work, contraction. Electrocardiograms (ECG) are the tracings produced by recording only the electrical action of the heart. In each heart cycle there are four major events: *stimulation* (firing), *depolarization* (spread of the impulse), *contraction,* and *repolarization* (recovery). Of these, contraction is mechanical and is therefore not seen on an ECG. Stimulation, depolarization, and repolarization are electrical events. Stimulation is also not seen on an ECG because it is not of sufficient magnitude to be recorded from the surface of the body. By the process of elimination, then, depolarization and repolarization are the electrical events which are recorded to produce the P, QRS, and T waves (see Fig. 4-1).

The P wave is due to atrial depolarization, the QRS complex is caused by ventricular depolarization, and the T wave results from ventricular repolarization. The electric currents of depolarization and repolarization are picked up and conducted to the electrocardiograph by electrodes placed on the patient's limbs and chest. These currents

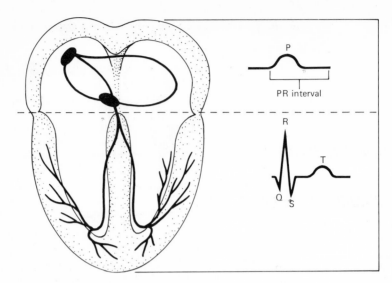

Figure 4-1 Anatomical basis for electrical activity.

are then amplified by the machine approximately 3000 times, and the positive and negative currents move a stylus which is in contact with moving heat-sensitive paper.

Most nurses are familiar with the way the resulting ECG patterns appear in only 1 of the 12 leads—lead II. The other 11 leads show the same electrical activity seen in lead II, but from different perspectives. A 12-lead ECG, then, provides more comprehensive information by showing electrical activity from 12 different directions. There are three major groups of leads within the 12-lead system: the standard leads, the augmented leads, and the chest leads.

STANDARD LEADS

The standard leads are *lead I, lead II,* and *lead III.* Once the metal electrodes have been attached to the patient's limbs, the ECG machine writes out each of these leads when the dial is changed. Lead I connects the right arm and the left arm, with the left arm being the positive or recording electrode. Lead II connects the right arm and left leg, with the positive end being the left leg. Lead III connects the left arm and the left leg, with the positive end again being the left leg. The custom is to label the positive end of each lead (see Fig. 4-2).

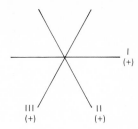

Figure 4-2 Standard leads.

AUGMENTED LEADS

The next group of leads is called the augmented leads and consists of *avR, avL,* and *avF.* Remembering these leads is much easier when the meaning of the letters is explained: avR simply means an augmented (amplified) voltage from the right. The "L" and "F" stand for "left" and "foot." These leads are represented in Fig. 4-3. The positive ends of each lead have been labeled.

Leads, then, can be defined as pairs of electrodes. Each pair has a positive end which is labeled. The reader may have heard of bipolar and unipolar leads. The standard leads are bipolar, meaning that both of the electrodes in the lead are subject to wide variations in electrical potential. The difference is recorded. The augmented leads are unipolar, and only one of the two electrodes has wide variation in electrical potential. Unipolar leads produce less amplitude, and it is this difference which requires the unipolar leads to be augmented. For a more detailed explanation, the reader should consult the bibliography.

Figure 4-3 Augmented leads.

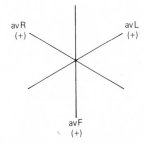

The standard leads and the augmented leads can also be called *limb leads* as the electrodes used to record them are placed on the patient's extremities. Combining the standard leads I, II, and III with the augmented leads avR, avL, and avF forms a circle of six leads. This is known as the *hexaxial* (six axes) *reference system* and is shown in Fig. 4-4. The practical application of the hexaxial reference system will be demonstrated later in this chapter when the QRS axis is discussed.

CHEST OR PRECORDIAL LEADS

The remaining six leads are called the *chest leads,* and they view the heart from a front-to-back (anterior-posterior) fashion. These leads are also called precordial or "V" leads, with "V" again meaning voltage. The correct position of the chest leads, V_1 through V_6, is shown in Fig. 4-5. V_1 is placed in the fourth intercostal space just to the right of the sternum. V_2 is placed in the fourth intercostal space just to the left of the sternum. V_4 occupies the fifth intercostal space in alignment with the midclavicular line, an imaginary vertical line drawn from the middle of the clavicle so that it intersects with the fifth intercostal space. The middle of the clavicle and the fifth intercostal space are located by palpation. V_3 is located halfway between V_2 and V_4. V_5 is placed at the same level as V_4 and the anterior axillary line. V_6 is located at the same level as V_4 and V_5 and the midaxillary line.

Some practical hints should be briefly discussed. Most nurses who have not done many 12-lead ECGs have some doubts about where the chest leads should be placed. If a wide variety of individuals with differing levels of expertise perform ECGs within an agency, a drawing of the kind shown in Fig. 4-5 should be placed in the machine for

Figure 4-4 Hexaxial reference system.

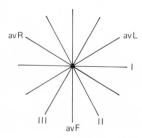

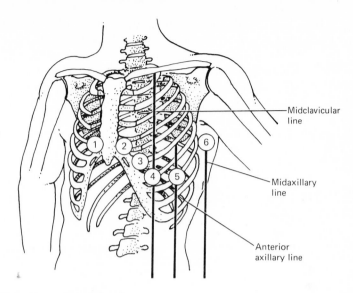

Figure 4-5 Placement of chest leads.

reference. If unusual difficulties such as dressings or massive breasts are encountered, a notation should be made for the person who interprets the tracing. It is best to locate the landmarks and place the amount of electrode paste desired on the six appropriate chest locations. By comparing the location of the paste to the reference drawing, mistakes can often be avoided. Some agencies have their personnel make ink dots on the patient's precordium so the subsequent ECGs will be consistent. This is an excellent opportunity for teaching if an experienced individual notices incorrect placement of dots.

DIRECTION OF ATRIAL DEPOLARIZATION

Earlier in this chapter, emphasis was placed upon the fact that the positive end of each lead should be labeled. The reason for that emphasis will now be explained. ECG machines are designed so that electrical activity moving toward the positive end of any lead is recorded as a positive deflection on ECG paper. See, for example, Fig. 4-6a. This shows lead II with the positive end labeled. Taking atrial depolarization as an example, one can see that it is moving toward the positive end of lead II and results in a positive or upright P wave on ECG paper. Conversely, electrical activity moving away from the positive end of any lead records a negative deflection on ECG paper. Figure 4-6b again shows lead II. Use of the same example of atrial depolarization demonstrates depolarization of the atria from below or retrograde. Since the electrical activity is moving away from the positive end of lead II, a negative P wave results. A third possibility exists. It has been seen that an impulse moving toward the positive end of any lead records a positive deflection in that lead, and that an impulse moving away from the positive end of any lead records a negative deflection, but what happens when an impulse is moving perpendicular to a lead? The answer is that the ECG machine either records a deflection which is equally positive and equally negative or records nothing. Figure 4-6c shows a *biphasic* P wave, which is one having two phases, one positive and one negative. Rarely, the positive and negative balance each other and the stylus does not move and no electrical activity is recorded.

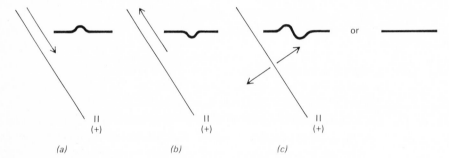

Figure 4-6 Direction of atrial depolarization. (*a*) Positive deflection. (*b*) Negative deflection. (*c*) Isoelectric.

The above example concerned atrial depolarization. The same principle applies to ventricular depolarization. The ventricular septum is the first structure within the ventricles to depolarize, with the wave of depolarization moving from left to right. The next area to depolarize is the ventricular muscle mass. Since the left ventricle is normally thicker than the right ventricle, all leads record a movement to the left. The posterior epicardial surface at the base (top) of the ventricles is the last area to depolarize. Figure 4-7a demonstrates this concept. A summary of the instant-to-instant wave of ventricular depolarization is diagrammed in Fig. 4-7b. This is frequently called a *vectorcardiogram.*

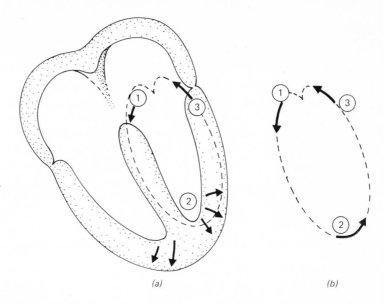

Figure 4-7 Direction of ventricular depolarization. (*a*) Sequence of ventricular depolarization. (*b*) Vector loop.

If this summary of ventricular depolarization is superimposed on lead I, the configuration of the QRS complex recorded in this lead can be determined (*see* Fig. 4-8). Remember that any lead records electrical activity moving *away* from its positive end as negative and *toward* its positive end as positive. The initial excursion (1) in Fig. 4-8 moves away from the positive end of lead I, and a negative deflection is inscribed. The impulse then moves back to the base line which is electrically neutral. Thus far, a Q wave has been formed. Ventricular depolarization now moves strongly toward the positive end of lead I producing a comparatively tall positive deflection (2) before returning to the base line. A tall R wave now follows the initial Q wave. The last portion of ventricular depolarization (3) moves away from the positive end of lead I to inscribe a final S wave. The QRS pattern seen in lead I has now been completed. This same process can be repeated for each of the 12 leads and explains the presence or absence of certain waves within the QRS complex and their relative height or depth in each lead. The characteristics of the QRS complex in each lead depend upon the summary loop of ventricular depolarization for individual patients.

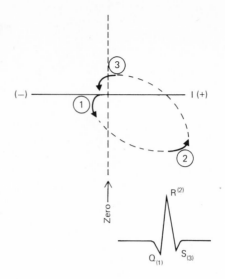

Figure 4-8 Sequence of ventricular depolarization in relation to lead I.

QRS AXIS

The official interpretation of a patient's electrocardiogram usually includes the determination of the QRS axis. This is a description of the major direction of ventricular depolarization. If a circle were placed over the ventricles as shown in Fig. 4-9, ventricular depolarization would be expected to take place in the quadrant containing the ventricular conduction system. For this reason, this portion of the circle is considered the normal QRS axis quadrant. Figure 4-10 shows the four labeled quadrants. This circle has been arbitrarily

Figure 4-9 Quadrant determination relative to the ventricular conduction system.

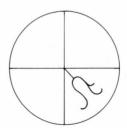

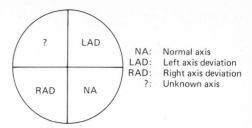

Figure 4-10 Labeled quadrants for axis determination.

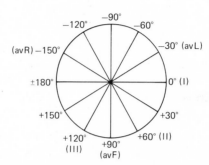

Figure 4-11 Relationship of degree designation of electrical axis and hexaxial reference system.

designated in degrees as shown in Fig. 4-11. A patient with a QRS axis of 0 to +90° is therefore considered to have a normal axis.

Diagnosing a patient's problem is often aided by determining the QRS axis as there are conditions commonly associated with left and right axis deviation (LAD and RAD). A few examples are given below:

Associated with LAD	Associated with RAD
Left bundle branch block	Right bundle branch block
Inferior myocardial infarction (MI)	Lateral MI
Left ventricular hypertrophy	Right ventricular hypertrophy

Various methods are available to determine the QRS axis. The simplest method involves looking at two limb leads and enables determination of the quadrant of the QRS. In other words, one should be able to determine whether the QRS axis lies within the normal, left, right, or unknown quadrant.

QUADRANT DETERMINATION OF AXIS

The two leads used in this method are lead I and avF. To begin, the QRS complexes are inspected to determine whether they are more positive, more negative, or isoelectric. Figure 4-12 gives examples of each.

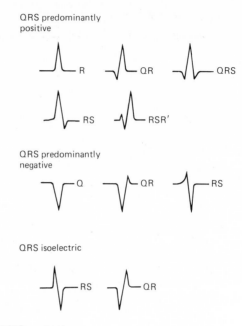

Figure 4-12 Examples of QRS variants.

Figure 4-13 shows lead I and the avF lead of a sample patient. To determine the quadrant of the QRS axis, several steps are performed. In the beginning it is advisable to do this on paper; after some practice these steps can be performed mentally. Lead I is clearly positive.

Figure 4-13 Leads I and avF.

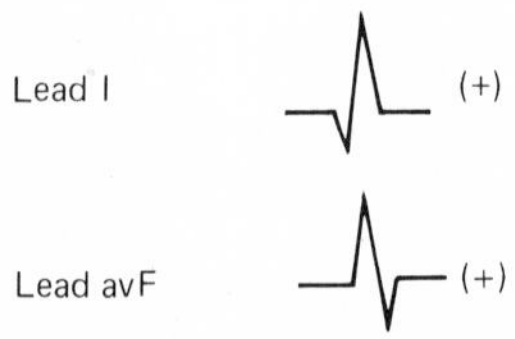

Lead I   (+)

Lead avF   (+)

This means that the main force of ventricular depolarization is moving toward the positive end of lead I as seen in Fig. 4-14a. The positive half of the circle for lead I is seen in Fig. 4-14b. Since the QRS in lead I is positive, the negative half of the circle for lead I can be eliminated as shown in Fig. 4-15.

Lead avF is now examined in the same manner. The QRS seen in avF was also clearly more positive than negative, showing that the forces of ventricular depolarization are also moving toward the positive end of avF. Figure 4-16a illustrates this concept. Figure 4-16b shows that the negative half of the circle for avF can now be elimi-

Figure 4-14

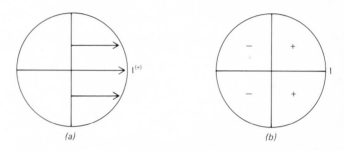

Figure 4-15

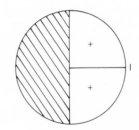

Figure 4-16

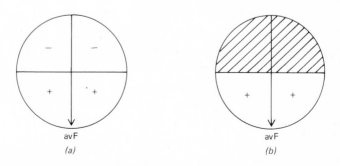

nated. Putting the information learned from lead I together with that from avF, we see that the only quadrant not elimi-

nated is the normal QRS axis:

Another example may help to clarify this method of QRS axis determination. As can be seen, a patient with the QRS complexes illustrated in Fig. 4-17 has a left axis deviation:

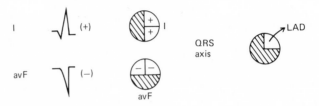

Figure 4-17 Summary of left axis deviation.

The axis of a patient with a QRS which is isoelectric in either lead I or avF is determined by using the same steps. Figure 4-18 illustrates the QRS complexes. Lead I shows the forces of ventricular depolarization moving toward the positive end of lead I. The negative half of the circle is therefore eliminated. Lead avF shows an isoelectric QRS complex which is not positive or negative but electrically zero. (Remember that an impulse traveling perpendicular to any lead may appear isoelectric.) The impulse must therefore be traveling in the manner depicted in Fig. 4-19. Combining the information learned from lead I and avF gives the result that the QRS axis is 0° or normal:

0° normal QRS axis (Refer to Fig. 4-11 for degree designation.)

Figure 4-18 Isoelectric QRS in avF.

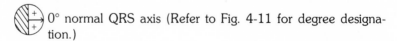

Lead I

Lead avF

The skills necessary to use this method of determining QRS axis are roughly comparable with learning the multiplication tables in that practice enhances memorization to make the information available when needed. The ECGs of the patients seen daily in the emergency room and the questions they provoke provide continuing education in basic 12-lead electrocardiography.

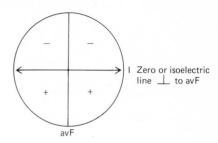

Figure 4-19   QRS axis of O°.

BIBLIOGRAPHY

Chung, Edward K., and Chung, Donald K., *ECG Diagnosis—Self Assessment*, Harper & Row, New York, 1972.

Netter, Frank H., *Ciba Collection of Medical Illustrations*, vol. 5, *Heart*, Ciba, Summit, New Jersey, 1969.

Vinsant, M., Spence, M., and Chapell, D., *A Commonsense Approach to Coronary Care: A Program*, Mosby, St. Louis, 1972.

Zalis, Edwin G., and Conover, Mary H., *Understanding Electrocardiography: Physiological and Interpretive Concepts*, Mosby, St. Louis, 1972.

CHAPTER 5
THE RESPIRATORY SYSTEM

JEANIE BARRY, R.N., M.S.

IN order to survive, humans must have a continuous supply of oxygen and adequate elimination of carbon dioxide. Providing them is the primary function of the respiratory system. The cardiovascular system works in close union with the respiratory system, transporting these gases to and from the cells.

Respiration is usually thought of in terms of alveolar gas exchange. This is often called *external respiration*. However, when the term "respiration" is viewed in its broadest sense, it encompasses not only pulmonary ventilation but also the metabolic reaction of O_2 and glucose within the cell.

This chapter is designed to provide the nurse with an overview of respiratory anatomy and physiology. Emphasis is placed on the microstructure of the alveolar-capillary membrane. In addition, oxygen transport and cellular respiration are discussed. Carbon dioxide transport is explained in Chap. 7.

THE RESPIRATORY TRACT

The respiratory tract begins with the nose and terminates in the alveoli which are the actual gas-exchanging units of the lung. All the other structures of the respiratory tract serve primarily as air conduits. The respiratory tract is divided into two parts: the *upper tract* consisting of the nose, pharynx, and larynx, and the *lower tract* consisting of the trachea, bronchial tree, and alveoli.

UPPER RESPIRATORY TRACT

As air passes through this tract, it is *warmed, moistened,* and *filtered.* Dirt, dust, and bacteria are entrapped by a blanket of mucus, and hair-like projections, called *cilia,* transport them back toward the nasal openings. It should be noted that air is warmed and moistened throughout the entire respiratory tract but the nasal mucosa performs the greatest amount of this humidification. When this structure is bypassed by a tracheostomy or an endotracheal tube, it is imperative that the air be humidified by artificial means.

LOWER RESPIRATORY TRACT

The lower respiratory tract is often conceptualized as a tree with the trachea as the trunk and the bronchial tubes as the branches (see Fig. 5-1).

The *trachea* is located in the midline of the neck and anterior to the esophagus. It is approximately 5 to 6 inches in length and 1 inch in diameter. The trachea is composed of smooth muscle and supported by C-shaped cartilagenous rings. At the second intercostal space, the trachea bifurcates into the right and left main-stem *bronchi.* The point of bifurcation is called the *carina.* The right main-stem bronchus is wider and more vertical than the left bronchus. If an endotracheal tube is passed to the point of the carina, it can easily slip into the right bronchus, and the left lung may collapse due to atelectasis. Furthermore, aspirated material such as foreign objects and vomitus more frequently enter the right lung.

Along with the pulmonary vessels, the main-stem bronchi enter the lung at a point called the *hilum.* They continue to subdivide into progressively smaller air passages until they terminate in the *alveoli.* Up to the point of the terminal bronchi, the bronchial tree is lined with smooth muscle, cartilage, and mucus-producing goblet cells. Bacteria, dust, and dirt are entrapped by the mucus and fanned upward by the wave-like movement of the cilia. Distal to the terminal

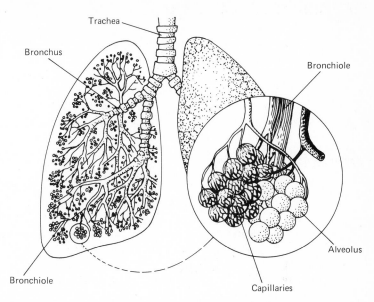

Figure 5-1 Right lung, cut away to illustrate dichotomous division of the respiratory tract. Insert shows a gas-exchanging unit with terminal bronchiole, dependent alveoli, and alveolar capillary meshwork. *(From Wade, Jacqueline, Respiratory Nursing Care: Physiology and Technique, 1st ed., Mosby, St. Louis, 1973, p. 3.)*

bronchi are the *bronchioles*. These structures differ from the bronchi in that they lack cartilage. The final portion of the air passages, the *terminal bronchioles*, lack goblet cells and cilia also.

LUNGS AND THORAX

The lungs are located within the *thoracic cavity* (see Fig. 3-1). The right lung has three lobes; the left has only two lobes due to the presence of the heart.

The lungs are separately encased by a thin membrane called the *pleura*. This membrane has two layers: the parietal pleura which adheres to the walls of the thoracic cavity and the visceral pleura which lines the lungs. A potential space exists between the visceral and parietal pleura. Within this space, a thin film of lubricating fluid is found. A *negative* or *sucking pressure* exists within the intrapleural space. (*Negative* indicates that the pressure is less than that of the atmosphere.) The intrapleural pressure counteracts the *elastic recoil* nature of the lung, and complete collapse of the lung with exhalation is prevented. A pneumothorax results when this negative intrapleural pressure is equalized to atmospheric pressure.

ALVEOLAR-CAPILLARY MEMBRANE

It has been noted that the terminal bronchioles are the final portions of the bronchial tree that are purely air conduits. Distal to these bronchioles are the actual gas exchanging units which include respiratory bronchioles (microscopic tubes with scattered alveoli), alveolar ducts, alveolar sacs, and the alveoli. The normal adult lung has approximately 300 million alveoli. Surrounding the alveolar structure is the pulmonary capillary network (see Fig. 5-1). In health, gases rapidly diffuse across this *alveolar-capillary membrane,* and arterial blood gas tensions are almost instantaneously achieved.

By use of electron microscopy, four distinct cells have been identified as components of this structure.

1. The first cell which forms the lining of the alveoli is a flat pancake-shaped structure known as the *type-I pneumonocyte.*

2. In addition to the type-I pneumonocyte, there exists a larger cell noted to have a microvillated surface, a great number of mitochondria, and a high metabolic rate. The cell has been named the *type-II pneumonocyte* and is believed to be responsible for *surfactant* production.

3. The *endothelial cell* forms the lining of the pulmonary capillary. The lumen of the capillary is wide enough to allow only one red blood cell to pass through at a time. Thus, anything which causes swelling of the endothelial cells greatly decreases oxygen uptake by the red blood cells.

4. The *mesenchymal cell* is unique in that it is capable of performing many functions. Physiologists have determined that it can become a fibroplast, a macrophage, or a smooth muscle cell.

A thin layer of interstitial fluid which exerts a slight negative pressure surrounds these fragile structures. Other than this fluid, there are no skeletal-like structures to support the alveolar-capillary membrane. It is critically important to appreciate the extreme delicacy of this membrane and thus its susceptibility to insult and consequent damage. For this reason, supportive respiratory care is one of the most important aspects in the emergency nursing care of the critically ill patient.

SURFACE TENSION AND THE ACTION OF SURFACTANT

It has been noted that the type-II pneumonocyte may be the site of *surfactant* production. Surfactant is a molecular compound containing a protein and a lipid (fatty) substance called *lecithin*. This compound reduces alveolar surface tension.

SURFACE TENSION   The alveolar surface is in essence a *gas-liquid interface* and thus possesses the physical property of *surface tension*. This tension is created by the molecular activity of the particles forming the liquid's top layer. These molecules are attracted inward and downward, and a force pulling toward the center of the liquid is created. The end result of this molecular attraction is surface tension. This tension tends to collapse alveoli and to resist alveolar expansion. Alveolar surface tension is also an important factor contributing to the elastic recoil nature of the lung. Since each of the 300 million alveoli has a gas-liquid interface, a great deal of inspiratory pressure would be needed to overcome the existing surface tension. Nature protects man from such a needless expenditure of energy by means of surfactant. It reduces surface tension at the gas-liquid interface, equalizing pressure within each alveolus and preventing alveolar collapse.

Any condition which injures the alveolar-capillary membrane may eventually damage type-II pneumonocytes, impairing surfactant production. The end result may be massive atelectasis and hypoxemia.

VENTILATION, BLOOD FLOW, AND DIFFUSION

Maintenance of arterial blood gases is dependent upon adequate pulmonary ventilation, pulmonary blood flow, and gaseous diffusion across the alveolar-capillary membrane.

PULMONARY VENTILATION

In order for external respiration to occur, a column of air must come in contact with the alveolar-capillary membrane. The movement of this column of air is known as *pulmonary ventilation*. It is dependent upon patent airways, an intact thoracic cage, and functioning respiratory muscles. If one of these factors is impaired, alveolar ventilation suffers, with hypoxemia and hypercarbia (CO_2 retention) resulting.

MUSCLES OF RESPIRATION The elastic recoil nature of lungs and thorax must be overcome by active muscular contraction during inspiration. The primary muscles which provide this respiratory force are the *diaphragm* and the *external intercostals*. The phrenic nerves which originate from C3–5 innervate the diaphragm; the nerves innervating the external intercostals arise from T3–6.

MECHANICS OF BREATHING Gas, just like fluid, flows because of *pressure gradients*. It moves from an area of higher pressure to an area of lower pressure. The process of breathing involves the creation of pressure gradients between the atmosphere and the lung. (See Table 5-1.)

Inspiration: When the lungs and thorax are in a resting position, there is no pressure gradient. Atmospheric and intrapulmonary pressures (pressure within the airways) are equal, measuring 760 mmHg at sea level.

With inspiration, the diaphragm contracts and the length of the thorax increases. In addition, the external intercostals lift the thorax up and out, increasing the anterior-posterior diameter of the chest. As the size of the thorax increases, intrapleural pressure becomes more negative. This is in accordance with *Boyle's law* which states that the volume and pressure of a gas are inversely proportional.

As the thorax enlarges, the lungs are expanded owing to the adherence of the parietal pleura to the thoracic cavity. The volume or size of the lungs increases; intrapulmonary pressure decreases. A gradient has been created, and air rushes into the lungs until pressure equilibration is reached.

Expiration: Expiration is passive because of the elastic recoil nature of the lungs. The diaphragm and intercostals relax; the thorax and lungs return to their preinspiratory size. Pressure elevates since volume has decreased and air flows out of the lungs.

Table 5-1 **Pressures within the thorax and lungs during the different phases of breathing.***

Pressures	Inspiration	Expiration	Chest at rest
Atmospheric	760 mmHg	760 mmHg	760 mmHg
Intrapleural*	752 mmHg	755 mmHg	756 mmHg
Intrapulmonary	757 mmHg	762 mmHg	760 mmHg

* The terms *intrapleural* and *intrathoracic* are synonymous.

LUNG VOLUMES   A knowledge of lung volumes helps the nurse to understand respiratory physiology and certain forms of pathophysiology. While pulmonary spirometry measures numerous lung volumes (see Fig. 5-2), this chapter discusses only vital capacity, tidal volume, and pulmonary ventilation.

Vital capacity: The volume of gas that can be forcefully expelled from the lungs following maximal inspiration is known as the *vital capacity* (VC). It ranges from 4500 to 6000 cc and is altered by size, posture, and position. Many clinical conditions can adversely affect the vital capacity and thus an individual's ability to increase alveolar gas exchange. Kyphoscoliosis, chest trauma, and abdominal distention are only a few of these conditions.

Tidal volume: The amount of air exhaled after normal inhalation is known as *tidal volume* (TV). For an adult, this measures about 500 cc per breath and can easily increase to 1.5 liters in times of stress. However, not all this air is available for alveolar gas exchange. Approximately 150 cc is wasted in the larger airways; these airways are appropriately called *anatomical dead space*. Anything which decreases the tidal volume or increases the amount of dead space adversely affects alveolar ventilation. Inadequate alveolar gas exchange and abnormal arterial blood gases are the end results.

Figure 5-2   Lung volumes and their subdivisions illustrated by spirograph tracing. (a.) Inspiratory vital capacity. (b.) The more common expiratory vital capacity. *(From Wade, Jacqueline, Respiratory Nursing Care: Physiology and Technique, 1st ed., Mosby, St. Louis, 1973, p. 18.)*

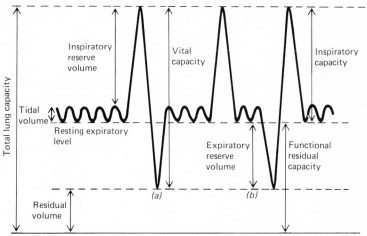

Pulmonary ventilation: Pulmonary ventilation (V̇E) is calculated by multiplying the tidal volume by the respiratory rate. For example:

$$500 \text{ cc} \times 15 = 7500 \text{ cc}$$
$$\text{(TV)} \quad \text{(Rate)} \quad \text{(VE)}$$

Of course, not all this air is available for alveolar exchange. If the amount of air lost in the anatomical dead space is subtracted (150 × 15 = 2250), the V̇E becomes *alveolar ventilation* (V̇A) which equals 5250 cc. This is the actual amount of gas which ventilates the alveoli. The reader should note that V̇A, and thus gas exchange, are increased by rapid, deep breathing. This type of breathing is a common sign in many emergency situations.

COMPLIANCE   Compliance is a measure of the elastic properties of the lungs and thorax. The term "elastic" implies that both the lungs and the thorax can be distended. However, muscular force must be utilized. Also, once this force is removed, the lungs and thorax demonstrate elastic recoil.

A decrease in compliance (often called *stiff lungs*) necessitates increased muscular force so that sufficient volumes of air can be delivered to the alveoli. Patients with diminished compliance also frequently have reduced tidal volumes. In order to maintain adequate alveolar ventilation, tachypnea results.

AIRWAY RESISTANCE   Just as blood encounters frictional resistance as it flows through the vascular tree, so does air as it flows through the bronchial tree. The pulmonary driving pressure is created by the gradients that occur between atmospheric and intrapulmonary pressures during inspiration and expiration. Caliber of airways and the nature of the airflow through them are important determinants of *airway resistance.*

As the caliber of airways decreases, greater pulmonary pressures are needed to force air through them. Decreased airway caliber is an important consideration when caring for patients with bronchospastic conditions because of its effects on pulmonary pressures and the work of breathing.

Airflow can be either *laminar* (streamlined) or *turbulent.* Laminar flow is smooth and occurs in the straight tubes like the trachea. As the airways become more irregular, turbulent flow develops. This type of flow normally is found in the small bronchi and bronchioles. It also develops when tidal volumes are elevated or when there are airway

obstructions. Large increases in driving pressures are needed to overcome turbulent flow, and the work of breathing also increases.

PULMONARY BLOOD FLOW

Pulmonary circulation's principal function is to change mixed venous
blood into arterial blood. In order to do this, adequate alveolar ventilation must occur. Thus, ventilation and pulmonary circulation are
related. The expression $\dot{V}_A/\dot{Q}$ is often used to express this relationship. $\dot{V}_A$ refers to alveolar ventilation, and $\dot{Q}$ refers to blood flow or
perfusion. If either of these factors is adversely affected, the body's
ability to arterialize mixed venous blood decreases.

PULMONARY PRESSURE AND RESISTANCE It has been noted that the pulmonary
vascular system is a *low-pressure, low-resistance* system. The blood
vessels are highly distensible, allowing the same amount of blood
which is circulated to the entire body to flow through the thorax in
1 minute.

Pulmonary capillary pressure measures approximately 6 mmHg.
If the pressure within these vessels rises above 25 mmHg, colloidal
pressure within the capillary is overcome; fluid begins to transude
into the pulmonary interstitium, and eventually alveolar pulmonary
edema develops. Left ventricular failure is a common cause of pulmonary pressure elevation.

Pulmonary capillary resistance can be elevated by alveolar
hypoxia, hypercarbia, and acidemia. These conditions cause vasoconstriction in the pulmonary bed, and pulmonary pressures must
increase to overcome this elevated resistance. If the hypoxia or
acidosis is chronic, pulmonary hypertension results. The work of the
right ventricle increases, and eventually right ventricular failure
develops. This condition is known as *cor pulmonale.*

DIFFUSION

Once alveolar air comes in contact with the pulmonary capillary
blood, rapid diffusion of gases occurs. This diffusion is a passive
phenomenon, dependent upon *pressure gradients* (see Fig. 5-3).
CO_2 is approximately 20 times more diffusible than oxygen and
leaves the plasma in less than 0.5 second. Oxygen is less diffusible,
entering the red blood cells in about 1 second.

Many things can affect the diffusion of the respiratory gases.
Jacqueline Wade has aptly described the diffusion pathway as an

"obstacle course through which gas molecules of O_2 and CO_2 must pass." [1] (See Fig. 5-4.) If any of the structures within the diffusion pathway are altered, the rate of diffusion can be impaired. Pulmonary edema and interstitial fibrosis are examples of diseases which alter the alveolar-capillary structures.

$\dot{V}_A/\dot{Q}$ BALANCE

Before proceeding to oxygen transport, one more important point needs to be made regarding the relationship between ventilation and perfusion. If adequate diffusion of gases is to occur, aerated alveoli must be surrounded by patent capillaries. If blood flows past hypoventilated pulmonary alveoli, inadequate gas exchange occurs. Emphysema is an example of this situation. Conversely, if well-ventilated alveoli are surrounded by obstructed pulmonary capillaries, diffusion is impaired. Pulmonary embolus produces this type

COORDINATED BODY FUNCTIONS

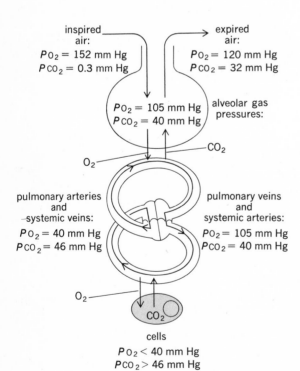

inspired air:
$PO_2 = 152$ mm Hg
$PCO_2 = 0.3$ mm Hg

expired air:
$PO_2 = 120$ mm Hg
$PCO_2 = 32$ mm Hg

$PO_2 = 105$ mm Hg
$PCO_2 = 40$ mm Hg
alveolar gas pressures:

CO_2

O_2

pulmonary arteries and systemic veins:
$PO_2 = 40$ mm Hg
$PCO_2 = 46$ mm Hg

pulmonary veins and systemic arteries:
$PO_2 = 105$ mm Hg
$PCO_2 = 40$ mm Hg

O_2

CO_2

cells
$PO_2 < 40$ mm Hg
$PCO_2 > 46$ mm Hg

Figure 5-3 Summary of carbon dioxide and oxygen pressures in the inspired and expired air and various places within the body. *(From Vander, A., Sherman, J., and Luciano, D., Human Physiology: The Mechanisms of Body Function, 2d ed., McGraw-Hill, New York, 1975, p. 298.)*

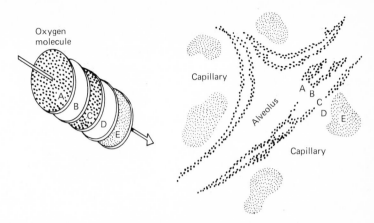

Figure 5-4 Diffusion pathway shown in stylized form (left) and as seen through an electron microscope (right). An oxygen molecule passes through the alveolar membrane and liquid lining (A), the interstitial fluid (B), the capillary membrane (C), the plasma (D), and into the red blood cell (E). The whole pathway is less than 1 μm long. *(From Wade, Jacqueline, Respiratory Nursing Care: Physiology and Technique, 1st ed., Mosby, St. Louis, 1973, p. 46.)*

of maldistribution of blood flow and ventilation. These diseases are known as ventilation/perfusion defects and can produce marked alterations in arterial blood gases.

OXYGEN TRANSPORT

After oxygen has diffused into the pulmonary capillary, a small amount dissolves in the plasma. However, more than 98 percent of the oxygen in the body is transported to the tissue in chemical union with the protein molecule, *hemoglobin.* The reaction between oxygen and hemoglobin is written as:

$$O_2 + Hb \rightleftharpoons Hb\ O_2$$

Since the number of oxygen sites on the hemoglobin molecule is finite, there is a limit to the amount of oxygen which can be transported. The most important factor determining the amount of oxygen which unites with hemoglobin is the *partial pressure of oxygen* (PO_2) in the blood. At the normal arterial PO_2 of 80 to 100 mmHg, approximately 97 percent of the hemoglobin is saturated. While

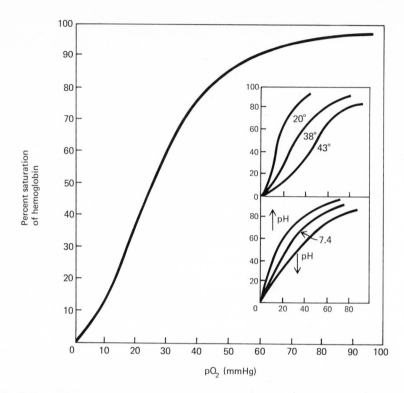

Figure 5-5 Oxyhemoglobin dissociation curve. The large curve applies to blood at normal temperature (38°C) and normal pH (7.4). The inset curves demonstrate the effects of abnormal temperature and pH on the relationship between PO_2 and hemoglobin saturation with oxygen. *(Adapted from Comroe, Julius, Physiology of Respiration, Year Book, Chicago, 1965.)*

arterial PO_2 can exceed 600 mmHg, the hemoglobin can never be more than 100 percent saturated.*

The relationship between PaO_2 and oxygen saturation is demonstrated in the *oxyhemoglobin dissociation curve* (see Fig. 5-5). The reader should note the S shape of this curve. The flat portion of the curve represents a critical safety factor in the supply of oxygen to the tissues. The PaO_2 can drop from 100 to 60 mmHg, yet the oxygen saturation remains above 90 percent. However, when the PaO_2 approaches 50 mmHg, the ability to saturate hemoglobin drastically decreases and marked tissue hypoxia may develop.

* A PaO_2 of approximately 600 mmHg can be reached when an individual with normal lungs is placed on a ventilator which supplies 100 percent oxygen. Note that 500 mmHg of this oxygen is unnecessary to adequately saturate the hemoglobin.

When oxyhemoglobin arrives at the tissue, the oxygen is rapidly unloaded from the hemoglobin and diffuses into the tissues (see Fig. 5-3). The speed of this reaction is accelerated by the enzyme *2,3-diphosphoglycerate* (2,3-DPG) which is synthesized within the red blood cells during glycolysis.

Under resting conditions, the hemoglobin is still 75 percent saturated when it reaches the venous side of circulation. In times of stress, tissues can extract greater quantities of oxygen from this reserve and meet increased metabolic demands. Current research indicates that the amount of erythrocyte 2,3-DPG increases to enhance the release of the additional O_2. Vasodilation in hypoxic tissues also contributes to the increased oxygen supply.

INTERNAL RESPIRATION

Once oxygen enters the tissue cells, *oxidative metabolism* occurs. While many foodstuffs are metabolized, only glucose is discussed in this chapter. Glucose metabolism can occur under both *anaerobic* (without oxygen) and *aerobic* (with oxygen) conditions.

In *aerobic* metabolism, glucose is initially converted to pyruvic acid. Following this, the glucose molecule is fully metabolized within the mitochondria to *carbon dioxide* and *water,* via the Krebs citric acid cycle (see Fig. 5-6).

Figure 5-6 A comparison of aerobic and anaerobic glycolysis. Note that the end result of anaerobic glycolysis is lactic acidosis and insufficient production of ATP.

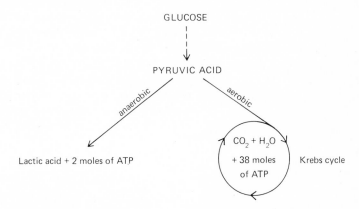

Anaerobic glycolysis occurs when the cells are hypoxic. Glucose is metabolized to pyruvic acid which is then converted to *lactic acid.* If hypoxia persists, a state of acidosis develops, and cellular functioning is adversely affected.

Both aerobic and anaerobic glucose metabolism involve the over-all production of heat and energy. Rather than allowing this heat to be randomly dissipated, the cell stores it as energy within the chemical bonds of adenosine triphosphate (ATP). The energy stored in the phosphate bonds of ATP can be selectively released to provide energy for biochemical enzymatic reactions. During anaerobic metabolism, only two moles of ATP are produced; aerobic metabolism of glucose produces 38 moles.

The cellular effects of hypoxia can now be more fully appreciated. Without sufficient quantities of O_2, cellular metabolism of glucose is incomplete. Increased quantities of lactic acid are produced and acidosis develops. In addition, anaerobic glycolysis produces insufficient amounts of ATP, and intracellular enzymatic reactions are adversely affected. The administration of oxygen to the hypoxic patient has important pharmacologic implications when the biochemical basis for internal respiration is understood.

NEURAL CONTROL OF RESPIRATIONS

Breathing is controlled through the integrated activity of several respiratory centers and receptors.

MEDULLA

The primary center for respiratory regulation is located within the *medulla.* Both inspiratory and expiratory neurons are located in this center. These neurons receive input from all the other respiratory centers and receptors within the body. Also located within the medulla are central chemoreceptors which are sensitive to carbon dioxide tension and hydrogen ion concentration within the cerebrospinal fluid. If the PCO_2 of the cerebrospinal fluid increases or the pH decreases, the respiratory center is stimulated and respiratory efforts are enhanced.

PNEUMOTAXIC CENTER

This center is located in the pons and is linked with the primary medullary center. The pneumotaxic center gives *rhythmicity* to respiration. Following stimulation of the medullary inspiratory neurons, impulses rapidly travel to the upper pons and the inspiratory muscles. The pneumotaxic center fires return impulses to the medulla, and inhibition of the inspiratory neurons occurs.

PERIPHERAL CHEMORECEPTORS

Within the carotid sinus and the aortic arch are *chemoreceptors* which are primarily sensitive to *reduced* levels of arterial *oxygen*. When stimulated, afferent impulses travel to the medulla, and ventilatory efforts are increased. These receptors are of particular importance in patients with chronic obstructive lung disease. With this disease, the medulla is less sensitive to elevated carbon dioxide levels, and the peripheral oxygen receptors become the primary regulators of respiration. The indiscriminate use of high-flow oxygen in these patients is absolutely contraindicated, since this would suppress the hypoxic drive to breathe.

HERING-BREUER REFLEX

Within the lung itself are stretch receptors which aid in controlling the *depth* of respiration. With inspiration, these receptors are stimulated; afferent impulses are sent via the vagus to the medulla, and further expansion of the lung is inhibited. Normal tidal volume is partially controlled by this pulmonary reflex.

CEREBRAL CORTEX

The cerebral cortex provides a *voluntary* center for respiratory control. Talking, laughing, breath-holding, or hysterical hyperventilation are examples of voluntary breath control. With voluntary breath-holding, an increase in the level of carbon dioxide stimulates medullary chemoreceptors, and spontaneous respirations occur.

This chapter has reviewed the basic principles influencing pulmonary ventilation, perfusion, and diffusion. This knowledge provides the foundation for the emergency assessment and treatment of pulmonary insufficiency.

REFERENCES

1. Wade, J., *Respiratory Nursing Care: Physiology and Technique,* Mosby, St. Louis, 1973, p. 46.

BIBLIOGRAPHY

Anthony, C. P., and Kolthoff, N. J., *Textbook of Anatomy and Physiology,* 9th ed., Mosby, St. Louis, 1975.

Comroe, J., *Physiology of Respiration,* Year Book, Chicago, 1974.

Ganong, W., *Review of Medical Physiology,* Lange, Los Altos, Calif., 1974.

Guyton, A. C., *Textbook of Medical Physiology,* Saunders, Philadelphia, 1976.

Hudak, C., Gallo, M., and Lohr, S., *Critical Care Nursing,* Mosby, St. Louis, 1973.

Langley, L., Telford, I., and Christensen, J. B., *Dynamic Anatomy and Physiology,* 4th ed., McGraw-Hill, New York, 1974.

Vander, A., Sherman, J., and Luciano, D., *Human Physiology: The Mechanisms of Body Function,* 2d ed., McGraw-Hill, New York, 1975.

CHAPTER 6
THE RENAL SYSTEM
DOROTHY A. BICKS, R.N.

KNOWLEDGE of the anatomy and physiology of the kidney is essential in the diagnostic evaluation of any critically ill patient admitted to an emergency department (ED) since the kidneys' major role is to establish the delicate balance of the body's internal environment. Although renal disease and failure are rarely encountered in the emergency department, the nurse is faced with circulatory, fluid, and electrolyte problems, which directly relate to kidney function. An important nursing goal is to help protect the patient's kidneys from insult and consequent injury which may jeopardize the homeostasis of the body's internal environment.

SURFACE ANATOMY

The two kidneys, each about the size of a small fist, are located just above the waistline, one on each side of the vertebral column. Because the liver presses down on the right kidney, it is usually lower than the left kidney. The location of the kidneys at the angle where the twelfth pair of ribs meet the twelfth thoracic vertebra is of diagnostic significance. This is known as the *costovertebral angle* (CVA), a significant landmark of physical diagnosis. *CVA tenderness* alerts the nurse to the possibility of kidney inflammation or obstruction. Capping the upper pole of each kidney is an *adrenal gland*. The inner concave surfaces of the kidneys, called the *hilum*, become the passageways for the renal blood vessels and nerves and the ureters which descend to the bladder (see Fig. 6-1).

A cross section of the human torso reveals that the kidneys are located near the posterior abdominal wall and lie outside the parietal peritoneum. They are described as retroperitoneal organs. The kidneys are well supported within a thick fat pad which helps to hold them in position and are encased in a fibrous membrane capsule. External injury to the kidneys requires either forceful blunt trauma or

Figure 6-1 Normal position of the urinary organs. *(From Francis, C. C., and Farrell, G. L., Integrated Anatomy and Physiology, Mosby, St. Louis, 1957.)*

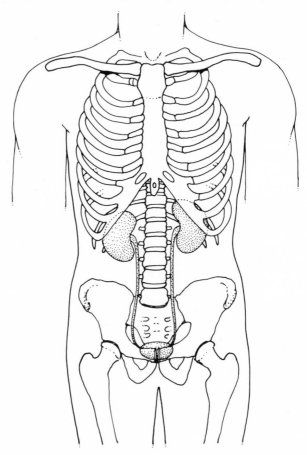

direct penetration because the kidneys are so well protected. Small bowel and peritoneum shield them in front, the vertebral column and thick muscles guard them in the back, and a thick fat pad encloses them in the center.

The protective fibrous *capsule* surrounding each kidney is non-elastic in nature. Diseases such as glomerulonephritis and pyelo-nephritis result in swollen and inflammed kidney tissue. The patient experiences severe flank pain because of the nondistensible nature of this capsule.

Under the fibrous capsule of the kidney is the outermost layer of renal tissue called the *cortex*. It is granular in appearance because it contains the glomerular tufts and the convolutions of the renal tubules. In contrast, the inner layer of renal tissue, the *medulla,* is striated in appearance due to its structures—the long loops of Henle and the collecting ducts. This tubular structure of the medulla is divided into 8 or 10 lobes or triangular masses called *pyramids.* Each pyramid converges into a cone-shaped *papillae,* whose ducts excrete urine into *calyces,* then the kidney *pelvis* and out through the *ureters*. The calyces and the pelvic walls are embedded with smooth muscle fibers which contract, propelling the urine into the ureters (see Fig. 6-2).

NEPHRON ANATOMY

The functional unit of the kidney is the *nephron,* a funnel-like struc-ture extending into a long tube (see Fig. 6-3). Each kidney contains about 1 million nephrons. Although the nephrons are basically similar in structure, about 85 percent of them are located within the cortex and have short-looped tubules. The remaining 15 percent of the nephrons are located at the border of the cortex and medulla (juxtamedullary nephrons), and extend long tubule loops into the medullary tissue. The important feature of the juxtamedullary nephrons is their ability to concentrate urine. Each nephron unit consists of a capillary tuft, the *glomerulus,* which is invaginated into a cup-like structure called the *Bowman's capsule.* The capsule ex-tends into a proximal convoluted tubule, the limbs of Henle, the distal convoluted tubule, and a collecting duct. Seventy-five percent of all the kidney tubules or nephrons can lose their function before gross abnormalities begin to appear. Amazingly, the remaining healthy nephrons can maintain the body's internal environment within normal limits.

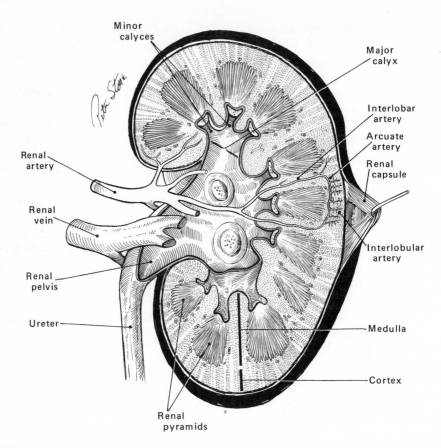

Figure 6-2 A kidney in longitudinal section. At the center are papillae of renal pyramids lying perpendicular to the plane of the section. *(Taken from Langley, L., Telford, I., and Christensen, J., Dynamic Anatomy and Physiology, 4th ed., McGraw-Hill, New York, 1974, p. 670.)*

Blood flows into the glomerulus, and part of it filters into the nephron tubule through the Bowman's capsule. The filtrate undergoes reabsorption and secretion changes along the length of the tubule until it is excreted as urine from the collecting duct.

GLOMERULUS

Blood enters the glomerulus through the *afferent arteriole* and leaves via an *efferent arteriole*. The walls of these two arterioles have specialized smooth muscle cells at the entry and exit points to the glomerulus. When changes occur in renal blood flow volume or renal artery pressure, these cells can constrict or dilate the arteriolar lumen size and ensure a constant blood flow into the glomerulus, despite systemic changes in blood flow volume or pressure. The specialized cells may be partly under the control of renal nerves, but they also are controlled by a unique system of *autoregulation*—a feedback mechanism which operates from conditions of the filtrate in the distal convoluted tubule of the nephron.

Three membrane layers separate the glomerulus from the Bowman's capsule and act as filtration barriers to both *blood cells* and *certain plasma proteins.* However, large volumes of fluid and smaller solute particles pass through readily as filtrate. The patient with glomerulonephritis has an infectious disease process which attacks the glomerular membranes and alters its ability to selectively filter. Consequently, this patient exhibits signs of proteinuria and hematuria.

Figure 6-3 Nephron anatomy, with increasing osmolar concentration of the interstitial tissue from the cortex to the medulla indicated by shading.

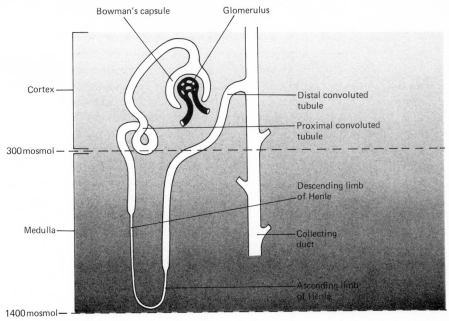

RENAL TUBULE

Differences in the size and shapes of the cells lining the tubule suggest that specific parts of the tubule have specific functions. For example, the cells that line the proximal convoluted tubule have fine long projections. This microvillated surface greatly increases the area in contact with the filtrate and enhances its *reabsorption.*

JUXTAGLOMERULAR APPARATUS

At the point where the ascending loop of Henle converges into the distal convoluted tubule, it makes contact with the surface of the afferent arteriole. The distal tubule wall has specialized cells called *macula densa;* in the smooth muscle wall of the afferent arteriole are specialized *granular cells* which contain an enzyme called *renin.* Together, this structure is known as the *juxtaglomerlar apparatus.* Via the release of renin, the juxtaglomerular apparatus appears to act as a feedback mechanism which controls renal blood flow and the amount of fluid that filters out of the glomerulus.

RENAL BLOOD AND CIRCULATION

Although the kidneys are small in comparison with other body organs, they receive 20 percent of the total cardiac output. This large volume of blood flow enables the kidneys to continually remove unwanted substances from the body fluid. The renal arteries branch off the *abdominal aorta,* enter each kidney, and subdivide into progressively smaller branches until each of the 2 million nephrons receives blood flow through its own individual vascular system.

Blood flow is supplied to each nephron unit via an afferent arteriole and a glomerulus. One-fifth of the delivered volume is filtered from the glomerulus into the nephron tubule, while the remaining volume exits from the glomerulus via the efferent arteriole. Blood flow to the remainder of the nephron tubule is supplied by two types of capillary systems: (1) the *peritubular capillaries* which supply the nephron's convoluted tubular structures, and (2) the *vasa recta* capillary loops which supply the long loops of Henle of the juxtamedullary nephrons (see Fig. 6-4).

The blood which has exited from the glomerulus via the efferent arteriole enters the peritubular capillary plexus. Along with this blood flow, the peritubular capillaries also pick up some of the filtrate that

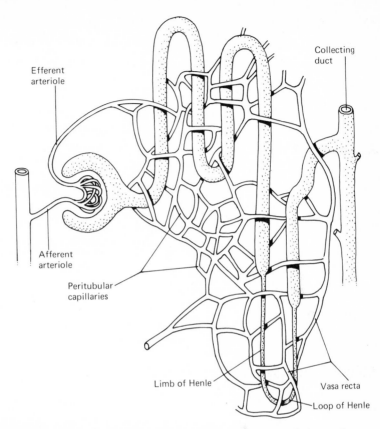

Figure 6-4 Relationships between vascular and tubular components of the nephron.
(Adapted from Vander, A., Sherman, J., and Luciano, D., Human Physiology: The Mechanisms of Body Function, 2d ed., McGraw-Hill, New York, 1975, p. 322.)

has been reabsorbed from the convolutions of the nephron and return the total volume to venous circulation. Blood flow from the efferent arterioles of the juxtamedullary nephrons continues into the long-looped vasa recta capillaries which accompany the loops of Henle of the nephrons into the medulla. Blood flow in the vasa recta proceeds at a very slow rate and in a direction which is opposite to the flow of filtrate in the loops of Henle. This arrangement of *counter-current flow* helps to maintain a concentration gradient of 300 mosmol/liter at the cortical boundary of the medulla to 1400 mosmol/liter at its apex near the kidney pelvis. The purpose of this gradient is to ensure the concentration of urine.

One of the most sensitive indications of pyelonephritis is a decrease in the concentration of urine. Pyelonephritis is usually the end result of an ascending urinary tract infection and is manifested by lesions localized in the medulla. The infectious lesions therefore affect the ability of the tubules in this area to maximally concentrate urine, and this results in a decreased urine osmolality (dilute urine).

RENAL PHYSIOLOGY

The main function of the kidney is to maintain the fluid environment of the body in a balanced state. More specifically, the kidney acts to regulate the balance of water, electrolytes, acids, and bases and to excrete metabolic wastes.

By the mechanisms of *filtration, reabsorption,* and *secretion,* the healthy kidney is able to adjust the quantities of water, electrolytes, acids, and bases to meet the body's requirements. Excesses of these substances together with metabolic wastes are excreted in the form of urine. Following is a progressive summary of these processes as they occur along the length of the kidney tubule from the delivery of blood flow to the glomerulus to the final excretion of urine.

GLOMERULAR FILTRATION

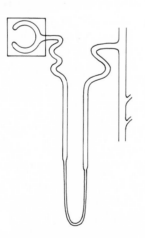

Blood flow to the glomeruli is supplied by the afferent arterioles at the rate of 650 cc/minute. This volume of blood is determined by (a) the total volume of the intravascular blood, (b) the force of the blood flow within the renal vascular system, and (c) constriction of the afferent and efferent arterioles.

Blood cells and *plasma proteins* are unable to cross the porous glomerular membrane owing to their large size. Water and the smaller particles filter into Bowman's capsule at the rate of 125 cc/minute. The amount and rate of filtration occur as the result of pressure gradients. A positive glomerular *hydrostatic pressure* of 70 mmHg is usually greater than the sum of the opposing pressures of plasma protein *osmotic pressure* (32 mmHg) and *Bowman's capsular pressure* (14 mmHg) which oppose filtration. Subtracting the negative forces from the positive leaves a net filtration pressure of 24 mmHg, which promotes filtration into the nephron complex (see Table 6-1). At this point, the volume of filtrate is large and its composition is identical to plasma. If it were to be eliminated at this point, the sudden drain of body fluids and metabolic substances would be fatal. Therefore, further processing is necessary.

PROXIMAL CONVOLUTED TUBULE

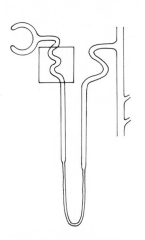

The glomerular filtrate passes from Bowman's capsule into the proximal convoluted tubule. Large volumes of fluid and solutes are reabsorbed at this point, and some substances are secreted into the tubular filtrate. The movement of fluid and solutes across the tubular membrane, both by *reabsorption* and *secretion,* is regulated by concentration and electrical gradients. Figure 6-5 summarizes the reabsorption and secretion of various substances in the proximal tubule. The reabsorbed substances pass out of the tubule into the surrounding interstitial space and diffuse into the peritubular capillaries.

Table 6-1	Summary of pressures influencing glomerular filtration		
	Type of pressure	*Amount of pressure*	*Effect on glomerular filtration*
	Glomerular hydrostatic	$+70$ mmHg	Favors formation of filtrate
	Plasma protein osmotic (colloidal)	-32 mmHg	Opposes formation of filtrate
	Bowman's capsular	-14 mmHg	Opposes formation of filtrate
	Net filtration pressure	$70-(32+14) = +24$ mmHg	Favors formation of filtrate

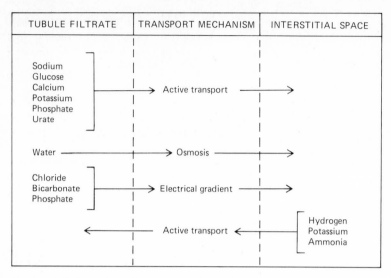

Figure 6-5 Summary of the renal mechanisms at the proximal tubule.

Ninety-eight percent of the filtrate which flows into the proximal tubule is reabsorbed. Though smaller in volume, the remaining filtrate retains an isoosmotic concentration and passes into the loop of Henle.

LOOP OF HENLE

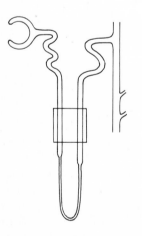

As the filtrate passes down the descending loop, it goes through a medullary interstitium which has a concentration of 1400 mosmol. By the process of *osmosis,* water is reabsorbed and the filtrate becomes hypertonic in concentration. The highly concentrated filtrate rounds the loop's curve and travels up the ascending loop toward the cortex. A unique mechanism operates here, whereby sodium is reabsorbed by *active transport* without water. The sodium ion is followed by chloride and bicarbonate. This reabsorption of sodium from the filtrate into the interstitium accounts for the highly concentrated medium of the medulla which in turn encourages the osmosis of water from the descending loop, which has been previously described. The concentration gradient is maintained because the blood flow in the vasa recta capillaries is too slow to remove much sodium, and thus this ion is retained within the medullary interstitium.

With the loss of solute, the now hypotonic filtrate has returned to the cortical area of the kidney and passes from the ascending loop into the distal convoluted tubule.

DISTAL TUBULE AND COLLECTING DUCT

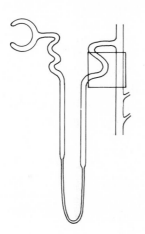

Within these last two structures of the nephron, the final modification of the filtrate takes place, primarily due to the influence of the *juxtaglomerular apparatus* and the *antidiuretic hormone* mechanism (see Fig. 6-6). As the filtrate enters the distal tubule, the macula densa cells are sensitized by the changes in sodium concentration of the tubular filtrate, as well as the rate or volume of filtrate flow. The macula densa cells stimulate the granular juxtaglomerular cells to secret renin. Renin activates a substance called *angiotensin I*, which then is converted into *angiotensin II*. This chemical stimulates the adrenal gland to release a hormone called *aldosterone*. Aldosterone acts directly on the distal tubule to reabsorb more sodium. One sodium ion is reabsorbed in exchange for a potassium ion which is excreted into the filtrate. If the body produces an excess of hydrogen ions, they compete with potassium ions for excretion. In addition to the stimulation of aldosterone, angiotensin II is also the most potent vasopressor in the body.

The tubular cells of these two areas are impermeable to water reabsorption, but the permeability is regulated by circulating levels of the *antidiuretic hormone* (ADH). The presence of ADH changes the permeability of the tubular cells, particularly those of the collecting ducts. More water is reabsorbed, and this helps to restore the plasma to an isosmotic or balanced concentration. The remaining fluid volume of filtrate is excreted as urine, at a rate of 1 cc/minute.

Along with hydrogen and potassium ions, the distal tubular cells also secrete ammonia and drug end products. One drug that is readily and rapidly excreted at the distal tubule level is penicillin. In order to prevent this and maintain an adequate plasma concentration, penicillin is often given in conjunction with a drug, Benemid, which blocks its excretion.

Figure 6-7 outlines the reabsorption and secretion of fluid and specific electrolytes at the level of the distal and collecting ducts.

Figure 6-6 Summary of hormonal action within the distal tubule and the collecting duct. *(Taken from Eli Lilly and Co., Kidney and Urinary Tract Infections, Indianapolis, 1971.)*

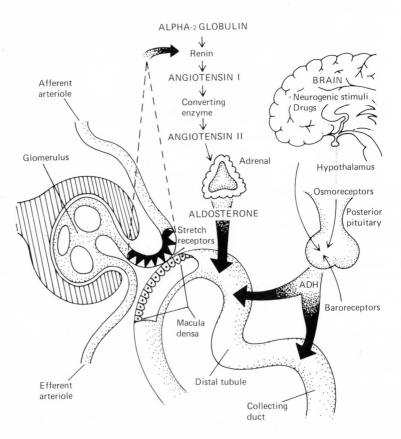

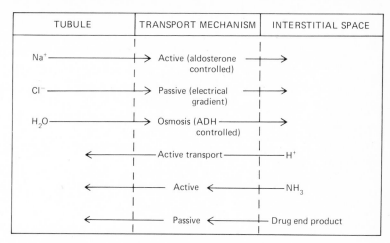

Figure 6-7 Summary of the renal mechanisms at the distal tubule and collecting duct.

SUMMARY OF KIDNEY FUNCTION

1. In health, the kidney receives 20 percent of the cardiac output. A unique method of autoregulation helps to maintain a glomerular filtration rate of 125 cc/hour despite changes in blood volume and hydrostatic blood pressure.

Although autoregulation can accommodate a wide range of change, severe hypovolemia or depressed hydrostatic blood pressure can result in diminished glomerular filtration and consequent nephron changes.

2. In health, the kidney tubule is able to reabsorb 99 percent of the filtrate and produce a concentrated urine volume of 1 cc/hour.

3. The tubule is also able to alter the concentration of acids and bases. When the body is acidotic, hydrogen ions are secreted in place of potassium ions, and bicarbonate and phosphate are conserved as buffers at the expense of chloride.

4. The kidney is able to excrete an average daily solute waste dissolved in a fluid volume that can range from a normal urine output of 1500 cc/day to a minimum obligatory output of 500 cc/day when it needs to conserve water to maintain an adequate extracellular fluid volume.

5. When nephron cells are damaged, they are no longer able to block the filtration of blood cells and plasma proteins at the glomerular level and are no longer able to reabsorb vital substances such as sodium bicarbonate and glucose, and the internal environment is jeopardized.

6. Another significant function of the kidney is its ability to produce a protein substance called erythropoietin. This substance acts on bone marrow to increase the rate of production of red blood cells. Patients with chronic types of renal disease exhibit anemia in response to the altered ability of the kidney to produce erythropoietin. In addition hypoxia stimulates erythropoietin production.

BIBLIOGRAPHY

Anthony, C. P., and Kolthoff, N. J., *Textbook of Anatomy and Physiology,* 9th ed., Mosby, St. Louis, 1975.

Guyton, A. C., *Textbook of Medical Physiology,* 5th ed., Saunders, Philadelphia, 1976.

Kidney and Urinary Tract Infections, Lily Research Laboratories, Indianapolis, 1971.

Metheny, N. M., and Snively, W. D., *Nurses' Handbook of Fluid Balance,* 2d ed., Lippincott Co., Philadelphia, 1974.

Reed, G. N., and Sheppard, V. F., *Regulation of Fluid and Electrolyte Balance: A Programmed Instruction in Physiology for Nurses,* Saunders, Philadelphia, 1971.

CHAPTER 7
ACID-BASE BALANCE
JILL D. HOLMES, R.N., M.S.

TO the uninitiated, the mysteries of acid-base balance seem complicated and involved. Confronted with laboratory results and a sick patient who depends on a rapid and accurate diagnosis, the novice may feel overwhelmed. Yet, the basic concepts are simple:

1. All cells, through daily metabolism, produce a variety of acids as an end product.

2. The metabolism of ingested foodstuffs, such as the proteins and fats, produce acids.

3. Therefore, man and mammalian family members are *acid-producing organisms.*

4. Cells, organs, body systems, hormones, and enzymes work best in a balanced environment which is slightly *alkaline,* or *basic.*

5. In order to keep the body from being overwhelmed by its acid products, there are systems which balance the acids and bases and keep the environment stable and steady. These are the *chemical* and *physiological buffer systems.*

6. Since a steady state is so important to the body, these buffer systems may be seen as lines of defense employed to defend and maintain the balanced environment.

REVIEW OF pH

The *hydrogen ion* (H^+) in the body is the acid ion. Actual concentrations of free H^+ in body fluids determine whether the fluid is strongly acid, moderately acid, neutral, or basic. In the body's extracellular fluids, concentrations of free H^+ are very low when compared with other cations such as sodium (Na^+). For example, Na^+ concentration is 145 meq/liter of body fluid while H^+ ion concentration is 0.00004 meq/liter. Obviously, it would be time-consuming to write out such a lengthy and minute number, so another measure of hydrogen ion concentration is used. The notation *pH* is commonly utilized to indicate the presence of free H^+ and its effect on the solution. The pH scale ranges from 1 to 14 (see Fig. 7-1). On this scale, a pH below 7.0 indicates relatively high concentrations of free H^+ ion; thus, the solution is an acid. A pH above 7.0 indicates relatively low concentrations of H^+. This solution is, therefore, called a base or an alkali. When a solution is tested and shows a pH of 7.0, it is said to be neutral, like water, because the H^+ ions are balanced by an equal number of basic hydroxyl (OH^-) ions.

Different body fluids have widely different pH ratings. For example, gastric acid (HCl) shows a pH of 0.8. Urine, usually acid, has a pH of 4.5, while pancreatic secretions lie at the alkaline side of the scale with a pH of 8.0.

The pH most often measured for overall assessment of the acid-base balance is that of arterial blood, which, in health, ranges from 7.38 to 7.45. Despite the end products of metabolism, increased physical activity, and varying dietary intake, the body's pH must remain within this narrow range for optimal cellular and enzymatic function. Deviation of a significant amount leads to cessation of normal body activity and death. The overall range of plasma pH is 7.0 to 7.8.

If a pH of the blood registers below 7.38, the patient is considered acidotic. If the pH exceeds 7.45, his status is alkalotic (see Fig. 7-2).

Figure 7-1 The pH scale, with 7 being a neutral solution.

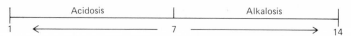

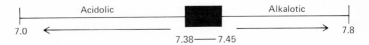

Figure 7-2 The pH scale for plasma, with normal and extreme ranges indicated.

Other descriptive words, such as acidemia and alkalemia, are used interchangeably.

REGULATORY SYSTEMS

As mentioned, regulation of the acids and bases of the body is handled by chemical and physiological buffer systems. The three regulatory mechanisms are: (1) body buffers; (2) the respiratory system; and (3) the renal system.

CHEMICAL BUFFERS

Chemically active body buffers are substances or compounds in body fluids and tissues which tie up free H^+ ions so that the pH in the solution changes very little. Buffers, it should be stressed, do not rid the body of H^+, but rather tie up the acid ion so that it is no longer free. Body buffers are:

1. Intracellular and plasma proteins

2. Hemoglobin

3. The carbonic acid–bicarbonate buffers

4. The disodium–monosodium phosphate buffers

Body buffers are composed of a *weakly ionized acid* or *base* and *its salt*. An example of an important body buffer pair is the carbonic acid–sodium bicarbonate buffer system. When a strong acid, like hydrochloric, is added to a solution containing this buffer pair, the following equation occurs:

$$HCl + Na^+ + HCO_3^- \rightarrow H_2CO_3 + NaCl$$

In this case, the H^+ ion in the strong acid, HCl, reacts with the sodium bicarbonate producing the weakly ionized carbonic acid

(H_2CO_2) and NaCl, a neutral salt. Since carbonic acid is mostly un-ionized and does not dissociate (break apart) in solution, the H^+ is contained and is not "free" to change the overall concentration of H^+. Therefore, the pH does not undergo a radical change.

PHYSIOLOGICAL BUFFERS

RESPIRATORY SYSTEM

The *lungs* are a major organ of excretion for two end products of metabolism, carbon dioxide and water. Carbon dioxide and water are constantly produced by the cell and transported to the lungs. Carbon dioxide is transported via the blood in three forms: (1) dissolved in the plasma; (2) chemically combined with unoxygenated hemoglobin as carbaminohemoglobin; and (3) in the plasma as the bicarbonate ion. The latter is the predominant means of CO_2 transport and is discussed below.

BICARBONATE TRANSPORT OF CO_2 Water and carbon dioxide, by-products of cellular metabolism, are released from the tissue cell into the capillary. Some of the carbon dioxide and water remain in the blood, but the greater amount enters the erythrocyte and forms *carbonic acid*. Within the erythrocyte, this reaction is sped up by the presence of an enzyme, *carbonic anhydrase*:

$$\text{H}_2\text{O} + \text{CO}_2 \overset{\text{carbonic}}{\underset{}{\rightleftharpoons}} \text{H}_2\text{CO}_3$$

carbonic
anhydrase

Carbonic acid then dissociates to form hydrogen ion and bicarbonate:

$$\text{H}_2\text{CO}_3 \rightleftharpoons \text{H}^+ + \text{HCO}_3^-$$

The free H^+ is promptly buffered by the *hemoglobin*, a very important body buffer, and the remaining bicarbonate ion is released to the plasma where it is utilized for further buffering activity. The chloride ion rapidly moves into the cell in exchange for the HCO_3^-, and so intracellular electrical neutrality is maintained.

Once the erythrocyte reaches the lung, the entire chemical equation reverses itself. CO_2 is once again formed and diffuses from the pulmonary capillary into the alveoli to be exhaled. Figure 7-3 illustrates the entire process of bicarbonate transport of carbon dioxide.

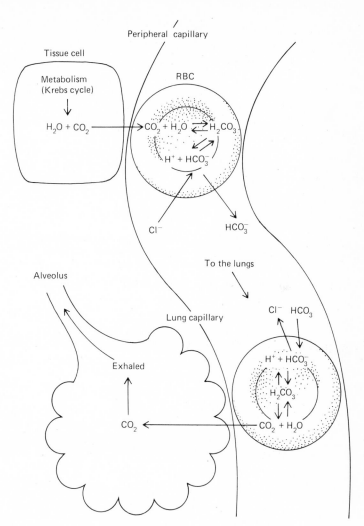

Figure 7-3 CO_2 transport via the bicarbonate ion.

When the two formulas are combined to represent the entire process, it looks like this:

$$CO_2 + H_2O \rightleftharpoons H_2CO_3 \rightleftharpoons H^+ + HCO_3^-$$

It is said that this equation demonstrates a state of *dynamic equilibrium*. In other words, carbonic acid is rapidly and constantly changing forms within the body. Yet in health, pulmonary function keeps pace with cellular activity; excess CO_2 is rapidly transported to the lung and exhaled, and thus a balanced hydrogen concentration is maintained in the body.

When the alveolar ventilation is impaired and excess carbon dioxide is not expelled via respiration, the addition of more CO_2 to the system drives the equation to the right. More carbonic acid is formed which then produces, by the process of dissociation, additional hydrogen ion concentration and lowered pH.

It is important to note that carbon dioxide and carbonic acid are directly related. Alteration of CO_2 elimination affects the concentration of carbonic acid in body fluids, and this affects the acid-base balance.

RENAL SYSTEM

Carbonic acid is considered a gaseous or volatile acid in that its concentration in the body is regulated primarily by the respiratory system. The kidney also aids in maintaining the correct concentration of this acid. In addition, fixed or nonvolatile by-products of metabolism such as sulfuric acid and bisodium phosphate are handled by the kidney.

As stated earlier, the body produces acids daily. The kidney must secrete this hydrogen load carefully so that living cells are not damaged by exposure to strong acids. It must also conserve, at the same time, important anions and cations which the body needs. By an exchange program, the kidney is able to do both.

Basically, hydrogen ion is secreted into the renal tubule in exchange for sodium, which is then returned to the body. Depending on the daily load of body hydrogen, the kidney excretes a urine which may range in pH from 4.5 to 7.8. Most of the time, urine is acid.

There are three mechanisms by which the kidney secretes hydrogen into the tubular lumen:

1. CO_2 present in the blood and in the cells lining the tubular lumen combines with H_2O to form *carbonic acid*, which then dissociates to form H^+ and HCO_3^-. The enzyme carbonic anhydrase facilitates this reaction. This reaction should be familiar to the reader. The hydrogen ion is actively secreted into the tubular lumen in exchange, electrically speaking, for another positively charged ion, usually sodium. Sodium is initially present in the tubular filtrate in combination with an acid by-product of metabolism such as sodium sulfate (N_2SO_4) or disodium phosphate (Na_2HPO_4). It is also in chemical union with the chloride ion (NaCl).

Once sodium is exchanged, it combines with the bicarbonate ion and is returned to the body for use as a buffer (see Fig. 7-4).

2. The *disodium phosphate buffer system* also aids the kidney in maintaining a normal pH. Na_2HPO_4 is a fixed acid present in the tubular filtrate. Hydrogen ion, produced within the renal cell, is actively secreted into the tubular lumen and combines with Na_2HPO_4 to form NaH_2PO_4. The sodium ion is reabsorbed in union with bicarbonate and further utilized as a buffer (see Fig. 7-5).

Both of the above buffering mechanisms are limited in their utility since they cease to function when urine pH reaches 4.5. The formation of the ammonium ion assists the kidney in the excretion of further hydrogen ion.

3. Through the formation of the compound *ammonium* (NH_4) from ammonia (NH_3), the kidney further promotes excretion of H^+ ion and conservation of Na^+ ion. Ammonia is formed from glutamine and other amino acids in the kidney tubular cells. It diffuses readily

Figure 7-4 The carbonic acid–bicarbonate buffer system in the kidney.

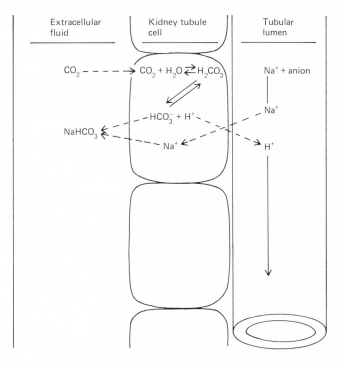

across the cell wall into the tubular lumen. H^+ ion, which is also secreted by the tubular cell, combines with the NH_3 to form NH_4, which is nonabsorbable. Na^+ present in the tubular filtrate is exchanged for the hydrogen ion and returned to the body. Chloride combines with NH_4 forming NH_4Cl and is excreted in the urine (see Fig. 7-6). Authorities estimate that 70 to 75 percent of the kidney's hydrogen ions are excreted via the NH_3 buffer system.

The three regulatory mechanisms just discussed, body buffers, respiratory system, and renal system, react to alterations in acid-base balance at different speeds. The body buffers react immediately at the cellular level, buffering added acids to prevent large swings in pH. The lungs take 2 to 3 minutes to respond after a sudden swing in pH, while the kidney requires up to 24 hours to respond fully. However, its response is a powerful one, and, as a buffering mechanism, it can maintain its activities for long periods of time. The lungs reach maximum buffering efficiency in approximately 1 hour.

Figure 7-5 The disodium–monosodium phosphate buffer system.

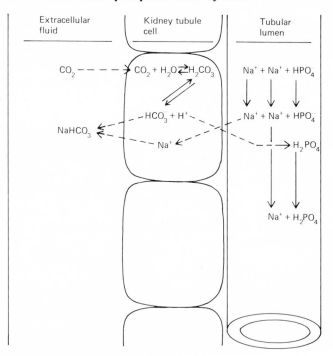

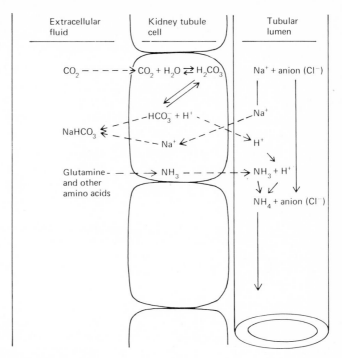

Figure 7-6 Excretion of ammonium.

pH, BICARBONATE, AND CARBONIC ACID

Before any discussion of alterations of acid-base balance, it is necessary to look at one final equation which shows the relationship that exists between pH, the bicarbonate ion, and carbonic acid. Without lengthy explanations, the simplified form looks like this:

$$pH = \frac{HCO_3^-}{H_2CO_3}$$

Basically, this formula for pH describes a ratio or balance which exists between the bicarbonate ion and carbonic acid. As long as the balance is maintained, the pH remains at the healthy level of 7.4. In health, the ratio should be:

$$pH = \frac{20}{1} = \frac{HCO_3^-}{H_2CO_3}$$

With disease, this ratio can be altered. For example, if the bicarbonate ion in the body were to decrease while the carbonic acid remained the same, the pH would be lowered and a state of *acidosis* would develop. The following equation is a simplified illustration of this concept:

$$\text{pH of } 7.2 = \frac{10}{1} = \frac{HCO_3^- \;\downarrow}{H_2CO_3} \qquad \text{Primary alteration}$$

However, if the body were to also lower the concentration of carbonic acid, via compensatory mechanisms, the overall ratio of bicarbonate to carbonic acid would be reestablished. The pH would return to normal despite the changes in actual concentrations of the chemicals:

$$\text{pH of } 7.4 = \frac{10}{0.5} = \frac{\downarrow \; HCO_3^-}{\downarrow \; H_2CO_3} \qquad \begin{array}{l}\text{Primary alteration} \\ \text{Compensatory mechanism}\end{array}$$

The significant point here is that the body, through use of its regulatory mechanisms, can alter concentrations of either bicarbonate or carbonic acid in response to a deviation in one of the chemicals. A normal or near-normal pH is maintained, which is the primary goal of the entire system. This mechanism is called *physiologic compensation*.

One further point needs to be made regarding the above formula. The denominator of the ratio, carbonic acid, is extremely difficult to measure directly in the body. Because it is in active equilibrium with dissolved carbon dioxide, at any given moment, it is present in the blood stream in extremely small amounts. Nevertheless, it is possible by laboratory test to measure the dissolved carbon dioxide.

Here is a familiar formula:

$$CO_2 + H_2O \leftrightharpoons H_2CO_3 \rightleftharpoons H + HCO_3^-$$

As can be seen, the amount of carbon dioxide is *directly proportional* to carbonic acid. Now the equation for pH can be rewritten to show the relationship of bicarbonate to carbon dioxide:

$$pH = \frac{HCO_3^-}{CO_2}$$

This equation is more meaningful for the emergency nurse since these values are frequently determined by arterial blood-gas analysis.

The above formula can be further expanded to show that:

$$pH = \frac{kidney}{lung} = \frac{HCO_3^-}{CO_2}$$

It is now evident that the bicarbonate ion is handled by the *kidney* while carbon dioxide is the responsibility of the *lungs*. Therefore, maintenance of an acid-base balance is the function of these two systems of the body.

ALTERATIONS IN ACID-BASE BALANCE

Alterations in acid-base balance may occur in a variety of ways, but the deviation is initially either acid or alkaline. The next step is to determine which system of the body is responsible for the deviation. It may be either a cellular problem (*metabolic*) or a *respiratory* one. Combining these two pairs gives four basic pathological situations: (1) respiratory acidosis; (2) respiratory alkalosis; (3) metabolic acidosis; and (4) metabolic alkalosis.

RESPIRATORY ACIDOSIS

PRIMARY ALTERATION   Any condition affecting the respiratory system that leads to *diminished alveolar ventilation* increases the concentration of carbon dioxide, which then produces an increased concentration of carbonic acid. Carbonic acid dissociates to form H^+ ion, and there is a decrease in pH. The state is acidosis, and the underlying cause is an alteration in the mechanics of respiration. Conditions such as chest trauma, emphysema, narcotic overdose, and paralysis of the muscles of respiration lead to respiratory acidosis.

In looking at the ratio:

$$pH = \frac{20}{1} = \frac{HCO_3^-}{CO_2} = \frac{kidney}{lung}$$

one can postulate that with a respiratory acidosis the overall concentration of carbon dioxide has increased with a decrease in pH resulting:

$$pH = \frac{20}{2} = \frac{HCO_3^-}{\uparrow CO_2} \qquad \text{Primary alteration}$$

The reader must remember that the measurement of carbon dioxide is in reality an indirect means of assessing the level of carbonic acid in the body.

COMPENSATORY MECHANISM   The body's first line of defense, the blood buffers, are utilized to buffer the additional H^+ ion. The respiratory center, stimulated by a rise in H^+, increases the rate and depth of ventilation. This action depends totally on an intact respiratory center and a healthy pair of lungs. These two responses, occurring within 5 to 10 minutes, may be all that is required to restore normal pH. However, if the pH remains low and the carbon dioxide remains high, the third line of defense, the kidney, begins to conserve bicarbonate. In addition, hydrogen ion is secreted in greater amounts into the urine, while the sodium ion is retained in exchange for the H^+. Sodium bicarbonate is produced and utilized by the body as an additional buffer. Ideally, the ratio between bicarbonate and carbon dioxide is reestablished, pH is stabilized, and the patient is said to be in *compensated respiratory acidosis*. "Respiratory cripples" with a chronically elevated carbon dioxide also show a chronically elevated bicarbonate level and a relatively normal pH. In other words, the kidney's compensatory mechanism is strong, constant, and complete.

RESPIRATORY ALKALOSIS

PRIMARY ALTERATION With this disorder, a deficit of carbonic acid occurs due to *alveolar hyperventilation,* with excessive loss of carbon dioxide resulting. The following equation illustrates this deviation:

$$\uparrow pH = \frac{20}{0.5} = \frac{HCO_3^-}{\downarrow CO_2} \qquad \text{Primary alteration}$$

Hyperventilation often is a self-induced reaction produced by anxiety or by strenuous exercise. Other etiologies may include central nervous system lesions, fever, and overventilation by mechanical respirator or with a bag-mask.

COMPENSATORY MECHANISM The compensatory mechanisms used by the body include, first, a slowing of the rate and depth of respirations to conserve CO_2 and, second, increased excretion of bicarbonate by the kidney. These mechanisms are not as efficient as those employed by the body in response to acidosis. Medical personnel must then assist these respiratory and renal mechanisms. By directing the patient to breath into a paper bag, alleviating anxiety, sedating the patient, and adjusting the respirator, the medical and nursing personnel assist the body to restore acid-base balance.

METABOLIC ACIDOSIS

All other conditions of acidosis not due to the concentration of CO_2 in the body are considered metabolic in origin. Some authorities refer to this type of alteration as *nonrespiratory acidosis*.

PRIMARY ALTERATION Metabolic acidosis can occur from: (1) increased concentrations of metabolic acids formed by the body as in diabetic ketoacidosis; (2) intravenous administration of acids such as ammonium chloride; or (3) increased intake of metabolic acids via the gastrointestinal tract such as acetylsalicylic acid (ASA). All these cause an overproduction of acids which the bicarbonate ion attempts to buffer. Eventually, the bicarbonate ion is consumed.

Another cause of metabolic acidosis is the loss of base from the body which then allows acids to predominate. The patient with severe diarrhea or a duodenal fistula demonstrates this type of acidosis since bowel secretion contains a large amount of sodium bicarbonate. Projectile vomiting of intestinal secretions would also lead to a loss of base with the same result.

No matter what the etiology, metabolic acidosis causes a decrease in pH and bicarbonate:

$$\downarrow pH = \frac{10}{1} = \frac{\downarrow HCO_3^-}{CO_2} \quad \text{Primary alteration}$$

COMPENSATORY MECHANISM   The body's chemical buffers are rapidly depleted and nonavailable to handle the acid load. The second line of defense, the respiratory system, attempts to improve the ratio by blowing off the respiratory acid—CO_2. The patient at this point demonstrates the well-known Kussmaul breathing. There is a rapid, partial compensatory response by the respiratory system. It should be noted that this respiratory compensatory response rarely elicits a total return to normal pH. In addition, the kidney attempts to excrete the additional acid load. Unfortunately, owing to the renal buffering mechanism used to handle these strong acids, sodium is also lost in urine. Without available sodium to combine with bicarbonate, the sodium bicarbonate buffer further decreases, and the ratio continues to shift to an acidosis.

Medical personnel assist the body to combat the metabolic acidosis by first correcting the underlying metabolic pathology. In addition, they support the kidney's effort to excrete the heavy acid load by supplying water. Also, NaCl must be provided to correct the existing deficit and to provide sufficient concentrations for the production of sodium bicarbonate, the body's base buffer. Extrinsic amounts of sodium bicarbonate can be administered to combat the acidemia.

METABOLIC ALKALOSIS

PRIMARY ALTERATION   Like respiratory alkalosis, metabolic alkalosis can also be self-induced. In this case, the alkalosis is the result of overdosage with alkaline medications such as sodium bicarbonate. Loss of a body acid through prolonged vomiting or suctioning of stomach contents

Acid (acidosis)	Base (alkalosis)
Respiratory acidosis	Respiratory alkalosis
Etiology: hypoventilation of the pulmonary alveoli	*Etiology*: hyperventilation of the pulmonary alveoli
Medical history may be: • Bronchial construction • CNS depression with a decrease in respirations • Trauma to the thoracic cage, airway conducting tubes or respiratory muscles	*Medical history may be*: • Hysteria or acute anxiety • Head trauma or lesion leading to hyperventilation • Hepatic coma
Signs and symptoms: • CNS changes such as disorientation, confusion, and stupor progressing to coma • Cardiac arrhythmias • Respiratory embarrassment	*Signs and symptoms*: • Deep, rapid breathing • CNS changes such as dizziness, facial twitching, seizures • Peripheral changes such as "pins-and-needles" sensation in fingers and toes, carpopedal spasm, or tetany • Cardiac arrhythmias
Lab studies (acute phase): • pH: less than 7.38 • CO_2: greater than 42 • Bicarb: 24 meq/liter	*Lab studies (acute phase)*: • pH: greater than 7.45 • CO_2: less than 38 • Bicarb: 24 meq/liter
Compensatory mechanism: • Kidney: retains $NaHCO_3$ and excretes H^+ ion	*Compensatory mechanism*: • Kidney: excretes $NaHCO_3$

Figure 7-7a Summary chart for respiratory acidosis and alkalosis.

can also produce an overall loss of body acid, altering the pH to an alkalotic state. Metabolic alkalosis can also be iatrogenically induced by overzealous administration of sodium bicarbonate during cardiopulmonary resuscitation efforts. No matter what the etiology, the result is:

$$\uparrow pH = \frac{40}{1} = \frac{\uparrow HCO_3^-}{CO_2} \qquad \text{Primary alteration}$$

COMPENSATORY MECHANISM The lungs in this condition provide a measure of compensation. More acid is needed, and so the respiratory rate and depth are decreased. At best, this mechanism is only partially effective since the patient must continue to breathe. Other measures might include administering drugs either to provide acid or to pro-

Acid (acidosis)	Base (alkalosis)
Metabolic acidosis	Metabolic alkalosis

Etiology: increase of body acids without excretion of concommitent H^+ ion or loss of body base without its replacement	*Etiology*: loss of body acids or increase of body base
Medical history may be: • Poorly controlled diabetes mellitus • Renal failure • Severe diarrhea (loss of bicarbonate from the bowel	*Medical history may be*: • Overtreatment with antacids for ulcer disease • Loss of gastric acids due to vomiting, gastric fistulas or nasogastric suctioning
Signs and symptoms: • CNS changes such as disorientation, confusion, stupor progressing to coma • Cardiac arrhythmias • Kussmaul breathing	*Signs and symptoms*: • Numbness of hands and feet • Muscular weakness • CNS changes such as nervousness, irritability, tetany, seizures
Lab studies (acute phase): • pH: less than 7.38 • CO_2: less than 38 • Bicarb: less than 24 meq/liter	*Lab studies (acute phase)*: • pH: greater than 7.42 • CO_2: normal or elevated, greater than 42 • Bicarb: more than 24 meq/liter
Compensatory mechanism: • Lungs: blow off CO_2 in attempt to reduce acids to base ratio • Kidney: if healthy secretes increased H^+ ions and conserves bicarbonate ion	*Compensatory mechanism*: • Lungs: retain CO_2 • Kidney: excretes bicarbonate

Figure 7-7b Summary chart for metabolic acidosis and alkalosis.

mote excretion of bicarbonate via the kidney. Ammonium chloride is an example of the former. Bicarbonate excretion is promoted by the drug acetazolamide, a carbonic anhydrase inhibitor.

In closing, Fig. 7-7 summarizes the signs and symptoms the emergency nurse may evaluate when assessing the patient for an acid-base imbalance. Final determination also depends upon a good medical history, clinical observations, and laboratory studies.

BIBLIOGRAPHY

Beck, William S., *Human Design Molecular, Cellular and Systemic Physiology,* Harcourt, Brace, Jovanovich, New York, 1971.

Beland, Irene L., *Clinical Nursing: Pathophysiological and Psychosocial Approaches,* Macmillan, 1975.

Davenport, Horace W., *The ABC of Acid-Base Chemistry,* 6th ed., University of Chicago Press, 1974.

Ganong, William, *Review of Medical Physiology,* Lange, Los Altos, Calif., 1974.

Guyton, A. C., *Textbook of Medical Physiology,* Saunders, Philadelphia, 1976.

Metheny, Norma Milligan, and Snively, William D., Jr., *Nurses' Handbook of Fluid Balance,* Lippincott, Philadelphia, 1974.

Mountcastle, Vernon B. (ed.), *Medical Physiology,* 13th ed., vol. 1, Mosby, St. Louis, 1974.

Reed, Gretchen Mayo, "Confused about Potassium? Here's a Clear Concise Guide," *Nursing '74,* vol. 3, no. 3, March 1974.

——— and Sheppard, Vincent F., *Regulation of Fluid and Electrolyte Balance: A Programmed Instruction in Physiology for Nurses,* Saunders, Philadelphia, 1971.

CHAPTER 8
BLOOD-GAS ANALYSIS
JEANIE BARRY, R.N., M.S.

AN in-depth understanding of the renal and respiratory systems and their regulation of acid-base balance is necessary for the proper interpretation of blood-gas results.* The emphasis of this chapter is on interpretation of laboratory values and arterial puncture techniques.

Emergency nurses customarily monitor the vital signs as a means to evaluate the changing pathophysiologic status of critically ill patients. Long before these parameters reflect an alteration, the body's internal environment may have deviated from normal. Blood-gas analysis (BGA) is a rapid method to assess the condition of the internal environment. A BGA includes a determination of *hydrogen ion concentration* (pH) and the *partial pressures of carbon dioxide* (PCO_2) and *oxygen* (PO_2) in the arterial or venous blood. These values can provide important information regarding "lung function, lung adequacy and tissue perfusion"[1] as well as the degree of compensation by the lung or kidney.

---

* The reader is urged to thoroughly review Chaps. 5 to 7 for the theoretical basis for blood-gas analysis. Chapter 8 provides only a few basic physiological concepts related to blood-gas analysis.

BLOOD-GAS VALUES

Only three parameters need to be measured in the usual analysis of blood gases—pH, PCO_2, and PO_2. Bicarbonate levels can be calculated after the pH and PCO_2 have been determined or can be measured directly (see Fig. 8-1). Base excess levels can also be analytically determined. Base excess refers primarily to the *bicarbonate ion* but also reflects the influence of the other body buffers (mainly plasma proteins and hemoglobin). Once the PO_2 is measured, oxygen saturation can be quickly calculated, utilizing the *oxyhemoglobin dissociation curve*. Hemoglobin type, pH, and temperature must be known for accurate calculation (see Fig. 5-5).

ARTERIAL AND VENOUS BLOOD GASES

OXYGEN EXTRACTION

The normal range of values for arterial and venous blood is listed in Table 8-1. A large difference between arterial and mixed venous blood is found in the *oxygen* levels. Several factors influence the

Figure 8-1 The pH-bicarbonate diagram with PCO_2 isobars. (*Adapted from Davenport, H. W., The ABC of Acid-Base Chemistry, 6th ed., University of Chicago Press, 1974.*)

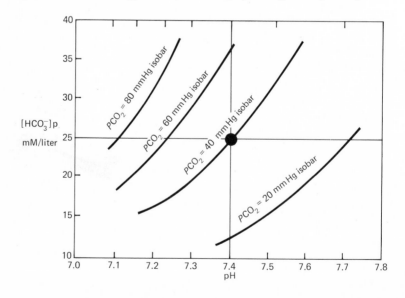

	Arterial	Mixed venous
Table 8-1	Normal values found in arterial and mixed venous blood-gas samples. (*From Davenport, H. W.: The ABC of Acid-Base Chemistry, 6th ed., University of Chicago Press, 1974.*)	

	Arterial	Mixed venous
pH	7.4	7.36
PO_2 (mmHg)	80–100	35–40
O_2 saturation	95 % or greater	70–75 %
PCO_2 (mmHg)	40	46
HCO_3^- (mM/liter)	25	26

amount of oxygen that is extracted by the tissues. Some of these include cardiac output, the integrity of the capillary membrane, cellular metabolism, and the adequacy of tissue perfusion. If any of these factors is abnormal, *tissue extraction of oxygen* may be altered.

The measurement and comparison of arterial and mixed venous blood gases may provide important information regarding the above factors. These data can be particularly helpful in the diagnosis and clinical management of the *shock* patient. For example, in low-flow shock states (i.e., hypovolemic or cardiogenic shock), the blood flow to the tissues is decreased. Since the peripheral blood supply is limited, the tissues attempt to meet their metabolic needs by extracting a greater amount of O_2. The amount of oxygen that returns to venous circulation is reduced. In septic shock, the capillary membrane is damaged, and O_2 extraction by the tissues is reduced. In this case, less oxygen can be extracted and venous PO_2 is greater than normal.

ACID-BASE BALANCE AND ARTERIAL OXYGEN LEVELS

The reader should recall that the ratio of HCO_3^-/CO_2 is proportional to the pH. Thus, these values are assessed when evaluating the *acid-base balance* of the patient. While maintenance of the arterial PO_2 within normal limits is essential for optimal cellular functioning, it must fall to critically low levels before acid-base balance is adversely affected. This critical level varies depending on which tissue is being adversely affected. For skeletal muscle, this level is an oxygen gradient of 67 mmHg between the capillary and skeletal muscle cell.[2] At this point, there is an insufficient oxygen gradient into the skeletal muscle cells, and cellular hypoxia develops. Anaerobic metabolism of glucose begins and lactic acid accumulates (see Fig. 5-6). If this cellular hypoxia is not promptly corrected, a *lactic acidosis* develops.

SITES FOR SAMPLE COLLECTION

For venous blood gases, peripheral venous blood should not be used since the true mixed central venous values are not indicated. [1,3] Mixed venous blood obtained from the *pulmonary artery* or *right ventricle* provides the most accurate measurement. If the patient does not have a pulmonary artery catheter in place, blood from a central venous catheter is often used. The nurse must realize that even the values from this central venous blood are not completely accurate. [1,3]

Arterial blood-gas values are the same no matter which major arterial vessel is used. The common sites are the *brachial, radial,* and *femoral* arteries. A temporary intra-arterial cannula with a heparin flush system may be used, or the sample may be obtained through an arterial puncture.

ARTERIAL PUNCTURE TECHNIQUES

The following is a brief summary of the steps necessary for a successful arterial puncture. This procedure is a rapid and relatively easy means to obtain a blood-gas sample, and all emergency nurses should know how to perform it. As with any technical procedure, repeated clinical practice is needed. In order to guarantee clinical proficiency, the emergency department should provide supervised classroom and clinical practice. The nurse must also be aware of the potential hazards of this procedure. There are reports in the literature of peripheral neuropathy, muscle ischemia, and hemorrhage occurring following arterial puncture in patients receiving anticoagulants. [4] Radial artery thrombosis and gangrene following radial artery cannulation have also been reported. [5,6]

EQUIPMENT

1. Five to ten cubic centimeter syringe: a glass syringe is preferred since there is a possibility of gas diffusion across a plastic syringe.

2. Vial of heparin, 1000 units/cc (10 mg/cc).

3. Disposable 20-gauge needle (in adults).

4. Local anesthetic (without epinephrine). *Make sure that the patient is not allergic to this drug.*

5. Blood-gas syringe cap (metal or cork).

6. Alcohol sponge and 4 × 4 pads.

7. Cup of ice.

8. Blood-gas request slip with notation of patient's name, clinical condition, temperature, percentage of inspired oxygen (F_IO_2), and route of administration. If patient has received bicarbonate, lactate, or ammonium chloride, time and dosage should be noted.

PROCEDURE

1. When possible, notify laboratory that a sample for a BGA will be drawn so technicians can calibrate machine for 15 to 20 minutes.

2. If patient is alert, prepare him or her for the procedure. Explain that many patients report a momentary deep throbbing pain with this procedure.

3. If patient is receiving supplementary O_2, he or she must receive an uninterrupted flow for a minimum of *10 minutes.* Suctioning, intermittent positive pressure breathing (IPPB), change in F_IO_2, turning, etc., will alter the PaO_2* reading.

4. An unclotted speciman is needed, so lubricate the barrel of the syringe with 0.5 cc heparin, ejecting any extra medication. Heparin has an acidotic pH, and excessive medication can falsely lower the patient's pH reading. It will also abnormally dilute the blood and distort any hematocrit readings.

5. Determine which artery to use (see Figs. 8-2 and 8-3). The radial and brachial arteries have the best collateral circulation and are preferred over the femoral artery in most cases. However, if the patient is hypotensive or peripherally constricted, the femoral artery may be the only available site. In addition, the brachial artery is contraindicated if the patient is on anticoagulants since Volkmann's contracture may develop.[4]

6. The radial artery will be used for the following explanation. Before choosing this site, collateral ulnar circulation must be assessed. Firmly compress the radial artery and have the patient clench his fist for 10 to 15 seconds. Maintain radial artery compression and instruct the patient to unclench his fist. The palm should "pink up" immediately. If not, ulnar circulation may be impaired (this is found frequently in elderly patients), and an alternate site must be chosen.

7. Carefully palpate the radial artery to determine its position.

---

* The letter "a" indicates that this is an arterial value.

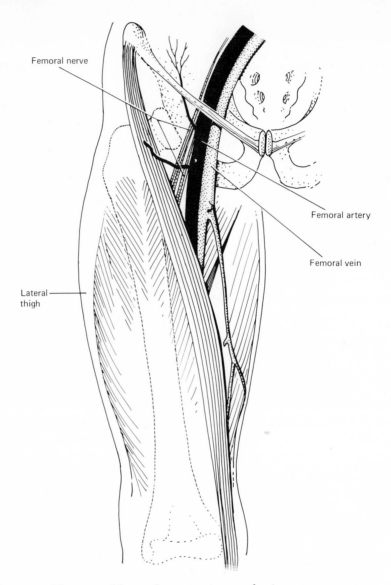

Femoral nerve

Femoral artery

Femoral vein

Lateral thigh

Figure 8-2 Anatomical location of femoral nerve, artery, and vein.

8. Place a rolled hand towel under the wrist to hyperextend the wrist.

9. Cleanse the skin with alcohol.

10. Inject local anesthetic intradermally. This numbs the skin and

Figure 8-3 Anatomical location of brachial artery and nerve and radial artery.

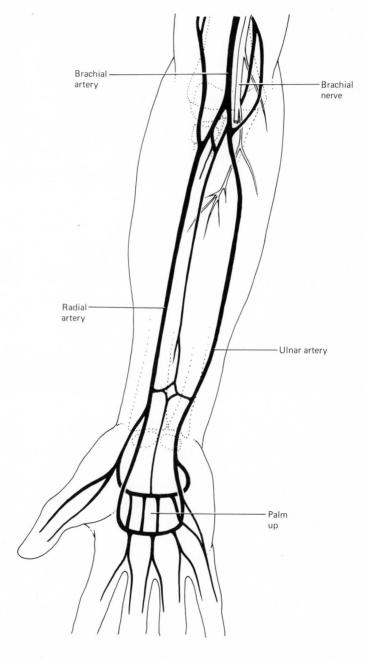

also decreases the amount of arterial spasm. However, the patient may still experience the deep throbbing pain referred to above.

11. Palpate for pulses and stabilize artery between first two fingers. Insert 20-gauge needle on the syringe into area of maximum pulsation. Frequently, the needle perforates both sides of the artery by passing completely through the vessel. If there is no pulsatile return of blood, slowly withdraw the needle.

12. Once there is a pulsatile return of blood, collect 2 to 4 cc. If the agency has a micro gas analyzer, as little as 0.5 cc is needed.

13. Hand the collected blood-gas sample to a second person, instructing the assistant to eject all air bubbles, cap the syringe, and immerse it in a cup of ice. If the sample is left uniced, it must be tested within 10 minutes, while a refrigerated, iced sample is good for several hours.

14. Even if the attempt is unsuccessful, apply direct pressure with a 4×4 pad to the puncture site for a minimum of 5 minutes (longer if patient has a clotting problem or is taking an anticoagulant).

15. When results are available, crosscheck the PaO_2 with the calculated O_2 saturation and $PaCO_2$, pH, and HCO_3^- with the bicarbonate nomogram. This provides not only a good check on laboratory accuracy but also a valuable repetitive learning experience for the emergency nurse.

16. Remember that arterial blood gases are only one parameter in the total clinical picture of the patient. A comprehensive history and repeated clinical assessments are also mandatory.

ASSESSMENT OF ARTERIAL BLOOD GAS RESULTS

When evaluating arterial blood-gas results, it is helpful to use an organized approach. To determine acid-base balance:

1. Look at the pH to determine if the patient is acidotic or alkalotic (see Fig. 7-2).

2. Check the $PaCO_2$ for a respiratory deviation.

3. Check the bicarbonate and base excess for a metabolic deviation.

4. A helpful fact to remember when evaluating acid-base balance is that any pH change fully explained by a change in $PaCO_2$ is a pure respiratory imbalance. There is a roughly equal but opposite relationship between these two values. For example, an increase in $PaCO_2$ of 10 units (40 → 50 mmHg) results in a decrease in pH of 0.10 units (7.40 → 7.30). If the pH deviation is not fully explained by the change in $PaCO_2$, a metabolic abnormality also exists. It should be noted that this equal but opposite deflection becomes less accurate the farther the $PaCO_2$ deviates from 40 mmHg, especially when the deflection exceeds 20 units.

5. Remember that there can be marked respiratory and/or metabolic deviations with the pH remaining within the normal range. This state, an attempt by the kidneys and lungs to restore the pH, is called *physiologic compensation.*

When evaluating the PaO_2, the following questions should be answered:

1. What is the normal oxygen value for this patient?

2. What is the concentration of inspired oxygen and how is it administered?

3. What is the level of hemoglobin? Remember that oxygen transport is dependent on adequate hemoglobin levels.

4. What are the temperature and pH? Remember that deviations in temperature and pH change the position of the oxyhemoglobin dissociation curve (see Fig. 5-5).

5. If the PaO_2 is low and the patient has been receiving supplementary O_2, did he or she receive an uninterrupted flow for at least 10 minutes?

Before evaluating the following case studies, an important point must be stressed. A normal BGA does not eliminate the possibility of a serious health problem, and an abnormal report could be due to laboratory error. An in-depth history and continuous clinical assessment are mandatory. *Remember to treat the patient, not the blood-gas report!*

ARTERIAL BLOOD-GAS CASE STUDIES

1. Mr. Philips is a 52-year-old man with a 10-year history of emphysema. During the last 4 days he has noted an increase in dyspnea and a productive cough of green tenacious mucus. He arrives in your emergency department, severely dyspneic, and belligerent. A stat blood-gas sample is drawn on room air.

Results		Interpretation
pH	7.28	Acidemia
$PaCO_2$	96	Respiratory acidosis
HCO_3^-	44	Metabolic alkalosis
PaO_2	46	Severe hypoxemia
O_2 sat.	73 %	Severe hypoxemia

This BGA is consistent with severe obstructive respiratory failure due to the presence of a severe hypoxemia and a marked respiratory acidosis. The metabolic alkalosis is a long-term compensatory response to the chronic respiratory acidosis caused by the emphysema. Remember that this emphysematous patient's respiratory drive is regulated in part by oxygen receptors located in the aortic arch and carotid sinus which are stimulated by decreased levels of oxygen. Supplementary low-flow oxygen (for example, 3 liters/minute) must be delivered with caution, and frequent arterial blood-gas samples must be drawn to monitor the response.

2. A BGA was made on a young woman with a 4-year history of diabetes and the results are summarized below. She had been well-controlled on diet and insulin therapy. Upon admission to your facility, she is stuporous, febrile (102°F), and hyperventilating. No oxygen has been administered.

Results		Interpretation
pH	6.96	Acidemia
$PaCO_2$	11	Respiratory alkalosis
HCO_3^-	2.4	Metabolic acidosis
PaO_2	98	Normal
O_2 sat.	93 %	Normal

This patient is in severe diabetic ketoacidosis with maximal respiratory compensation. The presence of fever suggests the possibility of an infection which may be the cause of the patient's sudden loss of diabetic control. She must be closely assessed for a site of infection. Intravenous sodium bicarbonate should be administered immediately since the pH has reached a dangerously low level.

3. A patient arrives in your emergency department reporting severe retrosternal pain of sudden onset. A 12-lead ECG and arterial BGA are done. The ECG shows an acute inferior MI. Results of the BGA, drawn on room air, are as follows:

Results		Interpretation
pH	7.57	Alkalosis
$PaCO_2$	23	Respiratory alkalosis
HCO_3^-	24	Normal
PaO_2	90	Normal
O_2 sat.	95 %	Normal

These data represent a pure respiratory alkalosis of very recent onset, since there is as yet no metabolic compensation. This patient is hyperventilating as a stress response to pain and increased anxiety. Analgesia and sedation must be administered promptly to diminish this stress response since an alkalosis may further increase the irritability of the damaged myocardium.

Measurement of blood gases is a common occurrence in most emergency departments. It is critically important that the emergency nurse be proficient in obtaining the blood-gas samples, aware of the possible hazards of this test, knowledgeable in the biologic effects of acid-base and oxygen imbalances, and skillful in the assessment and treatment of the patient.

REFERENCES

1. Betson, C., "Blood Gases," *American Journal of Nursing,* vol. 68, no. 5, May 1968, p. 1010.

2. Walthemath, C., "Oxygen Uptake Transport and Tissue Utilization," *Anesthesia and Analgesia,* vol. 79, no. 1, January–February 1970, p. 184–202.

3. Betson, C., "The Nurses' Role in Blood Gas Monitoring," *Cardiovascular Nursing,* vol. 7, no. 6, November–December 1971, pp. 83–84.

4. Macon, W., and Futrell, J., "Median-Nerve Neuropathy after Brachial-Artery Puncture and Anticoagulation," *New England Journal of Medicine,* vol. 288, no. 26, June 1973, p. 1396.

5. Katz, A., Birnbaum, M. Moylan, J., and Pellett, J., "Gangrene of the Hand and Forearm: A Complication of Radial Artery Cannulation," *Critical Care Medicine,* vol. 2, no. 5, September–October, 1974, pp. 270–271.

6. Gardner, R., Schwartz, R., Wong, H., and Burke, J., "Percutaneous Indwelling Radial-Artery Catheters: Risk of Thrombosis & Infection," *New England Journal of Medicine,* vol. 290, no. 22, May 1974, pp. 1227–1231.

BIBLIOGRAPHY

Comroe, J., *Physiology of Respiration,* Year Book, Chicago, 1974.

Hudak, C., Gallo, M., and Lohr, S., *Critical Care Nursing,* Mosby, St. Louis, 1973.

Wade, J., *Respiratory Nursing Care: Physiology and Technique,* Mosby, St. Louis, 1973.

TWO

THE
PSYCHOSOCIAL BASIS
OF
EMERGENCY NURSING

CHAPTER 9
COMMUNICATION WITH A PERSON AS A PSYCHOSOCIAL BEING

JEAN T. GRIPPIN, R.N., M.S.

A PERSON is more than a biological mass of cells which needs only to maintain itself in a state of physiological homeostasis. The total person is much more than the sum of his or her parts.

PSYCHIC FUNCTIONS

As a psychological being, a person is capable of performing four fundamental psychic functions. These are sensing, thinking, feeling, and using intuition.(1) Sensing is the process through which one gathers objective data (e.g., "I *smell* alcohol. I *see* an unconscious person who is dressed in dirty, worn clothing"). Thinking is the cognitive process through which one recognizes the *meaning* of the data (e.g., Alcohol is a central nervous system depressant. This person needs to be evaluated). Feeling is the *affective* aspect of all mental life (e.g., "I hate alcoholics!"). Intuition is the quick *perception of truth* without conscious attention or reasoning (e.g., "This person has no social support system and probably lives on skid row!").

These four functions are synthesized in an individual. Nurses frequently make the error of stating that what *they* sense is also sensed by another. This could be true if the other three functions of the psyche did not "contaminate" the function of sensing. However, once a person begins to think, feel, or use intuition, the sensing function is altered because each individual places meaning on an event, values an event, or has intuition about an event in a strictly personal manner. To understand another's psyche, the nurse must rely upon reports from that person. Such reports are given both audibly and silently.

People do not exist in a vacuum. From the moment of birth until death a person is either dependent on, independent from, or interdependent with others. People are social beings. Specific types of relationships with people are determined by the nature of the society into which a person is born.[1] That is, attitudes, values, and beliefs are determined by the culture. Everything a person does or does not do, every decision he or she makes or does not make is based on consciously or unconsciously held beliefs, attitudes, and eventually values. This fact is as true for the nurse as it is for the patient.

To know what a patient values, then, would help the nurse understand why that person behaves in a given manner (e.g., arriving in the emergency department every weekend with acute alcoholism). The nurse can know a patient's values by receiving reports from the patient. These reports are called, by Jourard, self-disclosure and are obtainable from the patient by listening to the silent and audible language.[2] Understanding the *why* of behavior is more often than not a prerequisite to deciding how to help. A person as a psychosocial being—a sensing, thinking, feeling, intuitive person whose every action is determined by the values he or she holds—can be understood only through the process called communication.

SILENT AND AUDIBLE LANGUAGES

You cannot *not* communicate! Sigmund Freud once wrote that "no mortal can keep a secret. If his lips are silent, he chatters with his fingertips; betrayal oozes out of him at every pore." All behavior has some meaning. All behavior is communication. Between 50 and 80 percent of every message is carried nonverbally. This being true, those who help others need to be aware of the communicative value of both the silent and the audible languages.

SILENT LANGUAGES

The silent languages encompass all the ways people use to communicate meaningfully in nonverbal, nonsymbolic ways. For example, communication occurs through the use of space, clothing, color, time, and gestures. It is critical for nurses to acknowledge that all the silent languages have meaning and influence the total message.

LANGUAGE OF SPACE   Many nurses are in positions which permit them to suggest or determine the use of the space that is called the emergency department. Where equipment is placed, how the furniture is arranged in the waiting area, and how physically closed the nursing station is, all communicate something to patients, their families, and physicians. *Where* the nurse sits when telling a family member that a loved one has died as the result of an auto accident, *where* one stands (behind the barrier of the desk or next to her) when reassuring a mother who has brought her sick child to the ED, and *how* one behaves (turning his or her back and walking toward another room or moving toward the patient with a nod of acknowledgement) when a patient arrives for a "shot" on the fifth consecutive night, all communicate something to the patient or relatives.

LANGUAGE OF CLOTHING   Nurses' choices of clothing tell patients and associates much about their conscious tastes and in addition give a portrait (which is largely unconscious) of the way they see themselves. The nurse who comes to work in jeans and changes to a scrub gown communicates something vastly different from the nurse who arrives in a neat, well-fitting uniform and clean, well-repaired shoes. Nurses working in scrub gowns have told the writer that their conscious reason for wearing the scrub gown is that "the uniform is constricting and it gets dirty." One can only speculate on the unconscious meaning of the scrub gown.

LANGUAGE OF COLOR   The "warm" colors—red, orange, and yellow—make people feel more responsive to others while the "cool" colors—green, blue, and gray—have a dampening effect on communication. Many nurses have opportunities to suggest the color the walls of the ED are to be painted. The color chosen may have important effects on the kinds of communication that occur in this department.

LANGUAGE OF TIME   Each person has a different sense of time. When a peer is late for work, what is communicated to the rest of the staff? How do they react to the nurse who always comes to work early? What do such phrases as "in a few minutes," "after a while," and "a short time ago" communicate to fellow workers and patients? When instructing patients to take one capsule of medication after each meal, are nurses telling patients to take the medication only if they eat a full meal or do they want patients to take a capsule at the time they, the nurses, eat meals? Both ideas are ridiculous, of course, but do the patients know what the nurse means?

LANGUAGE OF GESTURES   Gestures are expressive motions or actions. The most dramatic gesture is that of suicide. Subtle gestures include the way individuals use their eyes, where they place their hands, and how they move them when speaking to others. The nurse who sits and leans toward the patient communicates something vastly different than the nurse who stands and glances at a watch when speaking to a patient. It is important for nurses to interpret the gestures of patients and to also become aware of their own. A word of caution: To interpret another's gestures without validating that interpretation with the person is a mistake. Without validation one is likely to be communicating on the basis of wrong information about another.

A victim of rape once said that only one person in the ED communicated to her that she cared. The patient said the nurse's aide spoke no words, but communicated caring by bringing the patient a glass of water and by covering her exposed body parts with the sheet the nurse had "thrown over me." Gestures communicate!

AUDIBLE LANGUAGE

All are familiar with the audible languages. Some people are less familiar with the fact that when speaking, one is describing those interactions which happen inside oneself. No word or group of words has meaning in and of itself. Rather, each individual gives the words meaning.[3] Identical stimuli can never be experienced identically. Problems in communication often arise because this fact is forgotten.

Because each person experiences his or her world differently, nurses must become experts in listening. One may say, "Expert in listening? I listen to people all day every day." But does one really *hear* what people say? Hearing is not a passive activity. Everyone needs to work at "tuning in" to patients just as one tunes in to instrumental roles in an orchestra.

The values one holds often come into play to block the ability to listen. When the ability to listen to patients is blocked, one begins to think about the patient ("How stupid for him to overdose."), to think for him ("Next time try barbiturates and alcohol. That's a sure thing."), or to think ahead of him ("I know we saved your life this time, but you'll go do it again."). When the nurse realizes that she or he sees things a certain way and that the same things may appear different to others, the nurse is free to think with the patient. The nurse therefore gains an understanding of how things look from the patient's point of view and how this person feels about the issues. This is the goal of the process termed "good communication."

Some helpful hints for improving communication with patients include:

1. Identify yourself and your goal when interacting with a patient. "Hello, Mr. Smith. I'm Ms. Green, a nurse. I am here to help you." Patients often say they do not know one professional from another and are often confused about what to expect from them.

2. Assist the patient to identify what he or she is thinking and feeling. For example, "It must be frightening to think we do not care," is a reassuring response to a patient who complains, "I've been here 1 hour and you've treated everyone else first."

3. Seek validation for the assumptions made about a patient and his or her behavior. "Things must have been pretty bad for you to try suicide."

In conclusion, nurses frequently tell each other that in the ED they "don't have time" to be concerned with communication. Nurses are in some form of contact—and therefore, in communication—with every patient who comes to the department. The writer proposes that "not enough time" means "I don't (or won't) know what to say." If nurses care and let their patients know that they care, they will not often go wrong. There are no pat, surefire, sure-to-work "how to" methods in talking with patients. What has been presented here are some considerations about communication that ED nurses may find helpful in their professional practice.

REFERENCES

1. Hall, Calvin S., and Lindzey, Gardner, *Theories of Personality*, Wiley, New York, 1957, p. 89.

2. Jourard, Sidney M., *The Transparent Self,* Van Nostrand, Princeton, N.J., 1964.

3. Fabun, Don (ed.), *Communications: The Transfer of Meaning,* Glencoe Press, New York, 1968, p. 19.

BIBLIOGRAPHY

Adler, Alfred, *The Science of Living,* Pocket Books, Inc., New York, 1971.

Arnold, Helen M., "I–Thou," *American Journal of Nursing,* December 1970, pp. 2554–2556.

Bermask, Loretta S., "Interviewing: A Key to Therapeutic Communication in Nursing Practice," *Nursing Clinics of North America,* June 1966, pp. 205–214.

Fast, Julius, *Body Language,* Pocket Books, Inc., New York, 1971.

Goldsborough, Judith D., "On Becoming Nonjudgmental," *American Journal of Nursing,* November 1970, pp. 2340–2343.

Hall, Edward T., *The Hidden Dimension,* Doubleday, New York, 1969.

Hein, Eleanor C., "Listening," *Nursing '75,* March 1975, pp. 93–102.

Kalisch, Beatrice J., "What Is Empathy?", *American Journal of Nursing,* September 1973, pp. 1548–1552.

Mann, Floyd, "Handling Misunderstandings and Conflict," Center for Research on Utilization of Scientific Knowledge, University of Michigan (undated).

Murray, Jeanne B., "Self-Knowledge and the Nursing Interview," *Nursing Forum,* January 1963, pp. 69–78.

Veninga, Robert, "Communications: A Patients' Eye View," *American Journal of Nursing,* February 1973, pp. 320–322.

CHAPTER 10
STRESS AND ANXIETY IN THE EMERGENCY DEPARTMENT

JILL D. HOLMES, R.N., M.S.

EMERGENCY department! The very name conveys excitement, danger, high emotions, and activity. Unpredictable patients and crisis situations with dramatic medical interventions are all part of the ED scene. While the environment may be unpredictable, personnel in these critical care areas are expected to remain in control, working calmly under considerable stress. But sometimes even experienced personnel show signs of irritation or become less productive owing to the demands of the working environment. Responding to both physical and mental processes, staff can behave in different ways which may affect their work adversely. In addition, patients and families suddenly found in a crisis situation may also show an extensive repertoire of behaviors which may range from nervousness to irritation or anger to panic.

Behind all these observable behavioral changes is the fact that the ED is a stressful environment. Human beings, placed under stress, react in a variety of ways, but the response common to all is *anxiety*. While experienced nurses are certainly aware of their own anxiety and its effects on behavior, they must also be experts in assessing patients' anxiety and planning appropriate interventions. Therefore, this chapter defines and describes the concept of anxiety and outlines in a simple way various approaches nurses might use to lessen the negative effects of anxiety on themselves, hospital personnel, and patients and their families.

DEFINITION OF ANXIETY

There are many definitions of anxiety. For use in this chapter, anxiety is defined as a primitive emotional response with somatic components elicited by external and internal cues. Anxiety is frequently associated with three states of mind: a sense of *helplessness,* of *isolation-alienation,* and of *insecurity.* Each threatens an individual's identity. While the primary emotional response is subjective and not directly observable, the individual who is uncomfortable owing to anxiety often demonstrates a variety of behaviors or responses that can be assessed by others.

RESPONSES TO ANXIETY

What unique body responses make one uncomfortably aware of being under stress? What kinds of behavior do patients, families, and fellow staff members exhibit when they are anxious?

Physical reactions to anxiety are mediated by the *sympathetic division* of the autonomic nervous system. For some people, a cold sweat may break out; others report a feeling of "butterflies in the stomach." Other physical signs might include a rapidly pounding heart, a flushed face, dilated pupils, rapid breathing, and muscular tension along the spine, neck, and shoulders. Other people may be aware of a sudden need to void or to get a drink of water for an increasingly dry mouth. In the middle of a task which demands small motor coordination, some individuals may find their hands and fingers betray them by trembling. These physical responses may hamper work by interfering with coordination and task organization. All these physical sensations, if unchecked, tend to make one feel increasingly uncomfortable, and a spiraling cycle of increasing anxiety may ensue.

In addition, some individuals are aware that their thinking ability becomes more "scatterbrained." They may become tearful, more easily annoyed, or angry with events or people and find their emotions run high. In an attempt to regain composure and a state of equilibrium, individuals employ a variety of *coping mechanisms.* These mechanisms are habits or behavioral responses which have been developed by the ego for the defense of self-esteem and self-worth. Often these behavioral responses, when not recognized as coping mechanisms, may frustrate, anger, or appall others. It is important to remember that anxiety is a subjective personal response to a situation which threatens individual security or self. While nurses from their point of view may see that a situation is not truly threatening, the anxious person sees it as such and becomes even more anxious.

LEVELS OF ANXIETY AND NURSING INTERVENTIONS

Anxiety is part of living, and all human beings have experienced it. Depending on the degree, anxiety can either aid or disrupt efforts in getting through the day. At certain degrees or stages of anxiety, concentration and general alertness are enhanced. Tasks seem effortless, one's body does not tire as easily, and time seems to speed by. Yet at higher levels of anxiety, an individual may be unable to perform or act effectively.

Anxiety, therefore, can be viewed on a *continuum,* ranging from *mild* to *severe,* and its degree or level has a definite effect on a person's ability to think, perceive, cooperate, and learn. Nursing assessments and interventions are based on this concept.

MILD ANXIETY

Mild anxiety *motivates.* It is a rare, disciplined student who studies for an examination weeks ahead; most, faced with the threat of potential failure, open books and review notes only the night before the test. Because anxiety is slightly elevated, alertness, concentration, and retention of the necessary information are enhanced. Consider a patient in the ED who is not severely ill or injured but has come for treatment of a sprained ankle. Listening carefully to the nurse, this patient asks appropriate questions and seems to retain all information regarding the care of his or her ankle.

MODERATE ANXIETY

However, another patient with a routine sprained ankle may feel a moderate amount of anxiety and may not behave according to staff expectations. He or she demonstrates a heightened concern for self, focusing solely on the ankle with substantially reduced ability to see peripherally. He or she does not seem to hear everything that is said and asks the same questions repeatedly without comprehending the answers. The staff's attention and constant reassurance may be sought. This patient may act inappropriately annoyed or angry and is unable to pick up cues from family or friends that this behavior is embarrassing them. Faced with this situation, and not recognizing that the patient is moderately anxious and attempting to cope, a nurse or physician may react with exasperation, defensiveness, or anger.

The first step for the nurse is to recognize the patient's moderate anxiety level and not retaliate or become defensive in the face of this coping behavior. Intervention is aimed at helping the patient lessen the level of anxiety. With moderate anxiety, the patient may be able to focus but be unappreciative of peripheral cues or complex directions. Recognizing a decreased level of performance, the nurse can guide the patient by using simple words and short sentences. If convenient or appropriate, the patient may be engaged in a simple task such as going for a drink of water or holding a piece of equipment. The nurse should also provide the patient with a quiet, private space where he or she may talk, cry, or pace. If appropriate, a family member who is calm and knows the patient well could be asked to stay in the room. Remember to support the family members by briefing them about the situation, explaining simply that the patient needs to be with someone.

SEVERE ANXIETY

At still higher levels of anxiety, the individual's ability to focus, comprehend, and integrate environmental stimuli becomes compromised. No longer able to focus on any one thing, the severely anxious individual may see or hear scattered pieces of the environment, but the details are blown up, disproportionate to the real world. Unable to concentrate, this person may appear confused and unable to move toward any goals. Memory, too, becomes disarranged, and facts, commonly known, are forgotten or remembered incorrectly.

It is obvious that a patient at this point would misunderstand what is happening and would be unlikely to follow complex directions, or comprehend an important fact regarding treatment. Professionals, unfortunately, appear unaware of this when they continue to direct or teach this patient and react explosively to a patient's unresponsive behavior. "But I told him to take only one pill three times a day, not three pills once a day!" It may seem obvious, but staff also become anxious especially when a patient appears "deliberately" not to listen and gets into further trouble. Staff often will act out their anxiety by demonstrating anger or irritation.

Intervention by a nurse at this point is imperative. Nonverbal communication such as touch may work along with simple verbal directions such as "come" or "sit." Using the patient's first name along with an attempt to establish eye contact may reach through the patient's confusion. The nurse should remain with the patient, indicating acceptance. The presence of a calm, reality-oriented person provides a strong focal point for a patient in this state. The ED nurse is not being asked to begin in-depth therapy with the patient, but it is within his or her ability to listen to the patient, reflecting back stated feelings, and remaining responsive to physical needs.

PREVENTION OF ANXIETY

As a therapeutic person in the ED, the nurse not only *recognizes* and *intervenes in* anxiety states, but also actively works toward *preventing,* when possible, anything which would be likely to threaten an individual's self-identity or physical security. For example, most people have a fear of the unknown; this definitely affects an individual's feelings of security. Simple explanations, clear directions, and orientation to equipment surrounding the patient can be done by the nurse even while she or he is assembling supplies for a procedure. For example, "Mr. Smith, Dr. Jones will be looking at your hand in a few minutes. Meanwhile, I am going to set up some dressings and Band-Aids here. Have you ever had a cut sutured before? Let me explain what will happen."

Fear of isolation is also common; telling a patient that his or her family is in the waiting room and knows his or her general condition or will be meeting with one of the physicians ties the patient into a familiar relationship pattern. For example, "Mr. Smith, your son and your wife have arrived and know you are in the treatment room. Dr. Jones is with them now. As soon as Dr. Jones treats your hand, you may see them."

A patient may also be experiencing a real threat to his physical well-being, such as a serious accident or illness. Falsely reassuring a patient in the face of an obviously bad situation promotes the patient's distrust and heightens this sense of isolation from the staff. Remaining calm, providing pain relief, and recognizing and meeting the patient's physical and emotional needs promote an open, trusting relationship. For example, "I know your chest pain is severe, Mr. Jones. I am going to give you an injection for it, and I will stay with you until you feel better. You look concerned. All of this must be frightening for you." With this approach, nurses help patients say aloud thoughts or ideas they may have related to their physical status.

In summary, anxiety is a part of living, present in daily situations. Arising from situations which frustrate, threaten, or create conflict, it can either motivate or halt personal growth and achievement. In an anxiety-producing milieu such as an ED, the opportunities for nursing intervention are presented constantly. Nurses must first recognize the behavior for what it is, then decide how incapacitating it is for the individual, and plan their activity accordingly. Helping a patient through a difficult period of time can provide great personal satisfaction and growth for both patient and nurse.

BIBLIOGRAPHY

Chernus, J., "Finding Clues to Anxiety," *Consultant,* March 1974.

Cleland, V., "Effects of Stress on Thinking," *American Journal of Nursing,* vol. 67, no. 1, January 1967.

Luckmann, J., and Sorensen, K., *Medical-Surgical Nursing: A Psychophysiologic Approach,* Saunders, Philadelphia, 1974.

Peplau, H., *Interpersonal Relations in Nursing: A Conceptual Frame of Reference of Psychodynamic Nursing,* Putnam, New York, 1952.

Rickles, N., *Management of Anxiety for the General Practitioner,* Charles C Thomas, Springfield, Ill., 1963.

Selye, H., *The Stress of Life,* McGraw-Hill, New York, 1956.

Volicer, B., "Patients' Perceptions of Stressful Events Associated with Hospitalization," *Nursing Research,* vol. 23:3, May–June 1974, pp. 235–238.

CHAPTER 11
DEATH, DYING, AND THE GRIEVING PROCESS
JEAN T. GRIPPIN, R.N., M.S.

IN 1969 Dr. Elisabeth Kubler-Ross' book *On Death and Dying* reported her work with dying patients and their families.[1] Since that time much has been written for and by nurses on ways the nurse can help dying patients. Although nurses deal daily with dying patients and their grieving relatives and friends, little has been written specifically for ED nurses.

Kubler-Ross spelled out five psychological phases through which a dying patient may move, and she maintains that if nurses can accept, understand, and be comfortable with each phase, they can help the dying patient. The phases are: (1) shock and denial, (2) anger, (3) bargaining, (4) depression, and (5) acceptance. Patients in the ED and their grieving relatives also begin to move through these phases.

The nurse in the ED most frequently sees patients and their loved ones in the phases of shock and denial and anger. This chapter discusses ways the nurse can identify these two phases and intervene in a way that is helpful to patients and their relatives.

SHOCK AND DENIAL

DEFINITION

SHOCK   Violent impact of reality on the personality; an unwanted collision of reality with what the person consciously desires.

DENIAL   One of the ego defense mechanisms which automatically and unconsciously comes into action when the reality of a situation is too difficult for the personality to accept. (Perhaps one might think of it as one of nature's protections for the personality.)

IDENTIFICATION

SHOCK   The person seems "stunned." He or she may complain of "not feeling a thing." This person may say to the nurse that he or she cannot cry or "I know I should be frightened (or scared) but I'm numb."

DENIAL   The person may say "Oh, no, that's not true; this isn't happening to me." Upon hearing a diagnosis of life-threatening illness (e.g., "You've just had a massive myocardial infarction"), he or she responds with an intellectual acceptance and little emotion. Relatives and friends in denial after the death of a loved one often calmly initiate appropriate activities like calling the mortuary, other relatives, and their clergyman with little display of emotion. Patients and family members who respond in this way make it easier for the nurse to avoid feelings about his or her own mortality. The nurse denies also and calls the patient a "cooperative patient" and says about the family that "they sure took that well."

INTERVENTION

Before nurses can intervene in a helpful way they need to come to grips with what they think and feel about their own death. Gathered with a group process facilitator, nurses can assist each other to explore thoughts and feelings about mortality. Nurses have gained insights into themselves through planned weekly staff meetings where dying patients are the focus. There are no "right" or "wrong" things to believe. What is important is that all are consciously aware of what they think and feel because all will someday die.

SHOCK   Intervention into another's emotional shock is best done at a nonverbal level. The touch of a caring person, a look that says "I care," and simply being with the person without speaking a word communicate much. As the shock of the situation begins to be experienced, the nurse can be helpful by nonverbally directing a person to an out-of-the-way spot, bringing coffee or a glass of water, and staying nearby. In essence the nurse becomes a "shock absorber" in this situation. Many nurses are uncomfortable when not talking "at" a person— telling him or her how, why, when, and where; often a simple statement such as "This must be hard," or "It's sometimes difficult to know what you are feeling" (stated as a fact to which the person need not respond) is helpful when the nurse is uncomfortable with silence.

DENIAL   Nurses need to know that they cannot *make* a person who is denying reality "see the light." Often in one's vigor to use some newfound knowledge, valiant efforts are made "to point out reality" to people. This constant bombardment of the personality with overwhelming reality only causes people to use more denial.

If the nurse indicates to the patient that she or he will not be devastated by expressed feelings, the patient is then given the opportunity to express fear, anger, and pain; then the nurse can help this person. How can one indicate acceptance of a patient's feelings? The nurse can:

1. Make every effort to stay with the person for a time. Even a few minutes of just being there, of doing nothing but "being" with the patient, is helpful.

2. Say that if he or she were the patient (or the relative) he or she, too, would feel upset, scared, frightened, or whatever one's feelings might be in the same situation; then ask if the person is feeling this way.

3. Share with the patient what others in similar circumstances have shared with him or her. Tell the patient, for example, that patients with similar diagnoses have expressed fear and ask if he or she feels this way.

ANGER

DEFINITION

Anger can be defined as a feeling experienced when one's attempt to reach some goal has been frustrated by circumstances beyond one's conscious control.

IDENTIFICATION

Feelings are not subject to objective reading by the nurse as are, for instance, the vital signs. It is only as the nurse interprets the patient's subjective report, objectively views what the person does or is doing, and makes an assessment of the meaning of these, that she or he is in a position to say that the person is angry.

Most nurses have no problem identifying when a person is overtly angry. In the ED the person says that he or she has had to wait too long, that the diagnosis is wrong, or that hospitalization is not needed. Upon the death of a loved one the family sometimes tells the nurse that the staff did not do enough or call the doctor soon enough. Sometimes people cry when they are angry because being overtly angry does not fit with their self-image.

INTERVENTION

The behavior nurses frequently exhibit in such a situation is to defend themselves; i.e., they become defensive. Time is spent telling the patient or family that the staff did what they were supposed to do or that other patients also needed care. A nurse may remove himself or herself from these people and may ask another nurse to take over the care because the person is angry "at me." Actually, these people are angry with the situation in which they find themselves (dying, being afraid of dying, or having lost, in death, someone meaningful). However, it is difficult for the nurse who is being verbally criticized to understand this. The nurse must accept the fact of not being appreciated by all patients and, at times, will become angry and defensive with a patient. The nurse is human, too. A trusted colleague or superior can be helpful to the nurse if the person allows the nurse to discuss his or her angry feelings. In the process the nurse will be helped to identify the cause of these feelings. This process then becomes a growing experience for the nurse who, in future similar situations, will be more effective.

The way to help overtly angry people is to assist them to recognize their anger and to then talk about it. Several actions may help accomplish this goal:

1. Simply stating "you seem angry" if the person has not yet said this is helpful. The person will most often respond to this with "You're right, I am angry." This approach assists the person to know the nurse can accept the anger and help him or her with the feelings of rage at the reality of the situation.

2. Saying "I guess I would be angry also if I thought the nurses hadn't done everything possible." This does not say the angry person is right in assuming something was done improperly. It does imply that if the nurse thought what the patient does, she or he, too, would be angry.

3. Making an effort, which is sometimes very difficult, to stay with the person who is angry—to not leave him or her alone! Being willing to listen to another's anger is the most meaningful way to help that person.

4. Making a conscious effort to realize that the person is angry with the situation and not with the nurse, per se. For the nurse to become defensive is not helpful.

Nurses who feel compelled to "cheer up" the crying person are not as helpful as they might be. People ask "Why?" or "What did I do wrong?" or "Tell me it isn't my fault." They do not seek answers to such questions. When a person cries in anger, the best way for the nurse to help is to provide a private place and to be there to listen.

This chapter has explored ways in which ED nurses can be helpful to their patients who are dying or who believe they are dying and to the relatives and friends of patients who have died. Brief mention needs to be made of the nurse's feelings when, after working hard to "save" a patient, the patient still dies. The feelings discussed above may be experienced by the nurse as well. The nurse may deny that the patient's death meant anything (e.g., "It's all in a day's work, I'm used to it."), or may become angry at others (e.g., the doctor, supervisor, administration, family) for real or imagined lack of understanding of his or her difficult work. The nurse may become depressed or may accept the fact that people do die. True acceptance is possible only when one knows what one thinks and feels about one's own death. Gathering to explore their personal thoughts and feelings, attending seminars and classes, and discussing these problems with the multidisciplinary team in the ED are ways nurses can learn about themselves.

Because humans are biological, psychological, and social beings, it becomes vital for nurses to attend to more than their biological needs. The nurse furnishes the opportunity for those who are hurt to express their fears, anger, and pain to someone who will accept them and not be devastated by them.

REFERENCES

1. Kubler-Ross, Elisabeth, *On Death and Dying,* Macmillan, New York, 1969.

BIBLIOGRAPHY

Bernstein, Lewis, and Dana, Richard H., *Interviewing and the Health Professions,* Appleton-Century-Crofts, New York, 1970.

Browning, Mary H., and Lewis, Edith P. (eds.), *The Dying Patient: A Nursing Perspective,* The American Journal of Nursing Company, New York, 1972.

Cauthorne, C. V., "Coping with Death in the Emergency Department," *Journal of Emergency Nursing,* November–December, 1975, pp. 24–26.

Feifel, Herman (ed.), *The Meaning of Death,* McGraw-Hill, New York, 1959.

Rinear, E., "The Nurse's Challenge When Death Is Unexpected," *Registered Nurse,* December 1975, pp. 50–55.

THREE

PATHOPHYSIOLOGY: THEORY AND EMERGENCY TREATMENT

CHAPTER 12
EMERGENCY ASSESSMENT
JEANIE BARRY, R.N., M.S.

NO matter in what field of nursing one practices, the problem-solving process must be utilized continuously. Emergency nurses must be especially skillful in this process since they frequently deal with undiagnosed and potentially lethal health problems which need rapid interventions.

The problem-solving process includes five major steps:

1. Statement of problem: Immediate assessment and patient's chief complaint

2. Data gathering: History-taking, physical assessment, and crisis evaluation

3. Analysis of data

4. Plan of management

5. Evaluation of plan via patient outcome

No matter how brief the patient contact or how urgent the condition, when a person with a problem is brought to the emergency department, all five steps in the problem-solving process must be implemented. Steps 1 and 3 are discussed in this chapter; the remaining steps are covered thoroughly within the following chapters.

STATEMENT OF PROBLEM

In this step, two vital questions are answered: (1) What brings this patient to the emergency department (chief complaint), and (2) are there any life-threatening conditions present which require immediate care?

CHIEF COMPLAINT

The chief complaint should be stated in the *patient's own words*. One frequent mistake that health assessors make is changing a patient's complaint into a diagnosis. For example, a report of "crushing chest pain" is promptly changed into a diagnosis of "myocardial infarction." Before such a diagnosis is made, much supporting data must be collected. If the patient is unconscious, the family and transport personnel must be promptly interviewed. Medical information cards, bracelets, or tags should also be sought.

IMMEDIATE ASSESSMENT

In addition to determining the patient's chief complaint, the following conditions which may threaten survival must be quickly evaluated:

1. Airway obstruction

2. Inadequate ventilation

3. Active uncontrolled bleeding

4. Presence of shock

5. Coma

If any of these conditions are present, immediate resuscitation and stabilization must be started. The reader is directed to the appropriate chapters for a guide to specific interventions. During this initial contact with the patient it is essential that the nurse display an attitude of calmness, confidence, and reassurance. These first minutes of contact are crucial to the building of the open, trusting relationship which is essential to emergency care.

DATA GATHERING

HISTORY-TAKING

After discerning the patient's chief complaint and assessing and managing life-threatening conditions, the emergency nurse then proceeds to the history-taking phase of data-collection. Before discussing the specific points involved in this phase, a few basic interviewing techniques need to be reviewed. Emergency nurses should do the following:

1. Always introduce themselves by *name* and by *role*. Patients come to the emergency facility to receive help and thus have the right to know with whom they are dealing and what they may expect from this person.

2. Explain the *purpose* and the necessity of the interview. If the patient or family member does not understand the reason for the data-collection phase of problem solving, it is unrealistic for the nurse to expect cooperation.

3. *Provide privacy.* Patients frequently will be asked to share personal information, and attention to the provision of privacy is vital. If possible all patients should be interviewed in a *private* room. However, if this is not possible, the nurse can create a feeling of privacy by (a) pulling a curtain, (b) sitting close to the patient, shielding his or her face from others in the room, and (c) speaking in a quiet voice.

4. Avoid expressing surprise, shock, or disdain as the patient relates the history. While this history may contain facts or feelings contrary to personally held values, such expressions are counter-productive in that they block the sharing of information.

5. Avoid asking "why" questions. These often have a challenging character and may put the patient on the defensive.

6. Do not believe everything that is heard. If the information sounds conflicting, confusing, or even erroneous, attempt to clarify it with the patient or a family member.

7. Avoid expressing judgments over previous medical care. The nurse is hearing only one side of the story and thus has insufficient information. Also, such stated judgments are often the precursors of litigation.

8. Attempt to collect *quantitative* data when possible. Vague statements regarding the onset and current status of symptoms are often confusing and definitely less informative than precise quantitative facts.

9. Avoid the use of confusing medical jargon.

10. Always focus on not only what the patient is saying verbally but also on the nonverbal communication which accompanies it.

11. Utilize this time with the patient as fully as possible. In addition to focusing on the chief complaint, evaluate the patient's learning needs, emotional reaction to illness, and interpersonal behavior.

FOCUSED INTERVIEW TECHNIQUE This technique of history-taking focuses on the patient's *chief complaint.* Since rapidity, organization, and accuracy are the goals of this interview, the emergency nurse must have a structured plan in mind while interviewing the patient regarding the problem. Each problem can be broken down into four historical parts:

1. Details of *onset* which focuses on the first episode.

2. *Interval* history which focuses on the period of time between the onset and the patient's presenting in the emergency department.

3. *Current* status of the problem or what is happening *right now* in the emergency department.

4. Reason for seeking help *now.* This information assists in clarifying the current status of the patient's problem. The emergency nurse can also gain valuable insight into the patient as a *person.* For example, Mr. Jones arrives in the emergency department complaining of chest pain. The 12-lead ECG indicates an acute inferior wall MI. During the interview, Mr. Jones states, "My chest pain is not that bad, but my wife insisted I come." This statement may indicate the use of denial as a coping mechanism, and further assessment of the emotional reaction to this illness is indicated.

In addition to dissecting the problem into historical parts, the accompanying symptoms can be described in terms of:

1. Bodily location

2. Character

3. Severity

4. Duration

5. Influencing factors

Since pain is one of the most frequent problems presented in the emergency department, Mr. Jones and his chest pain will be used to illustrate the above factors.

Location: Have Mr. Jones describe as completely as possible the exact area of his body that is affected. Is the pain localized to just the sternal area or is it diffuse? Can he point to the pain with one finger? The nurse should also ask Mr. Jones if he perceives his pain as superficial or deep, i.e., can he touch the painful spot with his finger or is it too deep?

Character: Have Mr. Jones describe this pain in *his own terms;* for example, state "Tell me about your pain." Avoid using leading questions, such as "Is your pain sharp or dull?" It is critical, however, that the interviewer understands what the patient means by his choice of descriptive terms.

Severity: The severity of Mr. Jones' pain can be assessed in a number of ways. The interviewer can find out how it affects normal activities of living. For example, is this pain so severe that Mr. Jones cannot eat, sleep, walk? Another successful technique is to have Mr. Jones rate his pain at time of onset and at time of interview on a *rating scale* of 1 to 7 with 1 describing an absence of pain and 7 being the most severe pain possible. A history of chest pain rated as 7 that has little influence on activities of normal living provides a vastly different clinical picture than chest pain rated as 7 that prevents eating or sleeping.

Duration: Mr. Jones must be asked the length of each attack and the frequency of these attacks. The interviewer should assist the patient to be as specific as possible. Rather than accepting a vague description of frequent episodes of chest pain lasting a short time, the interviewer should strive for a quantitative statement such as: "Four episodes of chest pain in the last month rating 5 on the 1 to 7 pain scale. These episodes lasted 15 minutes each."

Influencing factors: Mr. Jones should be asked, "What makes your chest pain *worse;* what makes it *better?*" For example, a history of chest pain worsened by lying flat and deep breathing may indicate pericarditis.

Accompanying symptoms: Frequently the patient's chief complaint is accompanied by other signs and symptoms reflecting derangements in one or more body systems. Table 12-1 provides a guide to the review of systems; which systems are evaluated will, of course, depend on the nature of the patient's problem. Each ED should be equipped with a review-of-systems form, so that the nurse can quickly determine the presence of accompanying symptoms. Again, the reader is reminded to avoid medical jargon!

Table 12-1 Summary chart for the emergency review of systems. (*From Explanation Outline for Recording a History and Physical, University of Illinois Medical Center, 1972 (unpublished).*)

General
Present weight (loss or gain, period of time, contributing factors), weakness, fatigue, malaise, fever, chills, sweats or night sweats.

Skin
Pruritus, pigmentary and other color changes, tendency to bruising, lesions (location), excessive dryness, texture, character of hair and nails, use of hair dyes or other possibly toxic agents.

Head
Headache, head injury (how, when, where), dizziness.

Eyes
Pain, vision, glasses and recent change in acuity, diplopia, infection, glaucoma, cataract.

Ears
Earaches, hearing, tinnitus, vertigo, discharge, infection, mastoiditis.

Nose and Sinuses
Sinus pain, epistaxis, nasal obstruction, discharge, postnasal drip, frequent colds, sneezing.

Oral Cavity
Toothache, recent extractions, state of dental repair; soreness or bleeding of lips, gums, mouth, tongue, or throat; disturbance of taste; hoarseness; tonsillectomy.

Neck
Pain, limitation of motion, thyroid enlargement.

Nodes
Tenderness or enlargement of cervical, axillary, epitrochlear, or inguinal nodes.

Breast
Pain, lumps, discharge, operations.

Respiratory
Chest pain, pleurisy, cough, sputum (character and amount), hemoptysis, wheezing (location in chest), stridor, asthma, bronchitis, pneumonia, tuberculosis or contact therewith, date of recent x-ray.

Cardiovascular
Precordial or retrosternal pain or distress, palpitation, dyspnea (relate to effort), orthopnea,

---

Table 12-1 *(continued)*

---

paroxysmal nocturnal dyspnea, edema, cyanosis; history of heart murmur, rheumatic fever (enumerate the manifestations), hypertension, coronary artery disease, last ECG.

Gastrointestinal
Appetite, food intolerance, dysphagia (solids, liquids), heartburn, postprandial pain or distress, biliary colic, jaundice, other abdominal pain or distress, belching, nausea, vomiting, hematemesis, flatulence; character and color of stools (bleeding, melena, clay colored, diarrhea, constipation), change in bowel habits; rectal conditions (pruritus, hemorrhoids, fissures, fistula); ulcer, gallbladder disease, hepatitis, appendicitis, colitis, parasites, hernia; date of previous x-rays.

Genitourinary
Urinary: Renal colic, frequency of urination, nocturia, polyuria, oliguria, micturition (hesitancy, urgency, dysuria, narrowing of stream, dribbling, incontinence), hematuria, albuminuria, pyuria, kidney disease, facial edema, renal stone, cystoscopy.
Male: Testicular pain, change in size of scrotum.
Gynecological: Vaginal discharge or itching; intermenstrual or postmenopausal bleeding; dysmenorrhea; dyspareunia; urinary stress, incontinence (involuntary passage of urine on coughing, sneezing, stepping off curbs, etc.); uterine prolapse; date and character of last menstrual period; if menopausal, date of onset.
Venereal: Gonorrhea or syphillis—identify by common name and signs; note date, treatment, complications.

Extremities
Vascular: Intermittent claudication, varicose veins or complications, thrombophlebitis.
Joints: Pain, stiffness, swelling (note location, migratory nature, relation to known cardiac involvement); rheumatoid arthritis, osteoarthritis, gout, bursitis.
Bones: Flat feet, osteomyelitis, fracture.
Muscles: Pain, cramps.

Back
Pain (location and radiation, especially to the extremities), stiffness, limitation of motion, sciatica or disk disease.

Central Nervous System
General: Syncope, loss of consciousness, convulsions, meningitis, encephalitis, stroke.
Mentative: Speech disorders, emotional status, orientation, memory disorders, change in sleep pattern, history of nervous breakdown.
Motor: Tremor, weakness, paralysis, clumsiness of movement.
Sensory: Radicular or neuralgic pain (head, neck, trunk, extremities), paresthesia.

Hematopoietic
Bleeding tendencies of skin or mucous membrane, anemia and treatment, blood type, transfusion and reaction, blood dyscrasia, exposure to toxic agents or radiation.

Endocrine
Nutritional and growth history; thyroid function (tolerance to heat and cold, change in skin, relationship between appetite and weight, nervousness, tremors, results of previous basal metabolism tests, thyroid medication); diabetes or its symptoms (polyuria, polydipsia, polyphagia); hirsuitism, secondary sex characteristics, hormone therapy.

SIGNIFICANT PAST HISTORY In addition to assessment of the patient's chief complaint, any significant preexisting health problems must be identified. Special emphasis should be placed on:

1. Pulmonary disease

2. Cardiac disease

3. Hypertension

4. Stroke

5. Diabetes

6. Renal disease

The nurse should also question the patient regarding any *allergies* and current *medications.*

PHYSICAL ASSESSMENT

Just like the focused interview, the approach to physical assessment varies with the patient's problems as determined in the history. Again, organized, rapid yet accurate, physical assessment is the cornerstone of emergency nursing. The nurse must have a sound knowledge of normal findings, and this requires supervised practice and more practice. The nurse must become adept at using all senses to inspect and observe in an organized fashion so that even the subtle manifestations of a problem are eventually noticed.

TECHNIQUES OF PHYSICAL ASSESSMENT The four classic techniques include *inspection, palpation, percussion,* and *auscultation.* The techniques should be performed one at a time as each system is evaluated.

Inspection: In order to skillfully inspect a patient, the nurse must be aware of normal findings and then observe for deviations. Adequate lighting and exposure of the inspected area are essential for accurate inspection.

Palpation: This technique is used to elicit tenderness and to feel for organ enlargement, tumors, cysts, nodes, etc., temperature deviation, and presence or absence of vibration. Light intermittent palpation is preferred since sensitivity to touch can be dulled by deep, continued, or heavy pressure. However, deep palpation may be necessary during abdominal assessment (see Fig. 12-1). If local tenderness is suspected, this area should be palpated last.

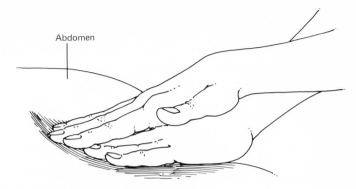

Figure 12-1 Position of hands for deep palpation.

Percussion: This technique is used to elicit pain and to demarcate underlying structures through variations in the number of vibrations heard when struck lightly with the examiner's finger (see Fig. 12-2). Basically the more solid the structure, the lesser the vibrations produced. There are four sounds which are elicited with percussion:

- *Flatness:* Normal sound heard if thigh percussed
- *Dullness:* Normal sound heard if liver percussed
- *Resonance:* Normal sound heard with lung percussion
- *Tympany:* Normal sound heard with stomach or colon percussion

The technique of percussion requires a great deal of practice on normal individuals before pathology can be readily detected.

Auscultation: One of the most important influencing factors in performing successful auscultation is using an adequate stethoscope that has:

1. Earplugs which fit snugly and comfortably

2. Short thick tubing approximately 10 in long to prevent damping of the sound

3. Both a bell-shaped chest piece for low-pitched sounds and a diaphragm for high-pitched sounds

Light contact with the stethoscope accentuates low-pitched sounds, and firm pressure accentuates high ones.

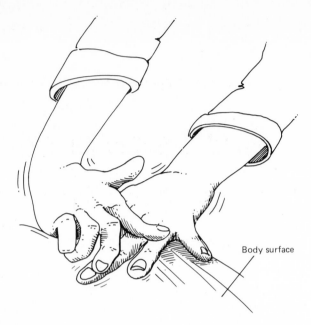

Body surface

Figure 12-2 Percussion technique. Note that the wrist movement is snapping in character.

As one embarks upon physical assessment, it is important to note that succinct *descriptions* of physical findings provide more information than just the word "normal." For example, in an evaluation of Mr. Jones' lung sounds, a complete explanation would include: "Good air entry bilaterally; no adventitious sounds heard."

GENERAL SURVEY This portion of the physical assessment includes an overview of the patient as a whole, rather than just the patient and the problem. Much of these data are collected in the first minutes of contact with the patient. Table 12-2 summarizes the various elements contained within this survey.

HEAD-TO-TOE EXAMINATION The goal of this section is to provide an organized head-to-toe assessment framework. Major parameters for each area of the body are listed. This list is not comprehensive but should be adequate for a rapid assessment of the emergency patient. The areas of the body to be evaluated will be determined by the presenting problem.

• *Head:* Hematomas, lacerations, active bleeding, tenderness; if infant, check fontanels

Table 12-2	Components of the general survey portion of the physical assessment.
	Race, sex
	Nutritional status
	Hygiene
	Apparent state of health
	Apparent age in relation to age stated by patient
	Posture and motor activity
	Behavior
	Odors: Acetone, urine, feces, alcohol
	Skin: Jaundice, cyanosis, pallor, diaphoresis

- *Face:* Symmetry, localized swelling, signs of infection or trauma

- *Eyes:* Inflammation, discharge, color of sclera, eye movements, size and reactivity of pupils, presence of normal corneal reflex, ptosis

- *Oral cavity:* State of oral hygiene, missing teeth, signs of trauma, color of mucous membranes, enlarged tonsils, ulcerations, ability to handle secretions

- *Ear: External auditory canal:* Discharge (blood, pus, cerebrospinal fluid), swelling, foreign body, cerumen. *Tympanic membrane:* Perforation, retraction, bulging

- *Nose:* Trauma, infection, discharge, deviated septum

- *Neck:* Midline trachea, quality of carotid pulses, bruits, neck veins (check both in flat position and at 45° angle), swelling of lymph nodes and salivary glands

- *Breasts:* Discharge or retraction of nipples, masses, tenderness, symmetry, ulcerations, or bruising

- *Chest: Thorax:* Chest wall configuration, scars, bruising, subcutaneous emphysema. *Respiratory:* Rate, rhythm, and depth of respirations, bilateral chest expansion, bilateral breath sounds (both air entry and adventitious sounds), use of normal and accessory muscles of breathing. *Cardiac:* Rate, rhythm, and quality of heart sounds (clear or muffled), presence of abnormal heart sounds, location of point of maximal impulse (PMI)

- *Abdomen:* Bruising, scars, distention, organ enlargement, voluntary guarding, rebound tenderness, vascular bruit, bowel sounds; if trauma patient, check lower abdomen for possible pelvic fractures

- *Extremities: General:* Swelling, bruising, lacerations, bilateral quality of pulses, obvious deformities, bilateral equality of sensory and motor function (deep tendon reflexes, hand grasps, leg pushes and foot pulls). *Upper:* Clubbing of fingers. *Lower:* Enlargement of inguinal lymph nodes.

• *Female Genetalia:* Abnormal discharge or bleeding, lacerations, lesions, state of hygiene

• *Male Genetalia:* Size, position, number, and consistency of testicles, discharge or bleeding from penis, cutaneous lesions

• *Skin:* Texture, color, temperature, scars, bruising, ulcers, turgor

• *Back:* CVA tenderness, curvature and mobility of spine

CRISIS EVALUATION

Oftentimes even what is considered a "minor" emergency by the staff can be an extremely threatening event for the patient and family. In fact, for some individuals, emergency illness or injury can precipitate an emotional *crisis.* Emotional reactions to illness are thoroughly discussed in Chaps. 9 to 11; this section will focus on the crisis evaluation as a vital component in the complete assessment of the emergency patient and family. Crisis theory as viewed by Aguilera, Messick, and Farrell is used as the framework for this evaluation. [1]

DEFINITION OF A CRISIS A person in crisis is faced with a problem which cannot be readily solved by using previous coping mechanisms. In this situation a person feels helpless and unable to problem-solve independently. As a result, *tension* and *anxiety* increase and a tremendous amount of energy is expended in an attempt to maintain a state of equilibrium. This further taxes the emotional and physiological resources of the individual, and a vicious cycle develops. Unless appropriate intervention is provided, a crisis situation may develop.

BALANCING FACTORS Aguilera, Messick, and Farrell have defined three balancing factors that can promote a return to equilibrium. These are: (1) a realistic perception of the event, (2) available situational supports, and (3) adequate coping mechanisms.

Realistic perception: If the situation is perceived realistically, the individual will be able to associate feelings of tension and anxiety with the particular situation. Once this cognitive association has occurred, the individual can be said to be reality-oriented, and problem-solving efforts can be directed toward a successful solution. However, if perception of the event is distorted, recognition of this relationship may not occur; attempts to problem-solve may be ineffective and tension may build. When assessing the patient or family for a realistic perception of the event, the following questions are helpful:

• What does the event mean to this individual?

• According to the patient or family member, what is the *worst* thing that can happen in this particular situation?

• How is this event going to affect his or her future?

• Can the individual connect bodily feelings of anxiety with the event?

Situational supports: Much has been written regarding the characteristics of the helping person, with such abstract concepts as empathy, sympathy, and self-awareness presented as mandatory attributes. While all this is important, the helping person can be described as one who:

1. Truly understands the other's position within the crisis situation. This of course necessitates that the helping person explores with the individual exactly what the crisis is and what the individual's role is within the crisis. For example, Mrs. G. is in the process of getting a divorce. She arrives in the emergency department acutely anxious and hyperventilating. After calming Mrs. G., the emergency nurse begins to interview her. Mrs. G. feels frightened and vulnerable; she states that she hates her husband for leaving and her children for depending on her. If the interviewer understands this message, conveying it can do much to allay Mrs. G.'s anxiety.

2. Acknowledges that the individual has the *right* to feel whatever way he or she does and communicates this to the individual. For example, the nurse could state to Mrs. G., "You've got a lot to be angry about."

It is important for the nurse to accept the fact that she or he may not always be able to understand the patient's position. To expect this is unrealistic! Also, the emergency contact with the individual is often short-term. Thus, assessment of the patient's family and friends for these supportive characteristics is essential. In addition, knowledge of community resources which may assist in providing this support is necessary. All emergency departments should have a comprehensive listing of available community resources which also describes the necessary referral procedures.

Adequate coping mechanisms: Through the process of daily living, all individuals develop a repertoire of methods to cope with anxiety and reduce tension. Available coping mechanisms can be simply described as "what people usually do when they have a problem." The selection of the mechanism is influenced primarily by past experiences. If the mechanism has worked (i.e., reduced anxiety), it will be repeated and may pass from conscious awareness to become a habitual response. Talking it out with a friend or professional, taking a quiet walk, and laughing or crying during a tense moment are a few examples of these responses.

When assessing the adequacy of the individual's coping mechanism, the nurse should consider these three questions:

1. Is the coping mechanism, whatever it may be, working; i.e., is it reducing anxiety and tension?

2. Does the person use a variety of coping mechanisms, or is he or she limited to a few? The healthy individual utilizes a vast repertoire of defenses to handle anxiety.

3. Does the patient need to utilize defenses *consistently* for one particular event? In other words, does one isolated event always arouse anxiety? For example, does Mr. A., an asthmatic patient seen repeatedly in the emergency department, *always* react angrily when the nurse begins to discuss discharge-planning? If so, this person may *not* be coping adequately in this particular situation, and further assessment of the situation is needed.

DATA ANALYSIS STAGE

When analyzing the data, the emergency nurse has three goals:

1. To identify the problem as clearly as possible

2. To further determine the problem's urgency (beyond the initial immediate survival evaluation)

3. To refer the patient to the appropriate health professional or agency for management

Depending on the nurse's level of expertise, this stage of problem-solving may result in a succinct diagnosis or simply a recognition of the urgency of the problem. No matter at what level one operates, the following steps should be followed:

1. Review and analyze abnormal findings, integrating any laboratory finding, ECGs, etc. The time and effort spent in performing an organized history and physical will facilitate this initial step.

2. Attempt to pinpoint which body system or systems are in disequilibrium. This may be very difficult if the patient's underlying problem is psychopathologic since symptoms are often too generalized or nonspecific (i.e., fatigue, increased gastrointestinal motility, tachycardia, headaches).

3. State the problem as clearly as possible. The nurse may be able to precisely state the problem as "chest pain secondary to acute anterior myocardial infarction" or may be limited to "substernal chest pain, etiology unknown."

4. Evaluate the urgency of the problem, using the principles of the *triage* system. Depending on the evaluation, the following actions may be indicated:

a. See MD stat.

b. MD evaluation needed.

c. Refer to other health professionals such as social worker or physician assistant, community health agencies, specialty clinics. The exact referral mechanism will depend on individual emergency department resources and procedures.

d. Further nursing evaluation needed to define problem.

For nurses to remain vital members of the emergency health team, their skills in history-taking and assessment as described in this chapter must be continually enhanced. This can be achieved only through supervised, repetitive practice and independent study.

REFERENCES

1. Aguilera, Messick, and Farrell, *Crisis Intervention: Theory and Methodology*, Mosby, St. Louis, 1974, p. 64.

BIBLIOGRAPHY

American Nurses Association and Emergency Department Nurses Association, *Standards of Emergency Nursing Practice,* ANA, Kansas City, 1975.

Continuing Education Curriculum, Emergency Department Nurses Association, East Lansing, Mich., 1975.

Cosgriff, J., and Anderson, D., *The Practice of Emergency Nursing,* Lippincott, Philadelphia, 1975.

Gedan, S., "This I Believe," *Nursing Outlook,* vol. 19, August 1971, pp. 534–536.

Goldin, P., "No Second Chance," *American Journal of Nursing,* vol. 72, no. 3, March 1972, pp. 477–479.

MacBryde, C., and Blacklow, R., *Signs and Symptoms: Applied Pathologic Physiology and Clinical Interpretation,* Lippincott, Philadelphia, 1970.

Sherman, J., and Fields, S., *Guide to Patient Evaluation,* Medical Examination Publishing Co., New York, 1974.

Stephenson, H., *Immediate Care of the Acutely Ill and Injured,* Mosby, St. Louis, 1974.

CHAPTER 13
EMERGENCY NURSING: A LAWYER'S SUGGESTIONS

RICHARD K. QUINN, ESQ.

HOSPITAL malpractice suits have recently increased to seemingly astronomical numbers. These suits have frequently involved emergency department activities and have sometimes named emergency nurses as defendants. This chapter will discuss some causes of malpractice suits and suggest ways that emergency nurses can prevent such suits or make the suits more defensible once filed.

LOST RAPPORT: AN OVERVIEW

Obviously, the multiplicity of malpractice cases is not due to a sudden increase in medical mistakes. In the past, the outpatient's only contact with medical science was in the family doctor's office or by way of a house call. The family physician was rarely sued because he or she was a caring and trusted friend whose mistakes were overlooked or accepted. Today, television serials depicting miraculous cures, technological advances, and higher costs have given patients unrealistic expectations of medical care. Furthermore, the practice of medicine has become depersonalized by clinic-oriented practice and increasing caseloads. Lost rapport with the patient and unfulfilled expectations together engender anger and suspicion which have, aside from actual medical negligence, become the root causes of malpractice litigation.

Emergency departments breed a high number of malpractice suits for at least two reasons. They are the first medical facilities to receive and treat cases of acute illness and trauma. Moreover, these units are often extremely depersonalized by the rush of emergent circumstances and by one-time patient contacts.

Emergency nurses usually make the first contact with patients and their family or friends. As a key step to preventing malpractice suits, emergency nurses must remain aware of the importance of creating *patient rapport* by constantly exhibiting friendliness, politeness, and caring concern. Additionally, since patients and those accompanying them are likely to observe emergency activities closely, all personnel should scrupulously avoid any word or deed which might cause suspicion of a medical mistake. A critical comment, a raised eyebrow, a headshake, or the utterance of a simple "tsk" might lead to a suit.

IMPORTANCE OF RECORD KEEPING

Record keeping plays an important role in both the prevention and defense of malpractice claims. The *detailed documentation* of events as they occur not only ensures the continuity of good care but also perpetuates evidence critically needed by defense attorneys at the time of trial.

The following record-keeping techniques are suggested:

1. Write legibly. This will not only help the physicians and nurses to give better care to the patient but also help the lawyer should a suit be brought. Be aware that the 8½- by 11-inch emergency sheet may someday be enlarged to a 3-by-4-foot exhibit in a courtroom. Every dot of one's i's and every cross of one's t's may be subject to close scrutiny.

2. Err on the side of too much detail. Record *everything* and more! Record negative as well as positive findings. Be aware that a malpractice suit naming the nurse as a defendant may be filed as much as 18 or 20 years from the moment of writing the record, that recall of today's events will be nonexistent so far in the future, and that one's defense will depend upon the specificity of this documentation.

3. Make the record contemporaneous. Carefully note the time of each event. A single time notation can mean the difference between winning and losing a malpractice case. If the nurse is monitoring vital signs at specific intervals, record *every* finding for *each* time interval. If the record is out of reach, write these findings on a separate paper or the palm of the hand and complete the emergency chart as soon as possible.

4. Fill in every blank and box on the record form. A missing notation can cause a lawsuit. In one case, a missing check mark after the word "tetanus" led to a suit. Keep in mind that 10 or 15 years from now this information may not be remembered.

5. Sign the record (legibly) where appropriate. *Never* forget to sign off and time each physician's order. It is essential that the nurse be identified and identifiable.

6. Do *not* lose lab slips, ECG strips, or other test results. A missing record will adversely affect the continuity of care and cause a jury to suspect malpractice.

7. In describing the patient or circumstance, use objective rather than subjective terms. Avoid making racial slurs or derogatory comments, like "He's a weirdo." Again, remember that a jury may someday read these words.

8. Miscellaneous recordings: Make sure the record reflects the emergency physician's parting instructions to the patient; e.g., "Pt. instructed to see personal M.D., Dr. Jones, tomorrow A.M." or "Pt. instructed to return if symptoms continue." If the patient refuses recommended treatment or hospitalization, note in detail what was recommended and refused. If the patient is given a "head card" or a referral slip to another physician, note these facts in the chart. If the patient is undergoing an operative procedure in the emergency department for which a consent form is signed, note in the record: "2:20 P.M. Dr. Smith explained nature and risks of procedure to pt. Consent obtained." Do not make reference to incident reports or the hospital's insurance company in the medical record.

9. Record in incident reports *every* event which might conceivably lead to a lawsuit. Each witness to the incident should prepare a separate report as soon after the incident as possible in a detailed and factual manner. Report all injuries, equipment failures, fights, complaints, etc. Incident reports should *never* be made a part of the medical record but should be kept in a separate administrative file.

CONSENT FORMS

Informed consent is often an issue in malpractice cases. Some informed consent suits allege that the physician negligently failed to disclose the nature of the condition to be remedied, the procedure necessary to remedy the condition, or the risks and consequences associated with the procedure. Other consent cases allege simply that the patient was "battered" or touched without authority.

An elective operative procedure can be performed only if the patient *knowingly, intelligently,* and *voluntarily consents* thereto. The patient must be informed of and understand the essential nature of the choices available to him or her and the risks and consequences of each choice. It is the physician's and *never the nurse's* duty to explain the options available and the necessity, nature, and risks of the chosen procedure. The nurse's job is to ensure that a proper consent form is signed, to witness the giving of consent, and to record that fact in the chart.

A consent form need not be signed in an emergency, when immediate treatment is imperative to avoid severe risk to the patient. However, even in an emergency, if time will allow, it is advisable to obtain the informed consent of someone who has authority to act for the patient, at least verbally, and preferably in writing.

The patient should sign the consent form if: (1) he or she is an alert, coherent, and otherwise competent adult (2) who is to undergo a surgical procedure in the ED and (3) the circumstances are not so emergent that medical care is immediately necessary to sustain life and health.

The medical records library should contain a guide listing all operative procedures by *code numbers.* If the procedure has a code number, then a consent form should be signed. If in doubt, obtain a signed consent.

A proper consent form should:

1. Be specific as to the condition that is to be remedied.

2. Name the physician(s) who will perform the procedure.

3. Describe the procedure in simple, layman's language.

4. State that different or additional procedures may be performed in the exercise of good medical judgment.

5. Identify the person who will administer the anesthetic and the method and type of anesthesia.

6. Itemize the risks and consequences attendant to the procedure.

7. Indicate that the patient has been informed that other risks may be involved, "including the loss of blood, infection, stopping of the heart."

8. State that the patient has been informed that medicine is not an exact science and that no guarantees have been or can be made.

9. Specify the date and time when the form is signed.

10. Include a *witness clause* to be signed by the nurse who witnessed the physician's explanation of the procedure and the patient's consent and signature.

Consent must be obtained from a *minor child's* parent or guardian or from an *incompetent adult's* spouse or legal guardian. If a minor or incompetent arrives unaccompanied and the circumstances are not too emergent, the physician should attempt to obtain the consent of the parent, spouse, or guardian by telephone. The physician's telephone conversation should be monitored by a nurse and memorialized in detail in the medical record.

OTHER FORMS

When applicable, the patient's signature should be obtained on one or more of the following forms:

1. Acknowledgement of Emergency Treatment Form wherein patients acknowledge that the treatment rendered was solely limited to emergency care and that they have been told to select and immediately see another physician for a complete work-up and treatment.

2. Physician Referral Slip wherein patients acknowledge that they have been referred to a particular physician for treatment.

3. Head Injury Information Slip wherein patients are instructed to call or return to the emergency department should dizziness, drowsiness, blurred vision, or other listed symptoms of head injury occur.

4. Refusal to Submit to Treatment Form wherein patients acknowledge that: (a) they have been advised by the physician of the nature and necessity for treatment and the possible consequences of refusing the same; (b) they still refuse the recommended treatment; (c) they assume the risks attendant to said refusal; and (d) they release the doctor, hospital, and staff from all liability.

ADDITIONAL SUGGESTIONS

(1) Do not give medical advice over the telephone. Advise the caller *politely* that such a practice is against hospital policy and invite him or her to the emergency department for appropriate work-up and treatment. (2) Do not talk to anyone inquiring about a patient or a particular case unless this person is a police officer acting in official capacity or a known family member. Refer all inquiries to the hospital administration for appropriate clearance. (3) If possible, call the police to handle combative or belligerent patients. (4) Finally, never discharge an emergency patient unless and until he or she has been examined by a physician. Examination by an intern is insufficient.

To avoid going to court, the emergency nurse should concentrate on good rapport, keep good records, and obtain signatures on all appropriate forms. If the nurse must go to court, these practices will be the key to a successful defense.

BIBLIOGRAPHY

Donahue, J. C., "Legal Aspects of Emergency Nursing," in Cosgriff, J., and Anderson, D., *The Practice of Emergency Nursing,* Lippincott, Philadelphia, 1975, pp. 37–51.

George, J. E., "The Legal Limit," *Emergency Nurse Legal Bulletin,* vol. 1, no. 2, 1975.

Goldie, R. R., "The Requirements of Informed Consent," *Hospitals Journal of the American Hospital Association,* vol. 46, no. 10, 1975.

Hospital Liability Litigation, 2d ed., Practising Law Institute, New York, 1970.

Medicolegal Forms with Legal Analysis, American Medical Association, Chicago, 1976.

CHAPTER 14
CARDIOVASCULAR EMERGENCIES

**JEANIE BARRY, R.N., M.S., MARY WIELAND, R.N., M.S.,
AND SANDRA GRESHAM, R.N., M.Ed.**

OVER 29 million Americans have some form of cardiovascular disease.[1] Some of the major diseases include hypertension, atherosclerosis, myocardial infarction, congestive heart failure, and cerebrovascular accidents. Over 23 million Americans are hypertensive; only 50 percent of these individuals realize they are afflicted. Atherosclerosis, as the underlying disease process, has caused almost 900,000 Americans to die annually from myocardial infarction and stroke. Prevention of these diseases is, of course, the ideal; however, complete eradication of cardiovascular disease is in the far-distant future. Until that time, emergency nurses will need to be knowledgeable in the pathophysiology and treatment of diseases affecting the heart and blood vessels. This chapter discusses the following diseases and their management: (1) Angina pectoris, (2) acute myocardial infarction, (3) pulmonary edema, (4) shock, (5) aneurysms, and (6) stroke. It also discusses many emergency cardiovascular drugs. Hypertensive crisis is discussed in Chap. 16, definitive cardiopulmonary resuscitation in Chap. 18.

ANGINA PECTORIS

Such terms as acute coronary insufficiency, intermediate coronary syndrome, and preinfarction angina have been used to describe the syndrome *angina pectoris*. The basic condition is coronary insufficiency which is commonly due to atherosclerosis. However, any entity decreasing the volume of blood that can be delivered to the myocardium can cause angina pectoris. Basically the oxygen supplied to the heart cannot satisfy the demands put upon the myocardium. Angina can be categorized as: (1) stress-induced, (2) Prinzmetal or variant, and (3) preinfarction or crescendo angina.

PATHOPHYSIOLOGY

STRESS-INDUCED ANGINA   Usually, these attacks are precipitated by factors which cause an increase in myocardial oxygen requirements that are inadequately met by the coronary arteries. Exercise, anxiety, or eating a heavy meal may precipitate an increase in heart rate, blood pressure, and stroke volume, giving rise to chest pain. The onset of compressive, retrosternal pain is sudden and usually relieved by rest, relaxation, and the administration of nitrates; all decrease the oxygen demands on the heart.

PRINZMETAL OR VARIANT ANGINA   This form of angina occurs in a cyclic fashion, usually at the same time each day. Unlike the stress-induced form, the chest pain occurs while the patient is *at rest*. Obstruction of a single coronary artery may be the major cause of Prinzmetal's angina; however, authorities differ as to the exact etiology.

PREINFARCTION OR CRESCENDO ANGINA   The most severe form of angina is the *crescendo* or *preinfarction* type. Patients experiencing anginal pain for the first time, angina unrelieved by rest and/or nitroglycerin, and post-MI victims with sudden onset of pain often develop this type of syndrome. Up to 40 to 50 percent of these patients may develop an MI within a few months after their initial attack.

SIGNS AND SYMPTOMS

Pain is the primary presenting symptom. Typical anginal pain, brought on by various precipitating events, is usually located retrosternally and may radiate to the neck and left arm. Patients may describe their discomfort as a heaviness, a squeezing or vise-like tightness in the midchest area. Relief of discomfort approximately 2 to 3 minutes after administration of *nitroglycerin* sublingually together with *rest* and relaxation is often diagnostic of a typical anginal attack.

Associated symptoms may include dyspnea, pallor, sweating, and a fear of impending death. Vital signs may be normal. However, initiating factors such as exercise may reveal an elevated blood pressure and a tachycardia. In addition, physical examination may reveal an S_4 gallop and an overactive cardiac apex impulse. The ECG may show evidence of myocardial ischemia, if it is recorded while the patient is experiencing chest pain. A *depressed S-T segment* might be recorded during the usual anginal attack. However, with variant angina it is not unusual for *transient S-T elevations* (see Fig. 15-4) and *ventricular tachyarrhythmias* to be noted with the pain attack. Serum enzymes drawn at this time will show no evidence of myocardial infarction.

EMERGENCY TREATMENT

1. Elicit a thorough *history* from the patient or the family including any initiating *events*, the location, character, and duration of the pain, associated symptoms, and medications taken prior to the patient's arrival in the emergency department.

2. Administer *oxygen* via nasal cannula or face mask, if the PaO_2 indicates hypoxemia. A sample for arterial BGA should be drawn to assess the need for and the effect of this supplemental oxygen. The head of the bed should be elevated if the patient is dyspneic.

3. Check *vital signs* every 5 minutes, noting carefully the pulse rate and rhythm and blood pressure while the chest pain is in process.

4. *Vasodilators,* usually one of the nitrates, administered sublingually every 3 to 5 minutes until pain is relieved, may be ordered. The main pharmacologic action of the nitrates is smooth muscle relaxation. Oxygen requirements of the myocardium are decreased owing to a reduction in ventricular volume and systolic arterial pressure. The drug of choice for anginal attacks is glyceryl trinitrate, commonly referred to as *nitroglycerin.* Dosage varies from 0.2 to 0.6 mg administered sublingually. Onset of action is within 1 to 2 minutes, with effects lasting up to 30 minutes. Fainting, headaches, and methemoglobinemia are recognized as adverse effects of nitrates. For its longer duration of action, nitroglycerin paste has recently been utilized by various physicians. If the pain is unrelieved by the nitroglycerin, the possibility of a myocardial infarction must be considered.

5. Evaluate the ECG during and after the pain attack.

6. Serum enzymes [serum glutamic oxaloacetic transaminase (SGOT), lactic dehydrogenase (LDH), and creatine phosphokinase (CPK)] may be drawn for diagnostic purposes.

7. Provide a relaxing, restful environment.

8. Assess the patient's understanding of etiological factors which predispose to coronary artery disease (CAD), myocardial infarction, and stroke (see Table 14-1), the modes of action of prescribed medications such as nitroglycerin and Inderal prior to discharge.

9. Provide information to the patient, if not under the care of a cardiologist, regarding (a) possible physician's referral, (b) recent advances in the detection of CAD such as cardiac stress treadmill testing, and (c) new treatments such as outpatient cardiac rehabilitation centers.

Table 14-1	Etiological factors predisposing to coronary artery disease, myocardial infarction, and stroke.

1. Positive familial history of heart disease

2. Sex—men are much more prone to MIs than women until onset of female menopause; the incidence of MIs is then equal for both sexes

3. Obesity

4. Diabetes mellitus

5. Hypercholesterolemia

6. Hypertension

7. Cigarette smoking

8. Psychological stress

9. Race—Black Americans are twice as likely to be hypertensive than whites; they also have a much higher incidence of strokes

10. Sedentary existence

11. Age—greatest number of myocardial infarctions occur after the age of 40

ACUTE MYOCARDIAL INFARCTION

Acute myocardial infarction (AMI) refers to the progressive development of ischemia and necrosis of a portion of the myocardium. In approximately 90 percent of AMI, coronary arteriosclerosis is the cause. Other causes may include severe hemorrhage, acute hypoxia, excessive doses of catecholamines, acute dissecting aneurysms, trauma, and myocarditis. While any area of the myocardium can be infarcted, the majority of AMIs occur in the left ventricle. Chapter 15 discusses the different locations of AMI and the changes that will be seen on the 12-lead ECG. This section deals primarily with the emergency management of the AMI patient.

PATHOPHYSIOLOGY

During the early phase of AMI, a number of profound local and systemic metabolic responses occur. The integrity of the myocardial cells in the anoxic areas is compromised, and intracellular ions such as potassium, calcium, and magnesium are lost. In addition, marked local lactic acidosis develops, and release of myocardial catecholamines occurs. In addition to these local changes, stimulation of the sympathetic nerve endings and the adrenal medulla occurs, with increased levels of circulating catecholamines resulting.

These local and systemic metabolic changes have been implicated as possible causes of two of the chief complications following AMI: serious arrhythmias and pump failure.[2] Alterations in the concentration of intracellular ions and enzymes, local acidosis, and increased levels of norepinepherine probably all combine to produce highly irritable areas in the damaged myocardium with cardiac arrhythmias resulting. Furthermore, elevated catecholamine levels increase myocardial oxygen requirements. Augmentation of myocardial oxygen requirements in already ischemic area leads to further ischemia, possible pump failure, and even extension of the infarction.[3]

SIGNS AND SYMPTOMS

AMI is diagnosed primarily on the basis of pain, acute 12-lead ECG changes, and serum enzyme levels.

Most AMI patients seek medical assistance because of a sudden onset of *chest pain*. Many terms are used to describe the pain such as vise-like, choking, or boring. It is most marked in the substernal region and may radiate to either or both arms, the neck and jaws, or to the upper abdomen. In contrast to most forms of anginal pain, this pain often occurs when the patient is at rest, often in the early hours of the morning. The pain is constant, and its intensity waxes and wanes and may last for hours. Nitroglycerin does not usually relieve it.

While pain is the primary symptom in most patients, so-called *silent MIs* have been reported, frequently in diabetic patients. If questioned closely, vague reports of indigestion or breathlessness may be elicited. In addition to AMI, severe chest pain may indicate a number of other clinical situations which are summarized in Table 14-2.

When examined, most AMI patients will be cold and clammy with ashen coloring. The pulse and respiration are usually rapid, and blood pressure is low. The patient is most often conscious (unless severe shock is present) but may be restless and most certainly fearful and apprehensive. Chest auscultation may reveal an S_4 sound and basilar rales. Heart sounds may sound less crisp and vigorous.

Table 14-2   Causes of chest pain other than myocardial infarction. These diseases must be considered when making a differential diagnosis.

1. Severe angina

2. Acute dissecting aortic aneurysm

3. Acute pericarditis

4. Pulmonary embolism

5. Pneumothorax

6. Acute abdominal conditions such as acute cholecystitis, peptic ulcer, esophagitis, Zenker's diverticulum, or pancreatitis

7. Rib fracture

8. Irritation of the lower cervical and upper thoracic spinal nerves from such causes as herpes zoster or disk disease

9. Bronchitis

10. Hyperventilation

11. Pleurisy

12. Tsetse's syndrome

13. Acute leukemia of the sternum

14. Intercostal or pectoral muscle pain

Peripheral pulses may be difficult to palpate, and neck veins are often abnormally distended. Cardiac arrhythmias are most common, occurring in as many as 80 percent of all AMI patients. In addition, the patient may report dyspnea, nausea, vomiting, and syncope.

EMERGENCY TREATMENT

Time is of the essence when providing emergency treatment for the AMI patient with prompt, safe transfer to the controlled environment of the coronary care unit one of emergency nursing's goals. Both the AMI patient and family will be acutely anxious during the stay in the ED. It is essential that the emergency nurse remain calm and explain all procedures quietly. If possible, a calm family member should stay with the patient as an additional situational support. Pending transfer to the coronary care unit, the following steps must be performed:

1. Evaluate the patient's *hemodynamic* and *respiratory* status. Level of consciousness, urinary output, skin temperature and color, blood pressure, pulse rate and rhythm, comparison of quality between central (carotid or femoral) and a peripheral pulse are excellent parameters for assessing the adequacy of cardiac output. Respiratory rate and depth plus auscultation for bilateral equality of air entry must be assessed. The presence of rales and rhonchi must also be noted. These assessments should be performed *every* 5 to 10 minutes and accurately *recorded* on a flow sheet (see Table 19-3a and b).

2. Start an *intravenous drip* of 5% dextrose and water with a *microdrip* chamber and infuse at a keep-open rate. This IV is used primarily as a *life line* if emergency cardiac drugs and analgesia are needed. Strict attention to intake and output records is essential— these records must be initiated in the ED.

3. At the time of IV insertion, draw blood for the following *tests:* serum enzymes (see Table 14-3), complete blood count (CBC), glucose, blood urea nitrogen (BUN) and creatinine, and serum electrolytes. Particular attention must be paid to the serum potassium level because of this electrolyte's profound effect on the electrical conduction system of the heart.

4. Place patient on *cardiac monitor* (see Fig. 14-1a and b) immediately. At least 80 percent of all AMI patients will have arrhythmias within a few days of the attack. Ventricular arrhythmias are most common during the first 3 to 4 hours (see Fig. 18-3). All emergency nurses should be highly trained in arrhythmia detection and treatment. In addition, they must understand the electronic monitoring equipment they are expected to use and be able to rapidly correct any malfunction of it.

5. *Relieve pain.* The drug of choice is morphine sulfate; the preferred route of administration is intravenous. The usual dose is 3 to 5 mg IV every 5 minutes until pain is relieved. Morphine sulfate causes both hypotension and respiratory depression, and so the nurse must carefully assess the vital signs.

Table 14-3   Analysis of serum enzyme measurements.

		Level			
					Other clinical conditions
				Returns	which can elevate serum
Enzyme	Action	Elevates	Peaks	to normal	enzyme level
CPK: Can fraction into *cardiac-specific isoenzyme*	Catalyzes a reversible reaction which provides *energy* for cardiac contraction.	Immediately	1–3 days	3 days	Acute alcoholism, primary muscle disease, CVA, diabetic acidosis, IM injections, and unaccustomed vigorous exercise
SGOT	Catalyzes a reaction which results in the synthesis of oxaloacetic acid, a key point for entry into the Krebs cycle; important in carbohydrate and protein metabolism.	8–12° post-AMI	18–36°	3–5 days	Any condition where there is injury or necrosis to transaminase-rich organs, i.e., skeletal muscle, liver, brain, and kidney
LDH: Can fraction into *cardiac-specific isoenzymes* with L_1 and L_2 *myocardial-specific*	Catalyzes the conversion of lactic acid to pyruvic acid. Pyruvic acid can then be converted to glucose or enter the Krebs cycle (see Fig. 5-6).	8–24° post-AMI	3–5 days	5–14 days	Anemia, liver and kidney disease, skeletal muscle injury, pulmonary infarction, and leukemia

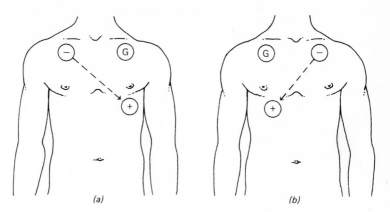

Figure 14-1 (*a*) Placement of lead II for cardiac monitoring. (*b*) Modified chest lead (MCL) I for cardiac monitoring; this is also called the Marriott lead. See Chap. 4 for a review of the standard and chest leads shown here. When placing leads on the chest, remember to (1) avoid large muscle masses, (2) avoid areas where defibrillator paddle will be placed or heart sounds auscultated, and (3) clean and dry the skin for good contact.

6. Take a technically accurate *12-lead ECG,* looking for changes indicating an acute AMI (see Chap. 15). It is important to note that many times acute ECG changes will not be immediately evident. It is vital for all emergency nurses to remember always to *treat the patient* and not the ECG.

Once these procedures have been completed, the patient should be safely transported to the coronary care unit. *Safe* transportation implies that:

1. The patient is monitored.

2. A portable defibrillator that *works* is taken.

3. A bolus of lidocaine and one of atropine are also taken.

4. A registered nurse highly skilled in arrhythmia detection, defibrillator technique, and cardiopulmonary resuscitation accompanies the patient.

Following the arrival at the coronary care unit, the emergency nurse should introduce the intensive care nurse to the family members. This provides a sense of security for the family who often feel forgotten during this initial stage of emergency care.

CARDIOGENIC PULMONARY EDEMA

Cardiogenic pulmonary edema is a syndrome which can be caused by a variety of diseases (see Table 14-4). No matter what the underlying cause, all have one thing in common: *alveolar-capillary membrane damage* due to impaired force of *left* ventricular contraction. Noncardiogenic pulmonary edema is also encountered. The alveolar-capillary membrane is damaged in all instances; only the cause differs. Table 14-5 is a partial list of diseases which may predispose a patient to noncardiogenic pulmonary edema; Chap. 17 presents necessary interventions.

PATHOPHYSIOLOGY

When the left ventricle fails, a variety of pulmonary and systemic changes occur (see Table 14-6). The end result is that venous return to the heart is augmented yet left ventricular output is decreased. Left ventricular end-diastolic pressure increases; this eventually leads to an increase in left atrial and pulmonary venous pressures. Once the hydrostatic pressure in the pulmonary capillary exceeds 20 to 25 mmHg (it is normally 7 mmHg), the colloidal pressure within the pulmonary capillary is overcome and edema results. Initially, this protein-rich fluid transudes into the interstitial lung spaces and finally into the alveoli. This fluid severely compromises lung function by causing:

1. Loss in compliance or stiff lungs

2. Bronchoconstriction

3. Damage to the alveolar-capillary membrane

4. Ventilation-perfusion defect which results in marked hypoxemia

SIGNS AND SYMPTOMS

The cardinal sign of cardiogenic pulmonary edema is *dyspnea*. In the early stages, this dyspnea may occur only with exertion. However, as the left ventricular failure progresses, the dyspnea may be present at rest. Paroxysmal nocturnal dyspnea is a classic finding and usually occurs 3 to 4 hours after retiring. The reason for this is that peripheral edema sequestered during the daytime is reabsorbed into circulation; the left ventricle is unable to handle this extra fluid load, and pulmonary congestion results. The patient awakens with marked res-

Table 14-4	Partial list of diseases causing cardiogenic pulmonary edema.
	Hypertension
	Coronary artery disease
	Acute myocardial infarction
	Aortic valvular disease
	Cardiomyopathy
	Mitral regurgitation/stenosis
	Rheumatic myocarditis
	Congenital anomalies

Table 14-5	Partial list of diseases causing noncardiogenic pulmonary edema.
	Chemical pneumonitis
	Drugs (e.g., heroin)
	Cardiac bypass
	Metabolic acidosis
	Shock of any kind
	Fat embolus
	Surgical interruption of blood flow
	Pancreatitis
	Crush injuries
	O_2 toxicity
	Hypoxemia
	Respirator lung syndrome
	Sickle-cell anemia
	Multiple transfusions
	Concussion to chest

piratory distress and often rushes to an opened window seeking additional oxygen.

In addition to dyspnea, the patient should be closely questioned regarding the presence of *orthopnea, fatigue* which reaches a peak in late afternoon, *nocturia,* and a recurrent hacking *cough.*

Many symptoms seen in the patient with cardiogenic pulmonary edema are due to sympathetic discharge: pale cold sweaty skin, tachycardia, and elevated blood pressure. The patient is often alert, restless, and acutely anxious. As hypoxemia and respiratory distress

Table 14-6 Systemic and pulmonary alterations which occur when the left ventricle fails. Note that normal adaptive mechanisms worsen the patient's condition; this fact is often referred to as the paradox of pulmonary edema.

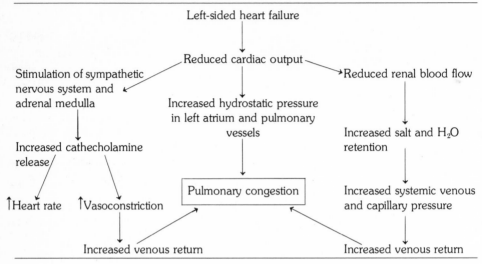

worsen, a depressed level of consciousness will result. Cyanosis may be present if hypoxemia is severe.

Upon auscultation, the examiner may hear wheezing (known as *cardiac asthma*) in the early stages of pulmonary edema when interstitial edema is present. When the fluid transudes into the alveoli, rales and rhonchi can be heard, and a productive cough of pink-tinged sputum develops. Cardiac auscultation may reveal an S_3 gallop; if valvular damage is present, murmurs may be heard.

Since right ventricular failure may also be present, distended neck veins, hepatosplenomegaly, and peripheral edema may also be seen. If the patient has been bedridden, the nurse must check for *sacral edema*. The ECG is nonspecific for heart failure itself, but may often show the cause such as AMI. Cardiac monitoring is essential since heart failure is often accompanied by acute and chronic *atrial* and *ventricular arrhythmias* (see Fig. 18-3a to d).

EMERGENCY TREATMENT

As with all critically ill patients, emergency treatment will involve prompt diagnosis, close monitoring and maintenance of vital functions, and providing meaningful emotional support for both the patient and family. In addition, the following treatment objectives must be kept in mind:

1. Improve ventilation

2. Retard venous return

3. Improve myocardial performance without increasing myocardial oxygen consumption

The following interventions will assist in attaining these objectives:

1. *Proper positioning* of the patient in high Fowler's position. This will increase vital capacity, allow for maximal use of respiratory muscles, and retard venous return to the heart. Allow the patient to lean forward on a Mayo stand covered by a pillow. When the patient is fatigued, this provides good support while still maintaining proper positioning.

2. *High-liter-flow oxygen* to correct hypoxemia secondary to the ventilation/perfusion defect. The mode of delivery will be determined by the clinical condition of the patient. For patients in moderate distress, oxygen per mask at 12 liters/minute can deliver an F_1O_2 of approximately 100 percent.[4] For patients in severe distress, intubation with assisted ventilation may be necessary. Of course, frequent serial BGA is necessary to monitor the patient's response. The goal of oxygen therapy is to maintain a PaO_2 of 60 mmHg with the lowest F_1O_2 possible.

3. *IPPB with 50 percent ethanol.* By using intermittent positive pressure breathing (IPPB) combined with an antifoaming agent, secretions are liquefied, oxygen is provided, and atelectatic areas are inflated. Venous return is also decreased by the inspiratory positive pressure. If ethanol is used as an antifoaming agent, IPPB nebulizations are often limited to 10-minute treatments to prevent elevation of blood alcohol levels and central nervous system depression. (See Table 17-3 for possible adverse effects from IPPB.)

4. *Morphine sulfate* IV is the drug of choice when treating cardiogenic pulmonary edema. It improves ventilation by decreasing the work of breathing; it causes a peripheral venodilation and thus retards venous return. In addition, its sedating effects help to relieve the patient's intense anxiety. Careful observation for hypotension and ventilatory suppression is necessary.

5. *Rotating tourniquets* can be used to retard venous return. Apply

to only three extremities, releasing one every 20 minutes and apply-ing it to the free extremity. Do not put a tourniquet on an extremity with an intravenous line. In the use of tourniquets, the goal is to *retard venous return, not arterial flow;* therefore, peripheral pulses should be checked frequently. When the tourniquets are discon-tinued, the nurse must remove them one at a time every 20 minutes. Removing all tourniquets simultaneously may suddenly overload the circulatory tree and cause pulmonary edema to redevelop.

6. *Diuretics:* Rapid-acting diuretics given intravenously are often administered during emergency care to reduce the cardiac workload, with many authorities recommending furosemide. In addition to reducing plasma volume, furosemide also decreases pulmonary artery pressure.[5] This decrease in pressure has been noted to occur 5 to 15 minutes following IV injection and thus is not due to a de-crease in plasma volume. Since hypokalemia may occur with rapid diuresis, stat electrolytes should be drawn. Careful monitoring of intake and output is essential.

7. *Laboratory aids:* Samples for blood work should be drawn for serum electrolytes and enzymes, CBC, BUN, and blood sugar. In addition, a stat ECG and portable chest x-ray must be performed.

The above therapy is generally recommended as initial steps in the emergency management of acute cardiogenic pulmonary edema. Definitive therapy will be determined by the underlying cause. Digitalis preparations may be given to enhance myocardial con-tractility. However, many authorities now agree that digitalis, when given to the AMI patient, may extend the infarcted area.[6] If digitalis is ordered, the patient must be questioned regarding any current outpatient digitalis regime since this will certainly alter the amount given initially in the ED. Aminophylline IV is often recommended for accompanying bronchospasm but must be used cautiously in the AMI patient due to the risk of ventricular arrhythmias. (See Chap. 17 for a further discussion of aminophylline.)

A new approach in the management of cardiogenic pulmonary edema is the use of *systemic vasodilators* such as nitroprusside. (See Table 16-1 for a summary of drug effects.) The theory is that if im-pedance to left ventricular emptying is decreased, abnormal end-diastolic volume and pulmonary venous pressure would also be reduced. This treatment should not be considered as a first-line approach in the management of acute pulmonary edema since close monitoring of pulmonary artery pressure and cardiac output is essential. Vasodilator therapy should be undertaken only in the intensive care unit.

SHOCK

Shock is not a single disease but rather a complex group of physiologic abnormalities that can be precipitated by a variety of factors. Thus, a simple, concise definition is impossible. Nor is it possible to define it simply by overt symptomatology such as hypotension. To understand shock, one must look beyond the overt signs and symptoms to the *cellular level*. With this perspective it is possible to provide a more comprehensive and clinically relevant definition. If a cellular frame of reference is used, shock can be termed a state in which perfusion is inadequate for metabolic needs of the tissue. Unabated, this generalized inadequacy of cellular metabolism leads to *anaerobic metabolism, cellular destruction, loss of organ function,* and finally *death*.

PATHOPHYSIOLOGY

Before proceeding to the diagnostic parameters and emergency interventions, a classification model for shock will be provided (*see* Table 14-7). This classification is based on five factors: (1) pathophysiology, (2) effects on peripheral resistance, (3) cardiac output, (4) central venous pressure, and (5) arteriovenous (AV) extraction ratios.*

HYPOVOLEMIC SHOCK   Hypovolemic shock can be caused by either frank hemorrhage or fluid loss from the gastrointestinal tract or into a third space. It is characterized by low cardiac output and an increased AV extraction ratio. Total peripheral resistance is markedly elevated; since extracellular fluid volume is lowered, central venous pressure is low. Treatment is directed toward stabilization through intravenous volume replacement. The specific fluids to be used will depend on the etiologic agent.

CARDIOGENIC SHOCK   This type of shock can be due to failure of *ventricular ejection* as with an acute myocardial infarction. It has a mortality rate exceeding 85 percent. In addition, cardiogenic shock can be secondary to a problem with *ventricular filling* as with a cardiac tamponade or a tension pneumothorax. Cardiac output is decreased and total peripheral resistance and the AV extraction ratio are increased. However, the CVP is elevated. With the first type of cardiogenic shock, treatment is directed toward improved myocardial functioning with-

---

* The reader should review the appropriate sections of Chaps. 3 and 5 for an explanation of these factors.

Table 14-7 Classification model summarizing four of the biological effects of four types of shock.

Type of shock	Effect on cardiac output	Effect on CVP	Effect on peripheral resistance	Effect on AV extraction ratio
Hypovolemic	↓	↓	↑	↑
Cardiogenic	↓	↑	↑	↑
Septic	↑	↑ Initially	↓	↓
Neurogenic	↑	↓	↓	No initial effect

out a concomitant increase in myocardial oxygen consumption. Cardiogenic shock secondary to cardiac tamponade or tension pneumothorax must be treated immediately; appropriate lifesaving interventions are discussed in detail in Chap. 19.

SEPTIC SHOCK: PRIMARY CELLULAR DEFECT Shock in association with septicemia results from both *gram-negative* and *gram-positive organisms*. The most common organisms by far are the *coliform* bacilli: *Proteus, Pseudomonas, Klebsiella, Aerobacter,* and particularly *Escherichia coli*. Septicemia and therefore septic shock are seen with far greater frequency in the debilitated, chronically ill patient and in association with diabetes, malignancy, chronic infection, immunosuppressive therapy, and urological surgeries.

This type of shock is often called a high output–low resistance syndrome. The AV oxygen extraction ratio is decreased. This may be a result of a cellular defect that prevents the cell from utilizing oxygen or a defect in the biochemical dissociation of oxygemoglobin at the cellular level. [7] Initially CVP may be elevated; however, as intravascular fluid is lost at the capillary level, it drops.

Depending on the underlying disease state as well as the particular organism involved, mortality approaches 30 to 40 percent in the major centers. However, particular organisms such as the *Bacteroides* species are associated with mortality rates of up to 60 percent even in the best of hands.[8] A high index of suspicion in susceptible patients will aid in lowering mortality rates if combined with early, vigorous treatment.

NEUROGENIC SHOCK   With neurogenic shock, there is a decrease in efferent impulses from the sympathetic nervous system to the smooth muscle of peripheral blood vessels. This type of shock may be secondary to *actual transection* of the cord or may be *functional* as with spinal anesthesia resulting in sympathetic blockage. Peripheral resistance is drastically reduced; to compensate, cardiac output is elevated. Little, if any, change is found in the AV oxygen extraction ratio in the early stages of this shock; central venous pressure is low. This type of shock is extremely rare in the spinal-injured patient; if this patient does present with signs and symptoms suggestive of shock, thorough assessment for other causes should be initiated immediately. If neurogenic shock is the diagnosis, intravenous administration of a sympathomimetic drug is the treatment of choice.

In addition to being categorized by its effects on certain cardiovascular parameters, shock may also be divided into two stages: *early* (reversible) shock and *late* (irreversible) shock.

EARLY SHOCK

SYMPATHETIC AND ADRENAL MEDULLA RESPONSE   When the body is threatened by a shock state, a marked sympathomimetic response is elicited. Peripheral resistance is increased due to *alpha-receptor* stimulation; *beta-receptors* are stimulated in the heart and lung, resulting in increased cardiac output and bronchodilatation. Filtration pressure at the precapillary sphincter is lowered; capillary colloidal pressure predominates, and fluid rapidly moves from the interstitial into the intravascular space (see Fig. 1-5).

Associated with the adrenergic response, the adrenal medulla secretes large amounts of *epinephrine* and *norepinephrine*. These catecholamines augment the alpha- and beta-mimetic responses. The end result is (1) increase in intravascular volume, (2) increase in cardiac output, (3) elevation of central blood pressure, and (4) diversion of blood flow from less vital stress areas (i.e., gastrointestinal tract, skin, muscle, and kidney) to the heart and brain.

Catecholamines also have a marked effect on *cellular metabolism*. Norepinephrine acts on adipose tissue causing the release of stored fat as free fatty acids and glycerol. Epinephrine works mainly on the liver and skeletal muscle to release glycogen as glucose. In addition, insulin release from the pancreas is suppressed. Thus, large quantities of glucose are made available for cerebral metabolism (the brain does not need insulin for glucose utilization), and the lipids can be readily metabolized by the heart. The goal of this metabolic response is to provide adequate nutrients for the survival of the vital stress organs.

ACTH AND GLUCOCORTICOIDS   The hypothalamus, via cortical releasing factor, stimulates the *anterior pituitary* to secrete increased amounts of ACTH which then acts upon the *adrenal cortex.* A rise in circulating glucocorticoids results. Glucocorticoids have a widespread effect on the body, but an in-depth analysis of their function is beyond the scope of this chapter. However, some of the most important effects are listed:

1. Inhibition of the inflammatory response to tissue injury with suppression of histamine release[9]

2. Stabilization of lysosomal membranes

3. Profound metabolic effects, including increased protein catabolism and conversion of glycogen into glucose

4. Enhancement of the catecholamine effect on adipose tissue

5. Possible maintenance of vascular reactivity to catecholamines[9]

In addition to the effects listed above, *aldosterone* and *antidiuretic hormone* are released; these hormones play a vital role in restoring plasma volume. (See Chap. 6 for complete explanation of their physiological action.)

LATE SHOCK

The systemic response to shock functions optimally during the early or reversible shock stage. Adaptive mechanisms maintain a state of homeostasis, and the vital functions of the heart and brain are sustained until the underlying pathophysiology is corrected. In fact, the body's compensatory reactions are so efficient that one can sustain a *substantial reduction in blood volume with no overt symptomology.* If a shock state is allowed to persist, a variety of disastrous physiological changes occur. These are listed below. These changes are associated with progressive cellular anoxia and destruction with subsequent loss of organ function.

1. *Breakdown of lysosomal membranes* (see Chap. 1 for a description of lysosomal function). As these membranes are destroyed, powerful proteolytic enzymes are released into the cell. These enzymes may be responsible for the release of certain vasoactive substances, the best known of which is bradykinin, a very potent vasodilator.

2. *Impaired cellular metabolism.* As cellular hypoxia worsens, there is insufficient oxygen for the complete metabolism of glucose via the Krebs cycle, and lactic acidosis develops (see Fig. 5-6). Initially hyperventilation stabilizes the pH. However, with continued inadequate blood flow, a combined respiratory and metabolic acidosis develops.

3. Anaerobic metabolism also leads to *insufficient synthesis of ATP.* Thus, energy production is decreased and cellular activity is further depressed.

4. As the shock state deepens, cellular membranes are further damaged. There is marked egress of potassium from the cells, and sodium and water enter the cell. *Resting membrane potentials are destroyed,* and major cardiac arrhythmias may develop.

5. Eventually the *cells* of the *capillary wall* begin to *swell* and *separate.* Intravascular fluid and proteins ooze into the interstitial spaces. Eventually venous return diminishes, cardiac output drops, and perfusion to the brain and heart suffers. Once blood flow to these two vital organs is inadequate for their metabolic demands, death follows.

6. Distortion of capillary dynamics fosters the *development of platelet aggregates* which interfere with local blood flow, produce pulmonary and hepatic emboli, and cause thrombocytopenia.

7. Stagnation of blood flow in capillaries, metabolic acidosis, and vasoactive substances can cause widespread clotting in the capillaries—*disseminated intravascular coagulation.*

SIGNS AND SYMPTOMS

As with any other emergency situation, maintenance of vital functions takes priority; Chap. 18 covers this topic in depth. In addition, correct diagnosis of the cause of the shock state is essential. Since shock is a life-threatening emergency, it is certainly appropriate at this time to reemphasize the need for an organized and rapid approach to history-taking and physical assessment. These techniques are explained in detail in Chap. 12. The following monitoring parameters should be assessed:

1. *Blood pressure.* The body may lose up to one-third of its circulating blood volume with little change in the cuff blood pressure (BP). If the nurse suspects shock in the presence of normotensive readings, the patient should be promptly checked for the presence of *orthostatic hypotension.* A drop in systolic blood pressure of 15 mmHg at 45 percent elevation is considered significant. The nurse must also watch for a *narrowed pulse pressure* since this is indicative of decreased stroke volume. BP should be checked every 5 minutes.

The ability to only palpate a blood pressure is a grave sign. In this case, the nurse is feeling a reflected pressure wave with little, if any, actual blood flow. It must also be noted that cuff pressure is often inaccurate when marked vasoconstriction is present. An unobtainable blood pressure usually indicates a systolic BP less than 50 mmHg, but 5 to 10 percent of shock patients may have a normal or even high BP.[10] If the BP is too difficult to palpate, an arterial line should be inserted so that accurate monitoring of BP is ensured.

2. *Pulse rate and quality.* Elevations in pulse rate are due to the sympathometic response of the heart; thready pulses are due to peripheral vasoconstriction and/or a decrease in stroke volume. Both *central* and *peripheral* pulses should be checked at least every 10 minutes for changes in quality. Of course, all shock patients will be on an ECG monitor so that arrhythmias can be rapidly detected. Heart sounds must also be assessed for quality and the presence of gallop rhythms and murmurs, any of which may indicate early heart failure.

3. *Respiratory rate, depth, and breath sounds.* Due to the development of hypoxia and metabolic acidosis, the patient will initially ventilate rapidly and deeply (see Fig. 8-1). This hyperventilatory response is frequently the earliest symptom of septic shock and is believed to be due to the endotoxins. Respiratory rate, rhythm, and depth must be assessed every 10 minutes. Frequent auscultation of the lungs is essential since the development of rales is often an early sign of left ventricular failure. Frequent BGAs are also necessary to monitor lung function since *respiratory failure* is a common complication of shock.

4. *Level of consciousness.* Most shock patients, even in the early stages, demonstrate a change in sensorium. Restlessness and apprehension are the most common signs and can be due to the massive catecholamine release and/or *cerebral hypoxia.* Too often, these early signs of decreased cerebral blood flow are overlooked, and the nurse is suddenly confronted with a stuporous patient. In fact, it is not unusual for sedation to be administered to relieve these symptoms of restlessness and apprehension. *This is a dangerous practice!* While sedation certainly reduces the cerebral response to hypoxia, it also eliminates a vital assessment parameter for reduced cardiac output. In addition, it predisposes the shock patient to respiratory depression and cardiovascular collapse.

5. *Central venous pressure.* The reader will recall that the CVP is determined by the interrelationship of blood volume, myocardial contractility, and the degree of venoconstriction. This pressure normally ranges between 3 and 15 cmH_2O and provides valuable information regarding venous return to the right side of the heart and the body's response to fluid challenges. Table 14-8a and *b* provides important information regarding CVP insertion and measurement techniques.

6. *Pulmonary artery pressure.* While CVP measurements do provide information regarding the right side of the heart, most authorities agree that they do not provide definitive data about the left side of the heart in acute situations. With the advent of the Swan-Ganz flow-directed *pulmonary artery catheter,* direct measurements of pulmonary artery and wedge pressures are now a reality. A pulmonary wedge pressure is a direct reflection of left atrial pressure which in turn reflects left end-diastolic filling pressures. This information is especially important when managing cardiogenic shock.

7. *Urinary output* is one of the most sensitive indicators of the adequacy of cardiac output. If urinary output is good (30 cc/hour), one may assume that perfusion to the kidney, heart, and brain is adequate. If the urinary outputs are low, then one must be concerned that cardiac output is inadequate and that blood flow to heart and brain is in jeopardy. While the patient is in the ED, urinary output should be measured every 15 minutes. The nurse must pay particular attention to the renal response when the patient is receiving fluid challenges. *Urinary outputs must be meticulously recorded.*

8. *Laboratory aids* include CBC, urinary analysis, BUN and creatine, blood sugar, serum electrolytes, and serial BGAs. If the patient is in

Table 14-8a Guide for CVP insertion, management, and measurement.

Site and catheter type	Advantage	Disadvantage	Nursing management
1. Subclavian vein; use an 8-inch, 14- or 16-gauge plastic needle with stylet	A. High level of accuracy B. Allows for free movement of arms C. Accurate as a CVP guide for a long period of time D. Preferred route for IV hyperalimentation E. Potential of being a fast percutaneous IV in emergency situations, i.e., codes, exsanguination	A. Difficult technique requiring a high level of expertise B. High incidence of pneumothorax, particularly in emphysematous patients and with inexperienced personnel	A. Suggest alternate route if personnel inexperienced B. Have chest x-ray taken after every insertion in attempt to rule out pneumothorax C. Securely anchor catheter (skin suture and tape) D. Heparinize solution E. Use sterile technique for insertion and dressing F. Defat skin with acetone and local antiseptic every third day G. Avoid injection of medication into tubing or blood infusion when possible to prevent contamination and clotting
2. Jugular vein (internal or external); use 8-inch, 14- or 16-gauge plastic needle with stylet	A. Same as subclavian vein B. Same as subclavian vein C. Same as subclavian vein D. Frequently used in pediatric emergencies	A. Same as subclavian vein B. External jugular vein: Easily visualized but has a curve preventing true CVP placement; vein rolls under skin C. Internal jugular vein: Hard to visualize but is a more direct route to superior venae cavae and does not roll under skin	A. Same as subclavian vein B. CVP readings more accurate if head turned to opposite side of insertion C. Same as subclavian vein D. Same as subclavian vein E. Same as subclavian vein F. Same as subclavian vein G. Same as subclavian vein
3. Cephalic vein (antecubital fossae; fourth finger side); use a CVP infusor set with 14- or 16-gauge needle*	A. Easier approach than subclavian and jugular veins B. Fewer complications	A. Interferes with arm movement B. May require cutdown to insert C. Less accurate than subclavian and jugular veins D. Cephalic vein narrows at deltoid muscle; 85% of the time catheter cannot be advanced beyond this point	A. Catheter placement must be checked by x-ray B. Abduct arm when taking CVP reading C. Same as subclavian vein D. Same as subclavian vein E. Same as subclavian vein F. Same as subclavian vein G. Same as subclavian vein H. Suggest that basilic vein insertion be attempted first

4. Basilic vein (antecubital fossae, thumb side); use CVP infusor set with 14- or 16-gauge needle*	A. Same as basilic vein	A. Same as cephalic vein	A. Same as cephalic vein
	B. Same as basilic vein	B. Same as cephalic vein	B. Same as cephalic vein
		C. Same as cephalic vein	C. Same as cephalic vein
			D. Same as cephalic vein
			E. Same as cephalic vein
			F. Same as cephalic vein
			G. Same as cephalic vein

* Unfortunately, the CVP catheter can be easily cut, partially or completely, by the insertion needle. To avoid this, be sure needle point is covered by needle guard; do not pull catheter back through needle. Also, following catheter removal, check to make sure *all* the plastic tubing has been withdrawn.

Table 14-8b   Precautions for CVP insertion, management, and measurement.

1. The patient should be flat while a CVP reading is taken. If the patient is unable to tolerate this position, the same degree of bed elevation should be used for each reading.

2. The column of water should fluctuate with respiration.

3. The manometer must be level with the right atrium. This level is found at the fourth inter-costal space, midaxillary line.

4. One CVP measurement, like one BP reading, tells little about the hemodynamic status of the patient. It is the trend of CVP readings that is important.

5. CVP measurements are not infallible. Therefore, treatment should never be based solely on this one parameter.

6. CVP catheters are frequently misplaced, and so proper placement must be confirmed by chest x-ray.

7. If the patient is on a positive pressure breathing apparatus, it must be temporarily discon-nected. If not, CVP readings are drastically distorted.

---

hemorrhagic shock, type and cross match for 10 units of blood. A portable chest x-ray and ECG must also be done.

EMERGENCY TREATMENT

FLUID MANAGEMENT   All shock patients will require early administration of *intra-venous fluids.* Both a central and a peripheral line must be inserted. If abdominal injuries are present, the peripheral line should be placed in an upper extremity since the inferior venae cavae may be dam-aged. Fluids from a lower extremity IV would then be lost in the belly. The type and amount of fluid are determined by many factors including (1) blood pressure, (2) pulse rate and quality, (3) urinary output, and (4) response of the CVP or the pulmonary wedge pressures to fluid challenges.

Fluids can be divided into two major categories: (1) *crystalloids* such as isotonic saline or Ringer's lactate, and (2) *colloids* such as whole blood, plasma, dextran, or albumin. The exact pathophysiology will determine the type of fluid used.

If multiple transfusions are needed, warming of the blood may help to reduce the incidences of cardiac arrhythmias.[10] The use of the newer blood filters may help reduce the incidence of respiratory failure secondary to pulmonary microembolization. If whole blood must be administered immediately, low-titer O-negative or type-specific can be used while additional blood is being typed and cross-matched.

Plasma and albumin can also be used as volume expanders; however, current research has demonstrated that these colloids may be detrimental in late shock.[10] These fluids may leak across the capillary membranes, worsening interstitial edema. If this happens in the lung, the chance of acute respiratory failure developing is greatly increased.

Dextran, another volume expander, is available in two forms, one with a molecular weight averaging 70,000 and a low molecular weight (LMWD) fluid of 40,000. The first type has been shown to coat red blood cells, making them difficult to type and cross-match, and LMWD has been shown to coat platelets, predisposing the patient to bleeding problems.[11]

Crystalloids are used for volume replacement. Controversy exists as to which crystalloid is best. Many authorities argue that using Ringer's lactate in the severely shocked patient worsens the lactic acidosis; however, there is little evidence to back this theory.[11] To facilitate the immediate management with fluids, EDs should decide upon a protocol regarding which crystalloid should be started immediately by emergency personnel.

The response of the CVP to a rapid infusion of fluid is an excellent emergency guide to volume replacement. This is known as a *fluid challenge,* and the amount of fluid infused is usually 200 to 300 ml over 5 to 10 minutes. If the CVP suddenly rises, with little change in arterial pressure, *fluid restriction* is necessary. Diuretics and a positive inotropic drug may also be considered. If the CVP remains low, hypovolemia is present, and *volume replacement* with crystolloids and colloids is essential. Frequent CVP measurements are essential to monitor the patient's hemodynamic response to the fluid challenge. It is important to note that if the CVP is already 20 cmH$_2$O or greater, a fluid challenge is of little value. It is helpful only if the CVP is low or within normal limits.

MAINTENANCE OF VENTILATION   *Respiratory insufficiency* is a frequent problem in shock patients. Hypoxemia is often present and generally indicates pulmonary congestion and atelectasis. Supplemental oxygen should be administered to maintain the PaO_2 above 60 mmHg. Carbon dioxide tension is often low owing to hyperventilation secondary to the metabolic acidosis, pain, or anxiety. If, instead, the carbon dioxide is elevated, the patient should be evaluated for progressive respiratory failure. Remember that the arterial PCO_2 is an excellent indicator of the adequacy of ventilation and that a respiratory alkalosis is the expected response to a shock state.

Some authorities recommend intubation for shock patients even in the light of normal blood gases because it does the following:[12]

1. Prevents sudden deterioration of blood gases secondary to atelectasis.

2. Provides ready access to the tracheobronchial tree for suctioning.

3. Decreases the work of breathing and thus decreases oxygen demands.

4. Permits sedation and pain control without accompanying worry of respiratory depression.

Since the best method of treating respiratory insufficiency is to prevent it, continuous monitoring of respiratory status through physical assessment and frequent BGA is essential.

ACID-BASE BALANCE   Adequate respiratory support and early vigorous efforts to improve tissue perfusion will prevent most acid-base problems. If the metabolic acidosis is severe, infusion of sodium bicarbonate may be necessary since a pH below 7.1 interferes with the body's ability to respond to catecholamines. Restoration of the pH should be gradual since a sudden change may lead to alkalosis and precipitate cardiac arrhythmias.

DRUG THERAPY IN SHOCK   The pharmacological management of shock may involve a variety of drugs. The major emergency cardiovascular drugs are summarized in the last section of this chapter.

SUMMARY OF TREATMENT FOR SHOCK

To summarize, shock is best thought of as *a complex disorder* in cellular metabolism. It is essential that emergency efforts be directed toward both the prompt diagnosis and treatment of obvious shock states and also toward actual prevention. All patients who fall into a high-risk category for the development of shock must be aggressively evaluated in the ED, and all data meticulously recorded. No high-risk patient should be allowed to linger in the ED or be sent to different areas of the hospital for diagnostic tests unless accompanied by an emergency nurse. Transfer to the intensive care unit should be prompt once a tentative diagnosis is made.

ANEURYSMS

PATHOPHYSIOLOGY

Arterial muscle wall weakness is most often due to *arteriosclerosis* with an associated hypertension. Syphilis, trauma, periarteritis, and congenital defects have been documented as other etiological agents. These conditions thin and stretch the arterial wall, leading to a dilatation or outpouching of an artery known as an *aneurysm*. It is important to note that these can occur in any artery throughout the vascular system. With each contraction of the heart, blood enters not only the artery, but also this dilated portion or aneurysm. Thus, the work load of the heart is increased greatly because of the reduced arterial mechanical efficiency. Four basic types of aneurysms may occur: (1) fusiform, (2) sacculated, (3) dissecting, and (4) pseudo-aneurysms. Figure 14-2 illustrates and describes each type. Aneurysms present as emergencies when either *rupture* or *dissection* occurs.

ABDOMINAL AORTA RUPTURE

Aneurysms secondary to arteriosclerosis are frequently located in the abdominal aorta. Males over 60 years of age may develop these aneurysms unaccompanied by any symptoms of discomfort. When ruptures (see Fig. 14-2d) of these aneurysms do occur (as in approximately 20 to 30 percent of these patients), a critically ill patient will present in the ED. A 30 to 50 percent mortality rate is associated with this vascular emergency.

Four basic types of aneurysms may occur:

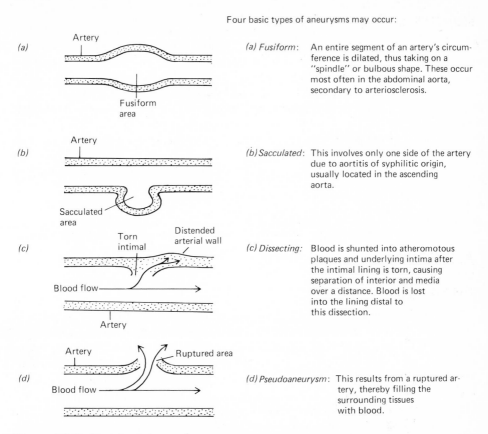

(a) Fusiform: An entire segment of an artery's circumference is dilated, thus taking on a "spindle" or bulbous shape. These occur most often in the abdominal aorta, secondary to arteriosclerosis.

(b) Sacculated: This involves only one side of the artery due to aortitis of syphilitic origin, usually located in the ascending aorta.

(c) Dissecting: Blood is shunted into atheromotous plaques and underlying intima after the intimal lining is torn, causing separation of interior and media over a distance. Blood is lost into the lining distal to this dissection.

(d) Pseudoaneurysm: This results from a ruptured artery, thereby filling the surrounding tissues with blood.

Figure 14-2 Four basic types of aneurysms.

SIGNS AND SYMPTOMS Often the histories of these patients vary. However, reports of sudden onset of excruciating abdominal, lumbosacral, groin, or rectal *pain* is common. A sudden onset of *syncope* may occur and is due to extravasation of blood into the retroperitoneal cavity. Due to this loss of circulating blood volume, *hypovolemic shock* may be present.

On physical examination, the abdominal assessment provides the most significant findings. A palpable, tender pulsatile mass generally in the umbilical area (to the left of the midline) will be noted. This will show as a calcified mass on abdominal films. Femoral pulses are usually present; those pulses distal to this area may be weak or absent.

EMERGENCY TREATMENT   Since shock is one of the primary complications of this emergency, the treatments outlined in the previous section should be implemented. Additional therapy includes:

1. Evaluate and compare the quality of bilateral peripheral pulses in the lower extremities (femoral, popliteal, posttibial, and dorsalis pedis).

2. Order a stat abdominal film. If the patient must go to the x-ray department for this film, an emergency nurse must accompany the patient.

DISSECTING ANEURYSMS OF THE AORTA

Although the occurrence is rare (only 5 to 10 patients per million each year), a *dissecting aneurysm* (see Fig. 14-2c) is the most common emergency involving the *aorta*. The majority of patients are middle-aged males with a history of hypertension.

The underlying pathology is usually due to cystic medial necrosis. The precipitating event which brings the patient to the ED is the tearing of the intima with blood directed into the already degenerated medial layer. Approximately 90 percent of the patients will have a history of *hypertension,* although blunt chest trauma and Marfan's syndrome have been associated with aortic dissection. Occlusion of aortic branches and rupture of the aorta leading to cardiac tamponade may result if these patients are not treated immediately.

SIGNS AND SYMPTOMS   *Pain* is the most common manifestation of dissection. A ripping or tearing substernal, chest, or interscapular pain is described by many patients. It is also common for the patient to report pain in the back or upper abdomen (due to the dissection along the course of the aorta). In addition, symptoms of orthopnea, dyspnea, CNS involvement (hemiplegia or paraplegia), and shock may be present.

Marked hypertension may also be noted. With subclavian artery involvement, blood pressure differences in the upper extremities may be discovered. Systolic precordial murmurs and aortic valve diastolic murmurs may be auscultated. Chest x-rays will reveal a widening of the mediastinum with a possible pleural effusion.

EMERGENCY TREATMENT   This patient may be treated both surgically and medically. Surgery may include resection, grafting, aortic anastomosis repair, or possible aortic valve repair. Emergency presurgical treatment is the same as that for aortic rupture or hemorrhagic shock.

If the patient is to be treated medically, the main focus will be on the *control* of the *hypertension*. A variety of antihypertensive drugs may be utilized (see Tables 16-1 and 16-2). Arfonad infusions are commonly used in the acute stage. This drug is extremely potent, and BP must be monitored every 2 minutes to prevent sudden and severe hypotension. *Reserpine* 1 to 2 mg IM every 4 to 6 hours, *Propranolol* 1 mg IM every 4 to 6 hours, or *Ismelin* 25 to 50 mg per os b.i.d. may also be ordered at a later time. The medical approach to treatment requires *continuous* hemodynamic monitoring by the nursing staff. Therefore, rapid transfer to the intensive care unit is essential.

CEREBROVASCULAR ACCIDENTS

Cerebrovascular accidents, apoplexy, or the layman's term stroke, follow heart disease and cancer as the leading disease entity in the United States. Estimates are that 1,650,000 Americans are afflicted by cerebrovascular accidents annually. Hypertension, atherosclerosis, increased blood cholesterol levels, smoking, and transient ischemic attacks have been recognized as predisposing factors to the development of these attacks. Knowing this, *prevention* of cerebrovascular accidents should be handled, as a top priority, in every ED.

TRANSIENT ISCHEMIC ATTACKS

PATHOPHYSIOLOGY   Up to 50 percent of all stroke patients will have warning signals prior to the actual emergency. These are *temporary,* focal cerebrovascular symptoms referred to as transient ischemic attacks (TIA). Platelet or cholesterol emboli from atherosclerotic plaques forming cerebral thrombi appear to be the mechanism behind such attacks.

SIGNS AND SYMPTOMS   This patient may present with a combination of symptoms such as vertigo, weakness, clumsiness, numbness, paralysis, dysarthria, aphasia, diplopia, or loss of vision. These symptoms are of short duration (½ to 24 hours) and may occur frequently. There have been rare reports of as many as 10 to 20 attacks a day. Because a TIA is often a forewarning of an actual cerebrovascular accident, any patient presenting with these symptoms should be evaluated thoroughly upon admission to the ED. Episodes of hypoglycemia, meningitis, Ménière's disease, cardiac arrhythmias, and a blood dyscrasia can produce similar symptoms and must also be considered as possible causes of the above symptoms.

With physical examinations, attention should be given to:

1. BP monitoring in both brachial arteries. With subclavian lesions, a systolic difference of 20 mmHg or more may be noted.

2. Funduscopic examination to detect cholesterol or fibrin platelets in the optic fundi.

3. Bruit detection in the carotid arteries. This is good indicator of atherosclerosis.

4. ECG monitoring since cardiac arrhythmias may be the initiating factor with these attacks.

5. Laboratory tests including CBC, blood glucose, uric acid, serum electrolytes, and cholesterol levels.

6. Lumbar puncture and skull x-rays may be done to rule out other CNS lesions.

7. Neurological testing to determine cerebellar, motor, and sensory functioning (see Fig. 22-2).

8. Neck flexion and temporal artery patency must also be evaluated.

EMERGENCY TREATMENT The main concern of the emergency department's health team when treating a TIA should be patient and family *teaching,* combined with a well-organized *referral system* within the health care system. Adequate amount of time must be spent in helping the patient and the family to gain knowledge of the role that anticoagulants, antihypertensives, a low-fat and low-cholesterol diet, cessation of smoking, and a possible endarterrectomy play in the prevention of these transient attacks and an actual cerebrovascular accident. Appointments to the referral clinics should be given so that this initial teaching will be reinforced, blood pressure and blood clotting factors (such as prothrombin times) will be monitored, and the diet will be evaluated.

It is hoped that the admission of actual cerebrovascular accident patients to the ED will be greatly reduced with such an organized system of health care and prevention.

Unfortunately, cerebrovascular accidents do occur despite preventive attempts by the health team. Basically, any interruption to the cerebral blood flow, whether it be due to a *thrombus, embolus,* or *hemorrhage,* results in a similar clinical presentation, indicative of cerebral dysfunction.

CEREBRAL THROMBOSIS

This is the most common cause of a cerebrovascular accident. Thrombosis which produces ischemia of the cerebral cortex may occur secondary to progressive cerebral atherosclerosis and/or a decreased cardiac output with hypotension. Generally, a gradual onset of unilateral weakness or paralysis is experienced, depending upon the area of the brain involved. Symptoms resembling those seen with TIA may also be present. Improving precipitating factors such as reduced cardiac output and hypotension often lead to recovery with these patients. However, cerebral thrombosis can progress to affect other areas of the brain, and permanent damage may result.

CEREBRAL EMBOLUS

Chronic atrial fibrillation, cardioversion, a patent foramen ovale, or cardiac surgery may be the initiating factor in the development of cerebral *emboli.* When interviewing the family, a history of headaches, an earlier MI, or subacute bacterial endocarditis may be elicited. The onset of symptoms is usually sudden with neurological findings generally indicating that the *middle cerebral artery* is affected. Contralateral weakness, paralysis and increased deep tendon reflexes, aphasia, sensory involvement, and the Babinski's sign may also be noted on the neurological examination. Frequently, these symptoms disappear as the occlusion is reduced; however, an intracerebral hematoma can develop as well.

CEREBRAL HEMORRHAGE

This event is often diagnosed by a history of hypertension, with a sudden onset of headaches, vomiting, vertigo, and clumsiness. The patient may suddenly collapse, oftentimes losing consciousness. On physical examination, unequal pupils, distended neck veins, contralateral facial droop and paralysis, and aphasia may be present.

EMERGENCY TREATMENT

1. As with any other situation, a patent *airway* must be established. Proper positioning of the patient is essential, not only in maintaining an airway, but also in *preventing aspiration.* If cervical spine injury has been ruled out, turning the patient on the side with the neck hyperextended is the position of choice.

2. Quick, thorough *neurological assessments,* including level of consciousness, mentation, pupillary size and reaction, eye movements, hand grasps, movements of extremities, and signs of incontinency must be evaluated every 5 minutes. Signs indicating increased intracranial pressure should be reported immediately (see Fig. 19-2).

3. Hemodynamic and respiratory assessments as outlined in preceding sections must also be performed every 10 minutes.

4. IVs and/or nasogastric tube may be inserted depending on the severity of the patient's condition.

5. An initial dose of 10 mg *Decadron* IV may be started in the emergency room. Many authorities believe this corticosteroid, with its low-salt-retaining properties, reduces cerebral edema which is a well-recognized complication of brain infarction.[13]

6. Laboratory work such as ECG, CBC, glucose, electrolytes, uric acid and cholesterol levels should be obtained for a differential diagnosis as well as for providing a base line for future comparisons.

7. If there are no signs of increased intracranial pressure or papilledema on funduscopic examination, a lumbar puncture may be performed for diagnostic purposes.

8. Although rarely ordered, arteriography may be performed to locate the occluded cerebral vessel.

PATIENT AND FAMILY SUPPORT

The diseases described in this chapter cause critical and often life-threatening emergencies. In addition, many patients and families fear a long period of rehabilitation and the possibility of permanent disability. Anxiety levels are high for all involved. The emergency nurse must function as a situational support, maintaining a calm, competent attitude. However, in an attempt to remain composed, too frequently the nurse is viewed as uncaring. Simple, yet caring, interventions help to avoid this misconception:

1. If the patient is alert, explain all procedures in simple terms. If unconscious, remember that hearing is the last sense to go, so talk to the patient. If the family can be in the room, urge them to also speak to the patient.

2. If the patient must go to surgery, have the operative permit signed *after* the health team has explained the need for the procedure and operative technique itself to either the patient and/or family in *understandable* terms.

3. Inform the family where they should wait while the patient is in surgery or undergoing a diagnostic procedure. Make sure the physicians know where the family is.

4. Since the majority of these patients need intensive care, introduce the staff of the intensive care unit (ICU) to the family prior to returning to the emergency department. Too frequently, the family is left in waiting rooms desperate for information and comfort while the patient is being cared for by the ICU staff. If the family at least knows that the ICU nurses are aware of their presence, this can make the waiting less painful.

CARDIOVASCULAR DRUGS

One of the most important functions of an emergency nurse is the knowledgeable administration of cardiovascular drugs. All remember the warning "Never give a drug without fully understanding its physiological effects!" This is often a challenging task since explanations of cardiovascular drug actions are often conflicting and confusing. This section discusses the pharmacologic actions, indications, side effects, and dosages of a number of cardiovascular drugs which work in two ways:

1. Via the autonomic nervous system (ANS)

2. Directly on the cardiac muscle

In addition, emphasis is placed on defining terms used to explain the effects of these drugs. If the nurse is familiar with these terms when looking up a drug, phrases such as "anticholinergic," "decreases slope of phase 4," or "sympathomimetic" will bring to mind an array of facts, and memorization will become less necessary.

DRUGS WHICH WORK VIA THE AUTONOMIC NERVOUS SYSTEM

Table 14-9 summarizes the anatomical divisions of the nervous system. From this table, the reader can see that the actions of sympathetic drugs are mediated via *alpha, beta* or *dopamine* receptors. These receptors are found throughout the body. For the purposes of this chapter, drug actions mediated via these receptors in the following areas of the body are discussed (Fig. 4-10*a* to *e*):

1. *Beta receptors:* Heart and smooth muscle of bronchial tubes and blood vessels

2. *Alpha receptors:* Smooth muscle of blood vessels

3. *Dopamine receptors:* Smooth muscle of the renal artery

As illustrated in Table 14-10, ANS drugs can either inhibit (block) or stimulate (mimic) the sympathetic or parasympathetic nervous system. Many terms are used to describe this phenomena; they are summarized in Table 14-11.

Numerous cardiovascular drugs act via the autonomic nervous system; eight drugs are discussed in this chapter. These drugs are listed under their appropriate category in Table 14-12.

Table 14-9   Major anatomical divisions of the body's nervous system.

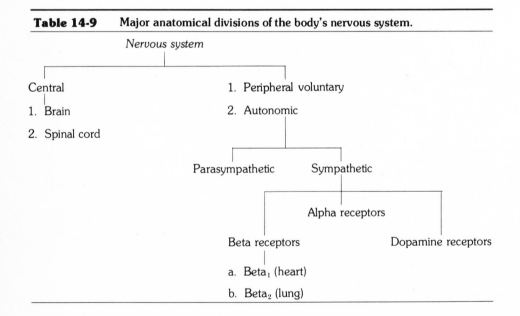

Table 14-10 Effects on the heart, bronchial tubes, and blood vessels when *beta, alpha,* and *dopamine* receptors are stimulated or inhibited. Common terminology used to describe these effects is provided.

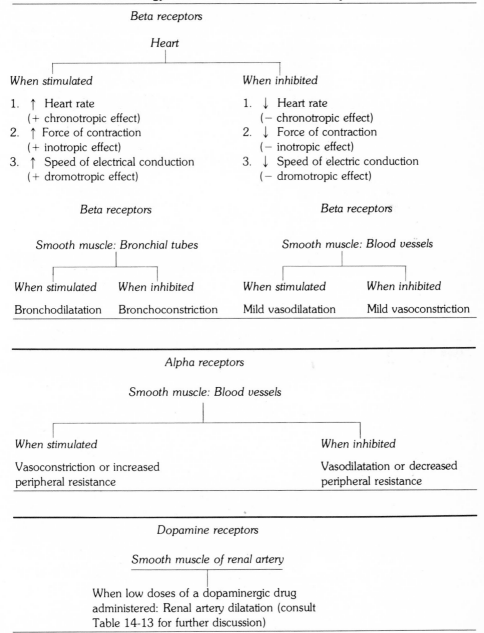

Beta receptors

Heart

When stimulated

1. ↑ Heart rate
   (+ chronotropic effect)
2. ↑ Force of contraction
   (+ inotropic effect)
3. ↑ Speed of electrical conduction
   (+ dromotropic effect)

When inhibited

1. ↓ Heart rate
   (− chronotropic effect)
2. ↓ Force of contraction
   (− inotropic effect)
3. ↓ Speed of electric conduction
   (− dromotropic effect)

Beta receptors

Smooth muscle: Bronchial tubes

When stimulated   **When inhibited**

Bronchodilatation   Bronchoconstriction

Beta receptors

Smooth muscle: Blood vessels

When stimulated   **When inhibited**

Mild vasodilatation   Mild vasoconstriction

Alpha receptors

Smooth muscle: Blood vessels

When stimulated

Vasoconstriction or increased peripheral resistance

When inhibited

Vasodilatation or decreased peripheral resistance

Dopamine receptors

Smooth muscle of renal artery

When low doses of a dopaminergic drug administered: Renal artery dilatation (consult Table 14-13 for further discussion)

Table 14-11   Specific terms used to describe a drug which either blocks or stimulates the sympathetic or parasympathetic divisions of the ANS. The italicized terms are used in this text.

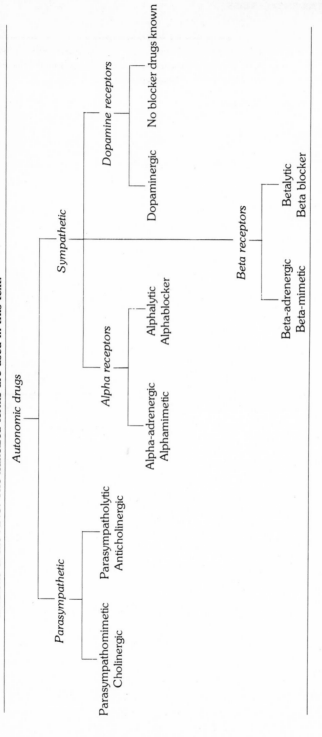

Table 14-12   Appropriate ANS classification for the eight drugs discussed in this chapter. Note that metaraminol, levarterenol, and epinepherine have both alpha- and betamimetic properties.

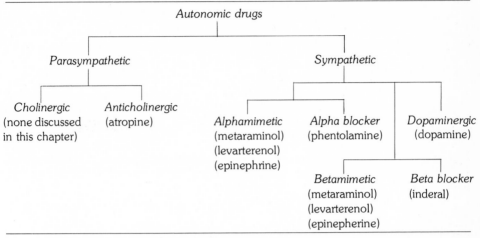

ATROPINE   Atropine is an *anticholinergic* drug that works on the parasympathetic nervous system by blocking the vagus nerve. It is used for its cardiovascular effect in sinus bradycardia and atrioventricular blocks due to excessive vagal tone. It is administered as an IV bolus in dosages varying between 0.4 and 1 mg (see Chap. 18). Possible side effects of this drug are:

1. Sinus tachycardia and increased ventricular irritability

2. Urinary retention, especially in older males

3. Increased intraocular pressure which is dangerous for patients with narrow-angle glaucoma (about 3 percent of all glaucoma patients)

4. Atropine psychosis

Many of the drugs discussed below are administered as intravenous infusions. The following nursing actions must always be followed when administering these infusions:

1. Always use a *microdrip* chamber.

2. Label the bottle indicating the *amount* and *type* of drug added. The *time* the infusion was hung must also be indicated.

3. Check *infusion rates* every 5 minutes by counting the number of microdrips per minute.

4. If the infusion is a vasopressor, take the blood pressure *every 2 minutes* until it has been stabilized by the drug.

METARAMINOL (ARAMINE)   Metaraminol is an alpha- and beta-mimetic agent. Its predominant action is *indirect,* releasing the body's own stores of norepinephrine from the nerve endings of sympathetic system. It elevates blood pressure by increasing peripheral resistance (alpha effect) and the strength of myocardial contraction (beta effect). For these effects it is used almost exclusively for *hypotensive states.* It is most frequently administered as an intravenous drip; common dosage is 100 mg metaraminol diluted in 250 cc D_5W. (Occasionally it is given intramuscularly; 5 mg IM is the common dose.) The medication should be infused at a rate to maintain blood pressure between a systolic of 80 and 100 mmHg. (If patient has a history of hypertension, it may be necessary to further elevate the blood pressure.) Possible side effects include:

1. No vasopressor effect. If this is the case, the patient's own stores of norepinephrine may be low (possibly because of chronic disease). Another vasopressor should be ordered immediately.

2. Rapid dangerous fluctuations in blood pressure. Careful, frequent monitoring of blood pressure will help to avoid this.

LEVARTERENOL (LEVOPHED) Levarterenol is *norepinephrine,* an alpha-beta-mimetic agent. It elevates peripheral resistance and increases coronary blood flow. Unlike metaraminol, it does not rely on the body's own stores of norepinephrine and will frequently work when metaraminol fails for this reason. Common dosage is 8 mg levarterenol diluted in 250 cc D_5W. Again, as with metaraminol, blood pressure must maintain between a systolic of 80 and 100 mmHg. Possible side effects include:

1. *Tissue sloughing* if the IV infiltrates; this is due to the marked vasoconstriction of the small vessels in the area of the leak. For this reason, this drug is best administered through a central venous line. If this is not possible or if the IV does infiltrate, *phentolamine* can be used to prevent sloughing. The proper dosage and administration techniques for this drug are discussed later.

2. Rapid, dangerous fluctuations in blood pressure

3. Reflex bradycardia

4. Marked renal artery constriction and renal ischemia

EPINEPHRINE (ADRENALIN)   Epinephrine is an alpha- and beta-mimetic agent used primarily in *cardiac arrest* situations, *anaphylaxis,* and *bronchial asthma.* It is not commonly used as a vasopressor (although it is one of the most powerful known) since it causes ventricular irritability, and its effects are transient. Dosages and routes of administration used in cardiac arrest situations are listed in Chap. 18; Chap. 27 lists those used during anaphylaxis; see Chap. 17 for those used for bronchodilatation. When administered, frequent monitoring of pulse and BP is mandatory. Side effects include:

1. Cardiac arrhythmias, especially sinus tachycardia

2. Rapid elevation of blood pressure

PHENTOLAMINE (REGITINE)   This drug is classified as a pure alpha-blocker and thus causes *vasodilatation.* It is used in three clinical situations:

1. Treatment and/or prevention of sloughing secondary to levarterenol infiltration

2. Pheochromocytoma

3. Occasionally for vasodilator therapy following an AMI

Only the first situation is discussed in this chapter.

To prevent sloughing, phentolamine can be administered in two ways. If infiltration occurs, stop levarterenol immediately and give 10 mg phentolamine locally into the infiltrated area. This must be done *immediately* to be effective. As a preventive agent, 2.5 mg of the drug can be added to the vasopressor infusion. This amount of phentolamine is adequate to prevent sloughing but does not act as a systemic vasodilator. With proper and prompt use of phentolamine, tissue sloughing secondary to levarterenol infiltration can often be avoided.

ISOPROTERENOL (ISUPREL)   Isoproterenol, a derivative of epinephrine, is a pure beta-mimetic drug and exerts its primary effect on the *heart* and *lung.* It also causes peripheral vasodilatation; this effect, combined with an increase in venous return, tends to improve peripheral blood flow.

This is in direct contrast to the marked alpha-mimetic effect of epinephrine and levarterenol. It is commonly used in:

1. Shock situations in which the patient's myocardium is healthy and the goal is to restore peripheral circulation

2. Advanced degrees of atrioventricular block

3. Bronchospasm secondary to bronchial asthma

For situations 1 and 2, isoproterenol is most frequently administered as an intravenous drip; 1 mg is diluted in 250 cc D_5W. For bronchodilatation, it is administered via nebulization (see Chap. 17 for dosage rates).

The onset of action of this drug is rapid, and so continuous monitoring of the cardiovascular status is essential. The toxic effects of the drug are usually due to overdosage and include:

1. Both supraventricular and ventricular tachyrrhythmias. If these arrhythmias require immediate control, propranolol can be used to competitively block the pharmacologic actions of isoproterenol.

2. Hypotension and angina in patients with diseased myocardiums. Owing to isoproterenol's vasodilating effects, aortic root pressure drops, causing a decrease in coronary blood flow. For this reason, isoproterenol is usually ineffective in treating cardiogenic shock.

PROPRANOLOL (INDERAL) Propranolol is a beta-blocking agent; its primary pharmacologic action is on the *heart* and *lungs*. It is used as an anti-arrhythmic agent for both supraventricular and ventricular tachyrrhythmias. This drug has also been used with varying degrees of success in patients with moderate to severe angina. Intravenous dosage is 1 to 3 mg given as an *IV bolus*. This drug must be given slowly and never administered to an unmonitored patient since its negative chronotropic and dromotropic effects are marked. Possible side effects include:

1. Marked slowing of the pulse. This drug is contraindicated in bradyrrhythmias and conduction defects.

2. Decreased myocardial contractility. Propranolol must be administered with great caution to patients with AMI and/or congestive heart failure. Hypotension may result, and so close monitoring of BP is essential.

3. Bronchoconstriction. While this bronchial narrowing is not a problem in patients with normal lungs, it is a problem in those with a history of asthma or chronic obstructive lung disease.

DOPAMINE (INTROPIN)   Dopamine is a precusor of epinephrine and norepinephrine (Fig. 2-18a); it is used primarily in the treatment of shock. It is commonly concentrated as 200 mg dopamine in 250 cc D_5W, and its pharmacologic action is dependent on the rate of administration (see Table 14-13). Many authorities agree that dopamine works best when administered in low to moderate dosages for its dilating effect on the renal artery. Adjunctive administration of an alpha-mimetic agent such as levarterenol will usually be required to increase peripheral resistance. The blood pressure, heart rate, and urine flow must be continously monitored. Adverse side effects include:

1. Hypotension and tachycardia

2. Possible renal artery constriction with high dosages

DRUGS WHICH WORK DIRECTLY ON CARDIAC MUSCLE

The following antiarrhythmic drugs are used primarily to control ectopic rhythms. Their predominant effect is directly on the action potential of the cardiac muscle rather than mediated via the autonomic nervous system. The reader should review the appropriate sections in Chap 1 for an explanation of the action potential and for

---

Table 14-13   A summary of dopamine's physiological effects. It is crucial to note that its predominant effects are determined by the rate of infusion. When the drug is concentrated as 200 mg in 250 cc D_5W, 800 micrograms (μg) = 60 microdrips. The patient's weight and the desired physiological effect must be known before this drug can be administered intelligently. Drug orders such as "infuse drug at a rate to elevate BP to 80 to 120 mmHg systolic" are inadequate and must be questioned by the nurse.

Dosage	Dopamine receptors (renal artery dilatation)	Beta receptors (heart rate)	Alpha receptors (vasoconstriction)
1–2 μg/kg/min	+ +	No effect	No effect
2–10 μg/kg/min	+ +	+ +	No effect
10–50 μg/kg/min	No effect	+	+ +
Greater than 50 μg/kg/min	No effect	+ +	+ +

clarification of terminology used in this section. Figures 1-7 to 1-9 and 3-10 illustrate important concepts relating to the action potential and should be referred to while reading about the following drugs.

QUINIDINE A derivative of quinine, quinidine has the following effects on the cardiac muscle and the surface ECG:

Action Potential
1. Decreases the slope of phase 4.

Surface ECG
1. Decreases ectopic beats.

2. Decreases the rate of rise of phase O which is depolarization. When phase O takes longer, so also does conduction.

2. Increases P wave duration because of prolonged atrial conduction time. Also prolongs QRS duration. When the QRS duration increases by 50 percent, stop giving it and report the finding. An example is a patient with a QRS of 0.06 second which increases to 0.09 second.

3. Prolongs phase 3 which is repolarization.

ST-T changes occur including increased duration, and inversion and notching of the T wave.

Quinidine has been used to convert supraventricular tachyrrhythmias and to control ventricular ectopics. Electrical conversion is generally preferable to conversion with quinidine. However, if this drug is used, the following procedure is recommended. When given by mouth, the common dosage is 200 to 400 mg doses every *4 hours* until conversion of the arrhythmia occurs or signs of toxicity appear. This drug is rarely given intravenously because of the increased risk of adverse effects. Toxic effects include:

1. Severe decrease in rate of ventricular conduction resulting in AV block, ventricular tachycardia or fibrillation

2. Marked decrease in myocardial contractility

3. Diarrhea, nausea, and vomiting

4. Tinnitus

5. General malaise

PROCAINAMIDE (PRONESYTL)   Procainamide works much like quinidine. It decreases the slope of phase 4 and prolongs phase 3, making the heart less able to respond to ectopic beats. Procainamide may also slow atrioventricular conduction and prolong intraventricular conduction time. It decreases myocardial contractility, particularly in higher doses. Both atrial and ventricular arrhythmias can be effectively controlled by this drug. When given intravenously, the rate should not exceed 25 mg/minute; up to 1000 mg can be administered by IV bolus. Side effects include:

1. Hypotension

2. Ventricular fibrillation or asystole

3. Nausea, vomiting, and diarrhea

4. A reversible lupus-like syndrome (when drug is given orally as long-term maintenance therapy)

LIPOCAINE (XYLOCAINE)   Lidocaine, another local anesthetic, is an antiarrhythmic agent which is primarily used to reduce ventricular irritability through reducing the slope of phase 4. In contrast to quinidine and procainamide, lidocaine is not known to have any significant effect on AV conduction or intraventricular conduction except that large doses have been seen to prolong AV conduction time.[14] It is commonly mixed as an intravenous drip, and the usual dosage is 1000 mg lidocaine in 250 cc D_5W. Drip rates should never exceed 4 mg/minute (60 microdrops/minute). When given as an intravenous bolus, 50 to 100 mg may be administered immediately. If ineffective, a second dose can be repeated in several minutes. Up to 400 mg of this drug can be given intravenously *within 20 minutes* for potentially lethal arrhythmias. Side effects include:

1. Drowsiness, confusion, or coma

2. In excessive dosages, respiratory arrest and grand mal convulsions can and *do* occur

3. Muscle twitching

DIGITALIS   Digitalis has been used medicinally for thousands of years and is presently a commonly used cardiac drug with a variety of complex actions. Basically, in therapeutic doses, digitalis:

1. Produces a positive inotropic effect which is thought to be due to increased availability of calcium in the cardiac cells

2. Decreases automaticity of ectopic foci

3. Decreases conduction velocity through the AV node

4. Prolongs the refractory period

The major therapeutic indication for digitalis is treatment of cardiac failure. A variety of digitalis preparations exist; each differs in its onset of action, time of peak effect, and half-life (see Table 14-14). Intravenous dosage varies depending on the type of digitalis preparation used (Table 14-15). Prior to administering intravenous digitalis, the emergency nurse should obtain electrolytes since *hypokalemia* predisposes the patient to digitalis toxicity. Since digitalis is predominantly excreted by the kidney, renal functions should also be assessed through a *serum BUN.* If the patient has been taking digitalis as an outpatient, a complete history of the drug regime must be determined prior to emergency digitalization.

Common side effects indicating digitalis toxicity include:

1. Cardiac arrhythmias, particularly paroxysmal atrial tachycardia, *with 2:1 conduction, ventricular bigeminy,* and *atrioventricular blocks*

2. Anorexia, nausea, and vomiting

DIPHENYLHYDANTOIN (DILANTIN) This drug has been particularly useful in the treatment of convulsions and digitalis-induced arrhythmias. It increases the speed of deplorization and increases the slope of phase 4. Diphenylhydantoin also stimulates conduction through the AV node. Like lidocaine, this agent is also particularly useful in the treatment of ventricular arrhythmias; it appears to have little therapeutic effect on supraventricular arrhythmias. As an intravenous bolus, 100 to 250 mg is the common dosage. This drug must be given *slowly,*

Table 14-14 Summary of four common digitalis preparations. The three factors described are based on intravenous administration. *(Adapted from Goodman, L., and Gilman, A.: The Pharmacological Basis of Therapeutics, 5th ed., Macmillan, New York, 1975.)*

Drug	Onset of action	Peak	Half-life
Digoxin	15–30 minutes	1–5 hours	3 days
Quabain	5–10 minutes	½–2 hours	1 day
Cedilanid-D	10–30 minutes	1–2 hours	3 days
Digitoxin	½–2 hours	4–12 hours	5–7 days

Table 14-15 Common digitalizing doses and times for two frequently used, rapid-acting digitalis preparations.

Timing	Digoxin	Cedilanid-D
Give immediately:	0.5 mg IV	0.4 mg IV
Give 1–2 hours later:	0.25 mg IV	0.2 mg IV
Wait another 1–2 hours, then give:	0.25 mg IV	0.2 mg IV

never faster than 25 mg/min! This drug precipitates with many other drugs, especially sodium bicarbonate and calcium chloride; flushing the IV line with *normal saline* prior to and following the diphenylhydantoin bolus will avoid this. This drug is a potentially dangerous agent and has many serious side effects:

1. Respiratory depression or arrest

2. Hypotension

3. Sinus bradycardia, ventricular asystole or fibrillation

4. Drowsiness, confusion, even coma

REFERENCES

1. *Heart Facts: 1975,* American Heart Association, New York, 1975.

2. Oliver, M. F., "The Metabolic Response to a Heart Attack," *Heart and Lung,* vol. 4, no. 1, January–February 1975, pp. 57–60.

3. Maskowitz, L., "Vasodilator Therapy in Acute Myocardial Infarction," *Heart and Lung,* vol. 4, no. 6, November–December 1975, pp. 937–946.

4. Goldberger, E., *Treatment of Cardiac Emergencies,* Mosby, St. Louis, 1974, p. 158.

5. Chung, E., *Cardiac Emergency Care,* Lea & Febiger, Philadelphia, 1975, p. 8.

6. Gunnar, R. M., and Loeb, H. S., "Use of Drugs in Cardiogenic Shock due to Acute Myocardial Infarction," *Circulation,* vol. 45, 1972, pp. 1111–1124.

7. Herman, C. D., *Advances and New Concepts in Shock,* Surgery Annual, Appleton-Century-Crofts, 1975, pp. 1–49.

8. Grubb, S., "Management of Sepsis," Lecture presented to the 8th Emergency Medical Services Nursing Class, Honolulu, August, 1974 (unpublished).

9. Ganong, W., *Review of Medical Physiology,* Lange, Los Altos, Calif., 1974, pp. 275–278.

10. Wilson, R., et al., "Shock in the Emergency Department," *Journal of American College of Emergency Physicians,* vol. 5, no. 9, September 1976, pp. 678–690.

11. Trunkey, D., "Review of Current Concepts in Fluid and Electrolyte Management," *Heart and Lung,* vol. 4, no. 1, January–February 1975, pp. 115–121.

12. Ayres, S. M., and Mueller, H., "The Over-All Approach to the Patient with Hypotension," *Heart and Lung,* vol. 3, no. 3, May–June 1974, pp. 463–475.

13. "Steroid Eases Pressure of Stroke," *Emergency Medicine,* August 1971, p. 104.

14. Gupta, P., et al., "Lidocaine-Induced Heart Block in Patients with Bundle Branch Block," *American Journal of Cardiology,* vol. 33, April 1974.

BIBLIOGRAPHY

American Heart Association, *Stroke—Risk Handbook,* Merck, Sharp & Dohme, 1974.

"Angina at the Brink," *Emergency Medicine,* vol. 7, no. 2, February 1975.

"Aortic Time Bomb," *Emergency Medicine,* vol. 7, no. 3, March 1975.

Ayres, S., Gianneli, S., and Meuller, H., *Care of the Critically Ill,* Appleton-Century-Crofts, New York, 1974.

Bevan, John A. (ed.), *Essentials of Pharmacology,* 2d ed., Harper & Row, New York, 1976.

Cosgriff, Anderson, *The Practice of Emergency Nursing,* Lippincott, Philadelphia, 1975.

Davis, K., and O'Boyle, C., *Emergency and Disaster Nursing Continuing Education Review,* Medical Examination Publishing Co., New York, 1975.

Eckert, Charles (ed.), *Emergency Room Care,* Little, Brown, Boston, 1971.

Gianelly, R. E., *Propranolol Hydrochloride Guidelines for the Management of Moderate to Severe Angina Pectoris,* Ayerst Laboratories, New York, 1975.

Hirshfield, John, et al., "Reduction in Severity and Extent of Myocardial Infarction When Nitroglycerine and Methoxamine Are Administered during Coronary Occlusion," *Circulation,* vol. XLIX, February 1974.

Keifer, C., and Wilkins, R. (ed.), *Medicine—Essentials of Clinical Practice,* Little, Brown, Boston, 1970.

Lawn, B., "The Diagnostic Traps of Angina Pectoris," in *Pitfalls in Cardiac Diagnosis and Management from Internist Observer,* Science & Medicine Publishing Co., 1973.

Meyer, J. S., and Marx, P., "Cerebral Autoregulation and Dysautoregulation and Their Relation to Cerebral Vascular Symptoms," in *Current Concepts of Cerebrovascular Disease: Stroke,* American Heart Association, vol. VI, no. 1, January–February 1971.

Sproul, C., and Mullanney, P., *Emergency Care,* Mosby, St. Louis, 1974.

Toole, J. F., *Diagnosis and Management of Stroke,* American Heart Association, New York, 1974.

Zelis, R., et al., "Angina Pectoris—Diagnosis and Treatment," *Postgraduate Medicine,* vol. 59, no. 5, pp. 12–18.

Zschoche, D. (ed.), *Mosby's Comprehensive Review of Critical Care,* Mosby, St. Louis, 1976.

CHAPTER 15
MYOCARDIAL INFARCTION AND THE 12-LEAD ELECTRO-CARDIOGRAM

SANDRA GRESHAM, R.N., M.Ed.

THE 12-lead electrocardiogram (ECG) is an excellent tool for the diagnosis of myocardial infarctions (MI), but realizing that it also has limitations is important. First, the tracing must be technically accurate. This requires eliminating electrical and movement artifact and ensuring that the correct lead is attached to the correct limb. Second, a normal resting ECG does not mean a normal heart. Nurses in critical care units are familiar with the statement, "I don't understand how he can have a heart attack! Just 2 days ago he had an ECG and everything was fine." The third limitation of a 12-lead ECG is that it is only one diagnostic tool and its findings should not be isolated from a careful history and physical examination. Its information must always be correlated to the patient, and when in doubt, the patient should be treated, not the ECG.

TYPES OF MIs

There are three basic types of MIs which should be briefly defined. Figure 15-1 shows a heart in which the atria have been removed and the exposed ventricles are seen from above. Area 1, which is shaded from the endocardium (inner wall) to the epicardium (outer wall), shows a *transmural* MI. "Trans" means through and "mural" means wall. Therefore a transmural MI is one which destroys the entire thickness of the heart wall. Area 2, which involves the epicardium and the tissue beneath it, shows a *subepicardial* MI. This type of MI can be due to trauma rather than arteriosclerotic heart disease. Area 3 shows an MI involving the endocardium and adjacent tissue and is called a *subendocardial* MI. Of the three types, the transmusal MI is most common.

LOCATION OF MIs

Although these three types of MI can occur in various locations within the heart, the vast majority occur in the left ventricle. Figure 15-2 shows a left ventricle as viewed from the left side. An MI can occur in the areas designated as *anterior, inferior, lateral,* and *posterior.* Combinations can also occur. For example, an MI in the inferior and lateral areas is called an *inferolateral* MI. There is a wide variation in terminology currently in use to describe these locations. For example, a commonly used alternative for the word inferior is *diaphragmatic* since the inferior surface of the heart is directly above the patient's diaphragm. If alternate terminology is used, ask for clarifica-

Figure 15-1 Three basic types of MI.

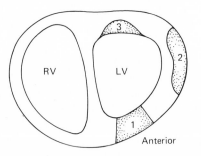

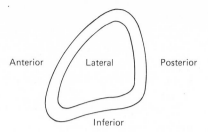

Figure 15-2 Locations of MIs.

tion. A labeled diagram often helps the nurse to relate the location of the MI to the word preferred by others on the patient care team.

In addition to specifying the type of MI and its location, approximating its extent is possible. For example, if the characteristic changes which accompany an MI are seen in just two leads with one patient versus five leads for another, the patient with changes in five leads has the larger MI.

ECG CRITERIA FOR MI DIAGNOSIS

The remainder of the discussion in this chapter concerning MIs is based upon two facts, that the majority of MIs occur in the left ventricle and the majority of MIs are transmural; therefore it deals with transmural MIs of the left ventricle. In determining whether a transmural MI of the left ventricle has occurred, what clues are sought? Two major criteria determine whether an MI can be diagnosed by electrocardiography. These are the presence of significant Q waves in any lead except avR and characteristic ST-T changes in any lead.

The term *significant Q wave* is defined as those Q waves which are 0.04 second or one small ECG block in duration or wider. Opinions differ currently as to the significance of the depth of the Q wave in addition to the width criteria. At present, the depth of the Q wave is not clearly of importance. Significantly wide Q waves, then, are looked for in all leads except avR. Recalling the hexaxial reference system (see Fig. 4-4), the reader should note that avR is in a much different position than the other five limb leads. Because of its placement, wide Q waves are frequently normal in this lead. Little emphasis is placed upon the ability to recognize the various waves which compose the QRS complex when arrhythmia recognition is the only task required of the nurse. However, now that MIs are being sought, it is important to be able to define the QRS variations accurately. Remember that a Q wave is always the initial negative deflection in the QRS complex. Subsequent negative deflections are referred to as S or S' waves. Figure 15-3 reviews five common types of QRS complexes.

Certain *characteristic ST-T* changes are associated with transmural MIs. Figure 15-4 describes these changes as well as the appearance of significant Q waves.

If significant Q waves and characteristic ST-T changes are noted on a particular patient's 12-lead ECG, the next step is to determine the location of the transmural MI. Figure 15-5 is the basis for determination of MI location. This 12-lead ECG is mounted to *approximate* the way in which the leads reflect electrical activity of the heart. The reader should notice that the six limb leads are arranged as if they were in the hexaxial reference system and the chest leads are superimposed anteriorly.

Look at these leads in relation to the location of transmural MIs which were anterior, inferior, lateral, or posterior. The leads which are able to provide the most information about the inferior surface of the heart are leads II, III, and avF. They will contain significant Q waves and characteristic ST-T changes when an acute inferior transmural MI occurs. Figure 15-6 shows an old inferior MI. The *location* is inferior since significant Q waves occur in leads II, III, and avF. The *age* is known because the ST segments are isoelectric and the T waves have returned to their upright position.

Again in Fig. 15-5, the leads which are able to give the most information about the anterior wall of the heart are in precordial leads. These leads will show the significant Q waves and characteristic ST-T changes when an anterior MI is seen. Figure 15-7 shows an old anterior MI with significant Q waves in V_1 through V_4.

Figure 15-3 Five common types of QRS complexes.

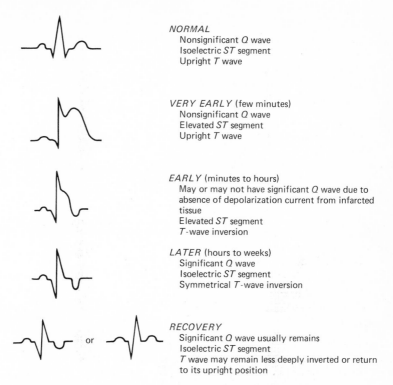

NORMAL
  Nonsignificant *Q* wave
  Isoelectric *ST* segment
  Upright *T* wave

VERY EARLY (few minutes)
  Nonsignificant *Q* wave
  Elevated *ST* segment
  Upright *T* wave

EARLY (minutes to hours)
  May or may not have significant *Q* wave due to absence of depolarization current from infarcted tissue
  Elevated *ST* segment
  T-wave inversion

LATER (hours to weeks)
  Significant *Q* wave
  Isoelectric *ST* segment
  Symmetrical *T*-wave inversion

RECOVERY
  Significant *Q* wave usually remains
  Isoelectric *ST* segment
  T wave may remain less deeply inverted or return to its upright position

Figure 15-4 ECG evolution of an MI.

Again consulting Fig. 15-5, the reader should note that a lateral MI may be best seen in leads I, avL, V_5, and V_6. Leads V_5 and V_6 can be thought of as partially anterior and partially lateral. Leads I and avL give information about the high lateral surface of the left ventricle where V_5 and V_6 show the lower lateral surface. The size and location of a lateral-wall MI determine whether it will be seen by all four of these leads.

Three of the four basic locations have now been discussed: inferior, anterior, and lateral. The remaining site is posterior. As might be expected, transmural MIs of the posterior wall of the left ventricle are somewhat difficult to diagnose. V_1 and V_2 provide helpful information about the posterior wall in an indirect fashion. These indirect changes are known as *mirror image* changes. Figure 15-8 shows that if an electrode were placed at the site of the posterior infarction, a significant Q wave would be present. However, the mirror image changes in V_1 are instead seen as a significantly wide R wave.

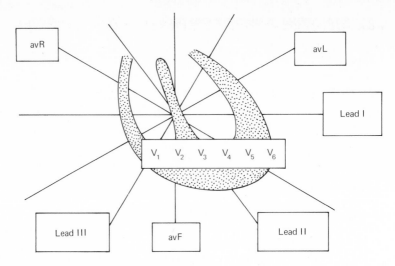

Figure 15-5 Anatomical mounting of a 12-lead ECG.

Figure 15-6 Old inferior myocardial infarction.

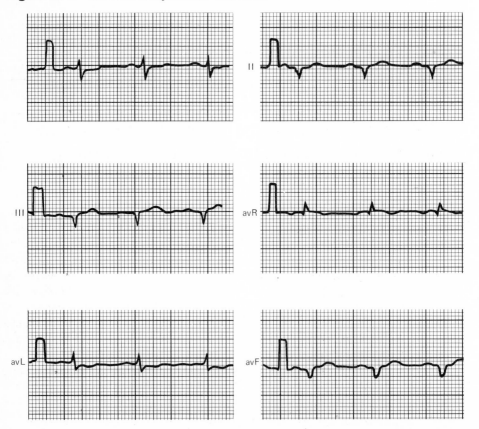

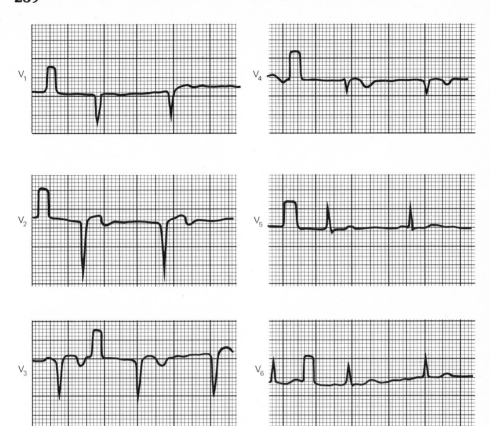

Figure 15-7 Old anteroseptal myocardial infarction involving V_1 through V_4.

In summary, transmural MIs are defined as those which have destroyed the entire thickness of the heart wall. They usually occur in the left ventricle. The location within this chamber can be inferior, anterior, lateral, or posterior or combinations of these. The leads which show direct or mirror reflections of significant Q waves tell the location of the MI. The Q waves appear within hours of the infarction and usually remain. The ST-T changes are more transient and usually disappear. Knowing the normal evolutionary patterns helps to determine the age of the infarction, but clinical correlation is essential.

In order to serve the best interests of patients cared for by critical care nurses, 12-lead ECGs should always be studied for the presence of MIs. Expertise can be attained only by frequent clinical exposure augmented by further reading, lectures, and practice workshops.

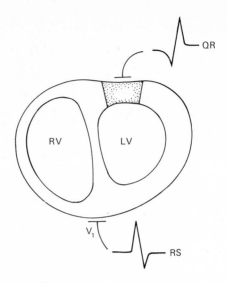

Figure 15-8 Posterior myocardial infarction.

BIBLIOGRAPHY

Chung, Edward K., and Chung, Donald K., *ECG Diagnosis—Self Assessment,* Harper & Row, New York, 1972.

Vinsant, M., Spence, S., and Chapell, D., *A Commonsense Approach to Coronary Care: A Program,* Mosby, St. Louis, 1972.

Zalis, Edwin G., and Conover, Mary H., *Understanding Electrocardiography: Physiological and Interpretive Concepts,* Mosby, St. Louis, 1972.

CHAPTER 16
HYPERTENSIVE CRISIS

CARL P. HOLLENBORG, M.D.

A *hypertensive crisis* may be defined as a clinical condition in which the degree of hypertension in a patient creates a life-threatening situation. Severe or malignant hypertension (a diastolic pressure greater than *130*) can by itself cause rapid deterioration of the brain, heart, and kidney function and lead rapidly to death. In the susceptible patient moderate hypertension (a diastolic pressure greater than *110*) may precipitate cerebral vascular accidents, myocardial infarction or failure, and renal failure. The purpose of this chapter is to alert one to those conditions in which one must institute immediate antihypertensive therapy and to tell how to use some of the many common medications.

PATHOPHYSIOLOGY

The precise etiology of mild, moderate, severe, or accelerated hypertension is not known. One may induce hypertension by stimulating the *alpha-adrenergic* endings of the *sympathetic* nervous system, thus contracting the smooth muscle linings of small arteries, increasing resistance, and raising the pressure of a closed system. Loading these smooth muscles with *sodium* results in a greater and more sustained hypertension. After repeated stimulation and salt-loading, the cardiovascular system resets the normal pressure "rheostat" at some higher level, and sustained hypertension results. Where these control mechanisms exist or how they are mediated for each patient is not known, but the central nervous system, reflex arcs in the cardiovascular system, and the various endocrine organs all play some part.

Hypertension destroys small blood vessels and places larger vessels at increased risk for damage. Autopsy data show fibrinoid necrosis of small arterioles in the brain, eye, kidneys, and other organs. Poor perfusion and edema about these areas, frank hemorrhage, and other effects to larger vessels are often found. The damage of hypertension may be expressed as the sum total of a relentless progressive process or the injury to an essential, weak vessel by high pressures. In the patient with malignant hypertension, this process is accelerated.

SIGNS AND SYMPTOMS

The clinical expression may be quite protean or sudden and localized. Weakness, fatigue, and weight loss are common. The effects on the *brain* may result in confusion, lethargy, nausea, vomiting, headache, personality change, stupor, or coma. *Papilledema* may be present, and *focal findings* such as hemiparesis, ataxia, and abnormal reflexes wax and wane. Blurred vision and *transient blindness* are common. *Renal insufficiency* is always present but may express itself as renal shutdown to changes in calculated function. A sustained diastolic blood pressure greater than *130 mmHg* with constitutional symptoms, affected mentation, and papilledema are the cardinal features of *hypertensive encephalopathy,* which is a medical emergency.

To a previously damaged circulatory system, however, moderately elevated pressures may be as life-threatening. Diastolic pressures greater than 110 may cause progression of cerebral vascular accidents, extension of infarction, worsening of heart failure, or further dissection of an aortic aneurysm. *Hypotensive therapy* must be employed without delay in many of these patients.

PHARMACOLOGICAL INTERVENTION

Many immediate-acting antihypertensive agents are available. Generally hypotensive agents lower the resistance offered by the peripheral blood vessels and are effective whether one's blood pressure is high or low. In the hypertensive patient, they somehow block the vicious cycle of *smooth muscle spasm, salt-loading,* and *higher pressures.* The pressure rheostat is lowered to usually a higher than normal range that is more easily controlled by lower dosages of milder medications. It is useful to classify six of the commonly used medicines into three categories by their general mode of action and effects on the circulatory system (see Table 16-1).

Table 16-1 Drug effects.					
Drug by mechanism of action	*Administration, IM or IV*	*Onset of action*	*Duration of action*	*Effect on cardiac output*	*Principle side effects*
Group 1 Sympathetic inhibitors					
Reserpine	IM 1.0–2.5 mg	1–2 hour	3–8 hour	None	Sedation, nasal congestion
Methyldopa	IV 250–500 mg	10–60 minute	1–8 hour	None	Sedation, nasal congestion
Group 2 Direct dilatation of arterioles					
Diazoxide	IV 300 mg	1–2 minute	3–24 hour	Increased	Sodium retention, hyperglycemia
Hydralazine	IV 10–40 mg	10–20 minute	1–6 hour	Increased	Reflex tachycardia, headache
Group 3 Ganglionic blockade					
Trimethaphan	IV 1.0–5.0 mg/minute	Immediate	During infusion	Decreased	Postural hypotension, renal insufficiency
Direct dilatation of arterioles and veins					
Nitroprusside	IV 35–560 mg/minute	Immediate	During infusion	Decreased	Postural hypotension, renal insufficiency
Adjuvant therapy					
Furosamide	IV 40 mg	1–5 minute	2–8 hour	Decreased	

Reserpine and *methyldopa* decrease sympathetic tone throughout the body, causing mental depression, but do not alter cardiac output. *Hydralazine* and *diazoxide* directly dilate arterioles, increasing cardiac output and maintaining perfusion to the kidneys. *Trimethaphan* and *nitroprusside* cause profound, immediate peripheral dilatation and postural hypotension. They decrease cardiac output and renal perfusion.

When encephalopathy, head injury, or cerebral vascular accident complicate the clinical situation, those drugs which effect *mentation*, group 1, should be avoided because if a patient becomes more lethargic under treatment, one does not know whether the medicine or disease is responsible. When *coronary insufficiency* is present, cardiac output must be maintained, and group 1 is preferred; hence, groups 2 and 3 should be avoided. When *renal insufficiency* is present, cardiac output should be maintained, and group 3 should be avoided. In order to properly evaluate the effectiveness of treatment and to avoid complications, the side effects of each drug should be known. Table 16-2 is included for reference.

Antihypertensive therapy is not a treatment of the disease but rather the effect of the disease, which can be fatal. The drugs so mentioned can lower the pressure to any level and so must be used with great caution to avoid the effects of hypotension to a body adjusted to hypertension.

Table 16-2	Preferred drugs in clinical situations.		
	Hypertensive emergency	*Drug of choice*	*Drug to avoid*
	Malignant hypertension without encephalopathy	Any	
	Encephalopathy Head injury Cerebral vascular accident	Hydralazine Diazoxide Nitroprusside Trimethaphan	Reserpine Methyldopa
	Coronary insufficiency	Reserpine Methyldopa	Hydralazine Diazoxide
	Renal insufficiency	Diazoxide Hydralazine Reserpine Methyldopa	Trimethaphan Nitroprusside

GENERAL THERAPEUTIC CONSIDERATIONS

With these thoughts in mind a general treatment approach may be formulated. The effect of severe and moderate hypertension on a given patient must be appreciated. An appropriate medication is selected with the competence of the patient's circulatory system in mind and the side effects of the medicine clear. Then the thoughtful performance of the treatment and observance of the clinical state are attended to in an intensive care unit.

When a patient presents with headache, nausea, vomiting, and markedly elevated diastolic blood pressure, a hypertensive encephalopathy must be considered along with cerebral vascular accident, pulmonary edema, and anxiety state. Treatment should begin immediately. Any sustained high blood pressure should be carefully evaluated, and hospitalization should be considered.

In any condition in which the blood pressure should be lowered immediately, a staff nurse should be assigned to that patient, and before treatment is begun blood pressures taken every 15 minutes.

An IV infusion must be started with D_5W, and preferably *furosamide* 40 mg IV should be given. The adequacy of cardiac output should be measured by an indwelling Foley catheter with recordings every hour. A CBC, UA, electrolytes, ECG, and chest x-ray are ordered in addition to any other laboratory diagnostic tests that may be helpful.

The position of the patient is important. A semi-Fowler's position is assumed for all patients so that if the medication selected for antihypertensive effect overshoots its mark, the health team can temporarily reverse the orthostatic effect by lowering the patient's head. When the medications in group 2 are used, a cardiac monitor is mandatory and would be useful in almost every situation.

When the antihypertensive medication is selected, continuous blood pressure monitoring is necessary either with an arterial line or by repeated cuff measurements.

Group 1 medications require close neurologic checks; group 2 medications require monitoring with 12-lead ECGs. Frequent checks of the serum blood glucose are recommended for the usage of diazoxide. One must closely follow the levels of the BUN and creatinine in the patient getting group 3 medications.

In the patient with elevated blood pressure, the health team must carefully assess the historical, physical, and laboratory findings to determine whether the patient is suffering a hypertensive crisis. In such a situation, the patient receives a fast-acting diuretic and appropriate additional fast-acting antihypertensives, while his or her clinical state and response to therapy are meticulously observed.

BIBLIOGRAPHY

Brunner, H. R., and Gavras, H., "Vascular Damage in Hypertension," *Hospital Practice,* March 1975.

Cohn, J. N., Limas, C. J., and Guiha, N. H.: "Hypertension and the Heart," *Archives of Internal Medicine,* vol. 133, June 1974.

Kincaid-Smith, P., McMichael, J., and Murphy, E. A., "The Clinical Course and Pathology of Hypertension with Papillaedema (Malignant Hypertension)," *Quarterly Journal of Medicine,* vol. 27, 1958.

Koch-Weser, J., "Hypertensive Emergencies," *New England Journal of Medicine,* vol. 290, no. 4, 1974.

Sandok, B. A., and Whisnant, J. R., "Hypertension and the Brain," *Archives of Internal Medicine,* vol. 133, June 1974.

Schmid, P. G., and Abboud, R. M., "Neurohumoral Control of Vascular Resistance," *Archives of Internal Medicine,* vol. 133, June 1974.

The Hypertension Handbook, Merck, Sharp & Dohme, West Point, Pa., 1974, pp. 104–112.

Tobian, L., Jr., "Hypertension and the Kidney," *Archives of Internal Medicine,* vol. 133, June 1974.

CHAPTER 17
ACUTE RESPIRATORY FAILURE
JEANIE BARRY, R.N., M.S.

ACUTE respiratory failure (ARF) is a syndrome which can accompany a variety of disease states. Prompt assessment and intervention are essential in the emergency treatment of patients with ARF. Therefore it is essential that all nurses working in the ED have a firm understanding of normal anatomy and physiology of the respiratory system (Chap. 5), arterial blood-gas analysis (BGA) (Chap. 8), the dynamics of ARF, and emergency measures to manage patients in acute respiratory distress.

This chapter provides an overview of ARF without going into detail about any specific diseases which may cause this failure. The reader can consult the table of contents for chapters which discuss specific causes of respiratory failure, such as respiratory arrest, acute epiglottitis, near-drowning, or pulmonary edema.

PATHOPHYSIOLOGY

ARF is a syndrome in which the pulmonary system is unable to maintain *adequate oxygenation* of the arterial blood. It is classically divided into two types:

1. Pure *hypoxemic* failure in which the PaO_2 is less than 50 mmHg and the $PaCO_2$ is decreased. This hypocarbia is due to hyperventilation secondary to the hypoxemic drive to breathe.

2. *Hypoventilatory* failure in which the PaO_2 is below 50 mmHg and the $PaCO_2$ is 50 mmHg or greater.

Many pathophysiological conditions can cause ARF (see Table 17-1). It is essential for emergency nurses to understand that even patients with *normal lungs* may suffer from ARF. A common example is central depression of the respiratory drive due to drug overdose or cerebral trauma. Better than studying each disease separately is understanding the physiological processes which maintain normal blood gases; this will assist in understanding the dynamics of ARF, reduce the need for memorization, and aid in the recognition of patients who fall into high-risk categories for developing respiratory failure.

DETERMINANTS OF NORMAL ARTERIAL BLOOD BASES

The lung determinants which maintain normal blood gases are:

1. Adequate *ventilation* which is dependent on (a) an intact thoracic cage, (b) functioning respiratory muscles, and (c) patent airways.

2. Adequate *pulmonary perfusion* which necessitates that (a) venous return to the right side of the heart is adequate; (b) the right ventricle functions well as a pump; and (c) the pulmonary vasculature remains a low-resistance system.

Table 17-1   Partial list of pathophysiological conditions leading to acute respiratory failure.*

Pulmonary and Thorax Configuration: Emphysema, bronchitis, pulmonary fibrosis, status asthmaticus, pneumonia, pulmonary edema, pneumothorax, flail chest, kyphoscoliosis
Neurologic: Myasthenia gravis, poliomyelitis, polyneuritis, cerebral vascular accident, tetanus, status epilepticus, meningitis, encephalitis, cerebral amyotrophic lateral sclerosis, central nervous system depression secondary to drug ingestion, hypoxia, trauma
Miscellaneous: Severe obesity, myxedema, cardiac, liver, and/or renal disease, systemic lupus erythematosus

*Consult Table 14-5 for additional causes of ARF.

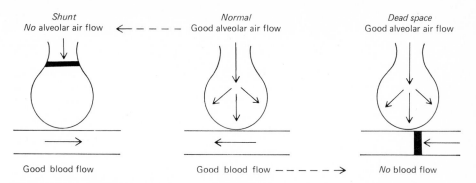

Figure 17-1 Ventilation-perfusion defects. Dotted arrows indicate progressive worsening in degree of dead-spacing or shunting.

3. *Diffusion* which is dependent on an intact alveolar-capillary membrane in which (a) the capillary lumen is adequate for RBC passage and (b) type-II pneumoncytes secrete adequate amounts of surfactant to prevent atelectasis.

4. Proper *distribution,* which implies that patent air-filled alveoli are surrounded by well-perfused pulmonary capillaries. If ventilation is adequate, yet perfusion impaired, this is known as a *dead-space abnormality.* Pulmonary embolization is an example. Conversely, if perfusion is normal yet ventilation inadequate, as in atelectasis, a *shunt* is said to exist. These dead-space and shunt abnormalities are known as *ventilation/perfusion defects,* and decreased ability to *oxygenate* the blood is the classic hallmark (see Fig. 17-1). Since carbon dioxide is far more diffusible than oxygen, the $PaCO_2$ will remain within normal limits until actual airway obstruction or hypoventilation occurs.

In addition to the above lung determinants, four other variables are important in maintaining normal BGAs:

1. Cardiac output

2. Hemoglobin (both its level and molecular configuration)

3. Oxyhemoglobin dissociation curve (has it shifted to the left or right?) (see Fig. 5-5)

4. Oxygen consumption

If any of these variables is abnormal, the patient must be placed in a high-risk category for developing ARF. Close observation for signs and symptoms of ARF then becomes essential.

SIGNS AND SYMPTOMS

When evaluating the ARF patient, primary attention must first be focused on *airway patency*. Once this patency is guaranteed, the nervous, cardiovascular, and respiratory systems must be evaluated since the nonspecific signs and symptoms of hypoxia and/or hypercarbia are usually manifested in these three systems:

1. *Pulmonary system.* The symptoms of ARF usually reflect an underlying lung disease and may include an increase in *sputum* production. Quantitative approximation of the amount of sputum produced, color, and quality (loose or tenacious) must be determined. If the patient reports that *dyspnea* is present, its relationship to exercise must be evaluated. Dyspnea on exertion should be quantified. For example, can the patient walk one block, two blocks, etc., before experiencing dyspnea? Remember, *dyspnea at rest* is always indicative of a serious problem. One good test for shortness of breath is to evaluate the patient's ability to speak. Can the patient tell the nurse about the symptoms in full sentences, or must he or she stop every few words for a breath? If the latter, this patient is probably experiencing acute respiratory distress.

The patient should also be questioned closely regarding the onset of *chest pain* or *hemoptysis,* as either may indicate pulmonary embolus. A past history of *chronic lung disease* is also of much significance as it will greatly influence oxygen administration. Respiratory rate, rhythm, and depth should be assessed every 5 minutes. Auscultation for rhonchi, rales, and diminished breath sounds should also be performed.

2. *Central nervous system.* The main symptoms manifesting hypoxemia and hypercarbia are related to this body system. They may range from headaches to restlessness to belligerence or even delirium and unconsciousness. The effects on the CNS may be so subtle that the family members may report only a gradual personality change. This is particularly true in progressive chronic lung disease. Level of consciousness should be assessed frequently to evaluate progressive and rapid CNS deterioration secondary to alterations in $PaCO_2$ and/or PaO_2.

3. *Cardiovascular system.* The circulatory manifestations of hypoxia and/or hypercarbia include tachycardia, cardiac arrhythmias, hypertension, and pale, cold, clammy skin. While these signs are usually present, if the *sympathetic nervous system* is not functioning adequately (as in the elderly or chronically ill patient), bradycardia and hypotension may be seen. If the PaO_2 is markedly reduced (50 mmHg), central cyanosis will be present. However, central cyanosis is an unreliable sign and should never be used as a primary determinant of oxygen saturation. Blood pressure, pulse rate, rhythm, and quality plus skin color and temperature should be assessed every 5 minutes. The patient must be placed on a cardiac monitor (Fig. 14-1a and b) since arrhythmias are common.

EMERGENCY MANAGEMENT

Emergency management of acute respiratory failure ultimately depends on the underlying pathophysiology. However, certain basic principles apply no matter what the etiology may be.

AIRWAY PATENCY

Maintenance of the airway may be achieved very simply through proper positioning of the head and neck or the insertion of an oropharyngeal or nasopharyngeal airway. In other cases, *endotracheal intubation* may be required (see Chap. 18). For patient comfort, nasotracheal intubation should be attempted when possible. Three criteria are used when determining the need for emergency intubation:

1. *Disease process.* There are three conditions which require immediate intubation. These are (a) a large flail chest (see Fig. 19-3), (b) a comatose patient who no longer has a gag reflex and therefore cannot protect his or her own airway, and (c) respiratory arrest.

2. *Disease course.* Observation of the patient's course centers on three parameters: (a) $PaCO_2$. If it is greater than 55 mmHg and *rising,* intubation is required. (b) F_IO_2. If the patient requires an F_IO_2 of 50 percent or greater using nasal cannula, catheter, or mask, intubation plus mechanical ventilation will be necessary. Ideally, the F_IO_2 can then be lowered and oxygen toxicity avoided. (c) PaO_2. If the PaO_2 is less than 60 mmHg while the patient is receiving supplemental oxygen, a significant right-to-left shunt is present and intubation is indicated.

3. *Ventilation reserve.* The patient's ventilatory reserve is assessed by two parameters: *respiratory rate* and *vital capacity* (VC). If the respiratory rate is greater than 36 or the VC is less than 15 mm/kg of

body weight, intubation is necessary. The reader will recall that VC is the maximal amount of air exhaled following maximal inhalation. The normal individual has a VC of 60 to 75 mm/kg. Thus a reduction to 15 mm/kg is indicative of serious respiratory distress. VC can readily be measured in the ED through the use of a Wright spirometer.

Once the endotracheal tube has been inserted, the emergency team must ascertain its position in the trachea. If the tube has been inserted to the point of the carina,* there is a definite possibility that the tube may slip into the *right bronchus*. Therefore, the following precautions are advised:

1. Check bilateral breath sounds immediately. If diminished on the left side, withdraw the tube approximately one-half inch and then reauscultate.

2. Observe the chest for equal expansion bilaterally. Again, if expansion is unequal, the endotracheal tube may have slipped into the right lung.

3. Take a chest x-ray immediately.

The three criteria for emergency intubation cited above cannot be interpreted as absolutes. They must also be considered in conjunction with the patient's clinical appearance.

Occasionally, prompt insertion of an endotracheal tube is not possible. An alternative for providing a temporary airway during a respiratory arrest is a cricothyroid puncture. Figure 17-2 provides an anterior view of the larynx with the cricothyroid membrane indicated. Since this membrane is relatively avascular, hemorrhage is not a problem. The procedure for a cricothyroid puncture is summarized in Table 17-2.

OXYGEN THERAPY

If hypoxemia is present, the general rule is to administer the lowest level F_1O_2 possible to achieve a PaO_2 of 60 mmHg (90 percent hemoglobin saturation). Remember that oxygen is a drying agent at high concentrations; therefore humidification is mandatory. Arterial

---

*This is the point where the trachea bifurcates into the right and left main-stem bronchi. This point is located at the second intercostal space (see Fig. 5-1).

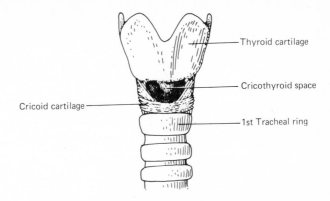

Figure 17-2 Anterior view of larynx with cricothyroid space illustrated.

blood gases should be checked immediately *before* administering oxygen (or *changing* the F_1O_2) and within 10 to 15 minutes *following* the *uninterrupted* flow of O_2. If chronic obstructive lung disease is an underlying problem, *low-liter-flow oxygen* (1 to 3 liters per nasal cannula) with serial monitoring of arterial blood gases and direct patient assessment is mandatory since rapid respiratory depression may occur. The rationale for this is that with the chronic lung patient, CO_2 is no longer the primary stimulant for breathing; *hypoxia* (PaO_2 of 60 to 70 mmHg) now stimulates respirations. If the PaO_2 is raised

Table 17-2	Procedure for a cricothyroid puncture.

1. Hyperextend the neck. If the possibility of cervical neck injury exists, the neck must remain in a neutral position.

2. Locate the cricothyroid membrane by running fingers down the anterior aspect of the neck. The first prominence felt is the thyroid cartilage; the second is the cricoid cartilage; the space between is the membrane.

3. Insert a large-bore needle, preferably 10 gauge. Currently, a 10-gauge polyethylene needle with a stylete is available. Ideally, all EDs are stocked with these special needles.

4. After fitting the needle with an appropriate adapter, attach the patient to a positive pressure breathing apparatus.

5. By utilization of this procedure, an adequate airway may be maintained until more definitive therapy can be instituted.

significantly above this level, the hypoxic drive to breathe is eliminated and *respiratory depression* occurs.

IMPROVEMENT OF VENTILATION

While a low PaO_2 can be improved by administration of oxygen, a respiratory acidosis ($\uparrow PaCO_2$) can be improved only by increasing effective ventilation. The following are some basic interventions:

1. Liquefy thick, tenacious secretions through humidification. If the patient has an endotracheal tube in place, frequent instillation of normal saline or sodium bicarbonate will assist in loosening secretions. Mucomist also liquefies secretions; however, it is irritating to the tracheobronchial tree and may cause bronchospasm. Administration of oral and parenteral fluids is also essential. The type of fluid and rate of intravenous administration will depend on the patient's age, cardiovascular status, preexisting fluid balance, and renal function.

2. Use frequent nasotracheal or endotracheal suctioning. Remember that suctioning removes not only secretions but also oxygen. If the patient is hypoxemic, increase the F_IO_2 to 70 to 100 percent for approximately 5 minutes prior to and following suctioning. Also, suctioning can be a *potent vagal stimulant,* and so careful monitoring of pulse rate is necessary. *Sterile, atraumatic* technique is essential when endotracheal suctioning is being performed. Each suctioning unit in the emergency department should be equipped with sterile gloves and an ample supply of the nontraumatic suction catheters now on the market.

3. Employ intermittent positive pressure breathing to assist in improving ventilation and loosening secretions. A saline nebulization can be given concurrently. If the patient has experienced IPPB previously and does not fear it, this treatment may also provide a much-needed opportunity for rest. While the IPPB treatment is being given, the nurse should frequently monitor the breath sounds, especially if the patient continues to be short of breath. Often, a small undetected pneumothorax will become a life-threatening tension pneumothorax during an IPPB treatment. This is especially true with emphysema where blebs often occur (see Table 17-3).

4. Other methods to improve ventilation include chest physiotherapy, postural drainage, and fibroptic bronchoscopy (especially popular for aspiration patients).

Table 17-3	Adverse side effects secondary to an IPPB treatment.

1. Possibility of developing a tension pneumothorax (see text).

2. Excessive oxygenation: air-mix dial on many IPPB machines provides an F_IO_2 varying between 40 and 90%.

3. Decreased cardiac output secondary to decreased venous return. This is not a common problem.

A word of caution should be made regarding rapid lowering of an elevated $PaCO_2$ in patients with chronic obstructive lung disease. As a compensatory mechanism to maintain a normal pH, these patients retain bicarbonate (metabolic alkalosis). If the $PaCO_2$ is *rapidly* corrected to a near-normal level, the pH may shift to an *alkalotic* level. Dangerous *cardiac arrhythmias* may result.

DRUG THERAPY

A comprehensive discussion of all the drugs used in the treatment of acute respiratory failure is beyond the scope of this chapter. Four categories of drugs are briefly covered: (1) sympathomimetics, (2) xanthines, (3) antibiotics, and (4) steroids.

SYMPATHOMIMETICS: Isoetharine (Dilabron),* epinephrine, and isoproterenol are three sympathomimetics used for bronchodilatation.

Isoetharine: This is a selective beta$_2$-receptor stimulant (see Table 14-9). Through its specificity for beta$_2$-receptors, this drug has a greatly *decreased* beta-mimetic action on the heart (see Table 14-10a), as compared with isoproterenol or epinephrine. Inhaled via aerosol or IPPB nebulization, it causes bronchodilatation promptly and remains *effective* for approximately 4 hours. Common IPPB nebulization dosage ranges are 0.25 to 0.5 mm 1 percent isoetharine dissolved in 2 mm normal saline. Side effects include nervousness, weakness, and tremors.

Epinephrine and *isoproterenol:* The pharmacological actions, in-

---

*Other selective beta$_2$-receptor stimulants include metaproterenol (Alupent), salbutamol (Ventolin), terbutaline (Bricanyl), and ritodrine (Premar).

dications, and side effects of these two drugs have been covered in Chap. 14. Only dosages and routes of administration used for bronchodilatation are discussed here. Epinepherine is most commonly given *subcutaneously*. The dosage ranges from 0.1 to 0.5 mg. Isoproterenol is often administered via IPPB nebulization. Eight drops of either a 1:100 or 1:200 isoproterenol solution dissolved in 1.5 mm normal saline is the common dosage.

Both epinephrine and isoproterenol are available in hand-nebulizers. The uses of these is controversial.[1]

XANTHINES   Caffeine and theophylline are two xanthine compounds. They are *central nervous system stimulants*. Their actions include relaxation of smooth muscle (notably in bronchial tubes and blood vessels), cardiac stimulation, and a diuretic effect. *Aminophylline,* a derivative of theophylline, is the widely used xanthine and is utilized primarily for its bronchodilatating effect. It is available in several forms: intravenous solutions, tablets for oral administration, and rectal suppositories. Intravenous dosage varies between 250 and 500 mg. Aminophylline can be given as a bolus; if administered in this manner, it must be given *slowly* as its side effects can be quite severe. Another method of administration which is preferred by this author is dilution of the drug in 50 to 100 cc IV solution and dripped in slowly over 15 to 20 minutes. As with any intravenous drip, a microdrip chamber must be used. The rate of administration is far more controlled when this method is utilized. The side effects associated with aminophylline can be quite severe, particularly in the AMI patient. These side effects include:

1. Cardiac arrhythmias, palpitations, and angina

2. Hypotension

3. Nausea and vomiting

ANTIBIOTICS   There are numerous antibiotics that can be used when treating pulmonary infections. The reader is referred to the bibliography for a complete discussion of these drugs. The only point to be made here is that a *sputum* for *culture* and *sensitivity* must be collected prior to initiating antibiotic coverage.

STEROIDS   The many physiologic effects of steroids (see p. 202) are discussed in detail in Chap. 14. Their use in noncardiogenic pulmonary edema (see Table 14-5) is controversial; however, many authorities recommend using pharmacological doses of steroids for a palliative anti-inflammatory effect when treating patients with *aspiration pneumonitis.* The recommended dosage for *methylprednisolone* (Solu-Medrol) is 30 mg/kg.

LABORATORY AIDS

The nurse should order an arterial BGA (this should be performed immediately), serum electrolytes, hematocrit and hemoglobin, white blood cell count with differential, chest x-ray, and an ECG.

WHAT NOT TO DO

1. Because of possible respiratory depression, *no sedatives* should be given to patients with ARF unless they are receiving mechanical ventilation. This rule is of great importance for patients with chronic lung disease.

2. Do not correct acid-base imbalances without careful monitoring of *serum electrolytes.*

5. Do not *overcorrect* the PaO_2. Excessive use of oxygen damages the alveolar-capillary membrane.

4. Do not leave a patient *alone* while *oxygen* therapy is initiated. The nurse may return to find an unconscious patient since the hypoxic drive to breathe has been depressed.

Perhaps one of the single most important elements in the emergency care of the patient with, or the potential for, acute respiratory failure is the skillful observation and prompt, knowledgeable intervention of the emergency nurse. This nurse must constantly monitor the respiratory status of the patient, watching for subtle changes as well as the very obvious ones of respiratory depression. In addition, the nurse must know when endotracheal intubation is indicated and be willing to take the initiative to mobilize the emergency team when lifesaving measures are needed. Once this patient is stabilized in the ED, safe yet rapid transport to the intensive care unit is necessary.

REFERENCES

1. Goodman, L., and Gilman, A., *The Pharmacological Basis of Therapeutics,* Macmillan, New York, 1975, p. 509.

BIBLIOGRAPHY

Hudak, C., et al., *Critical Care Nursing,* Lippincott, Philadelphia, 1973.

Hudson, L., "The Acute Management of the Chronic Airway Obstruction Patient," *Heart and Lung,* vol. 3, no. 1, January–February 1974, pp. 93–96.

Pierson, D., "Respiratory Stimulants: Review of the Literature and Assessment of Current Status," *Heart and Lung,* vol. 2, no. 5, September–October 1973, pp. 726–732.

Wade, J., *Respiratory Nursing Care,* Mosby, St. Louis, 1973.

Wilson, R., "The Diagnosis and Treatment of Acute Respiratory Failure in Sepsis," *Heart and Lung,* vol. 5, no. 4, July–August 1976, pp. 614–620.

Winslow, E., "Visual Inspection of the Patient with Cardiopulmonary Disease," *Heart and Lung,* vol. 4, no. 3, May–June, 1975, pp. 421–430.

Zschoche, D., *Mosby's Comprehensive Review of Critical Care,* Mosby, St. Louis, 1976.

CHAPTER 18
CARDIOPULMONARY RESUSCITATION
SAMUEL C. GRESHAM, M.D.

THIS chapter includes patient selection criteria for cardiopulmonary resuscitation (CPR), the major points of CPR technique,
the initial steps of drug therapy, and finally an overview of the
more definitive aspects of therapy. It is assumed that the reader has
been trained in basic life support, including an hour-long film and
supervised mannequin practice.

Although the current CPR technique was rediscovered and
applied at Johns Hopkins 15 years ago, the implementation of an
effective program across the nation and in the community hospital
has occurred only in the last 4 to 5 years. Prior to this time, patients
who developed sudden collapse, particularly if due to ventricular
fibrillation, might have been given a face mask with oxygen. In
general, the attendant personnel stood by helplessly and watched
the patient die.

To emphasize the utility of this technique, a statistical review of a
year's (1971) activity in CPR at the Queen's Medical Center in
Honolulu, Hawaii, will be shared. During this time there were 241
CPR attempts on 203 different patients. Of these patients, 38 (18.7
percent) survived to be discharged from the hospital. Another 70
resuscitations were temporarily effective, but these patients eventually succumbed before discharge from the hospital, either from
underlying disease or from extensive hypoxic brain damage.

The CPR approach used at Queen's Medical Center is that of a *team response,* utilizing the first-year resident and the two medical interns on call as the nucleus of the resuscitation team. These individuals are the most medically knowledgeable personnel available on a 24 hour a day, 7 day a week basis. In addition, the team consists of a nursing supervisor, an emergency department nurse, an inhalation therapist, a nurse anesthetist, and a surgical resident. However, even with this high-powered team, the most important person remains the *nurse* who decides that the patient needs resuscitation and begins the manual CPR.

In summary, approximately one out of five patients, who would have almost certainly died, recovered and was discharged from the hospital because of the application of this potent therapeutic tool.

PATIENT SELECTION

The basic recommendation is *nonselection.* This means that if there is any question whether the patient can be resuscitated or not, the technique should be applied. Many are concerned that this approach to CPR may leave a number of people with severe brain damage because of the resuscitative effort. This is, by and large, a fallacy. In the above series of the 38 patients who were discharged, there were only two with significant brain damage. One was a 2-year-old girl with asthma who vomited, aspirated, and had a prolonged episode of hypoxia. Her brain damage consists of some residual spasticity, but her intellect remains intact. Both her mother and the pediatrician caring for her, in retrospect, affirm that they would still want the resuscitation effort. The second patient is a 50-year-old man who remains in a vigil coma; he is able to open his eyes and look around, but what he sees apparently does not register. A number of the 70 patients who were temporarily resuscitated suffered severe brain damage, but the majority succumbed within 24 hours of the resuscitation attempt. On balance, one patient out of 38 with severe brain damage seems a small price to pay for saving the lives of the other 37.

INITIAL PATIENT ASSESSMENT

On initially assessing the patient, what criteria should one use to determine whether to perform CPR? In some patients it obviously will be of no avail. Examples are the patient with rigor mortis and the terminal cancer patient found without signs of life. Many other cases are less obvious. All remember the admonition that the brain is damaged after a 4- to 6-minute period without circulation or oxygen. This is probably true, but with a 20-minute history of collapse there is no way of knowing when the ventricular fibrillation seen on the oscilloscope started. The initial collapse may have been due to hypotension with bradycardia or a tachycardia, either supraventricular or ventricular, which eventually deteriorated into ventricular fibrillation. Perfusion to the brain may have been adequate until the onset of ventricular fibrillation.

Since the history is not always reliable, what other criteria can be used to determine the need for CPR? The *carotid pulse* is the first parameter to be assessed and should be felt for midneck, alongside the trachea. If it is not obvious on one side, the other side can be felt, but not simultaneously, since one stops cerebral blood flow that way. If a faint throbbing of the fingertips is felt, it may be one's own pulse. Whether it is or not is irrelevant because if the patient's own heart beat is that weak, cerebral perfusion is probably inadequate. The carotid pulse is assessed rather than other pulses (radial or femoral) since these pulses may be absent while the heart is still pumping quite effectively.

The second parameter to be assessed is the *state of consciousness*. If the blood flow to the brain is inadequate, the patient will be confused, if not comatose. If the patient is fully conscious, perfusion to the brain must be adequate. Usually, it takes less than 30 seconds for the patient to become unconscious when blood flow ceases to the brain.

Many ask whether *pupillary size* should be checked. The pupils become fixed and dilated between 20 seconds and 2 minutes after the circulation to the brain stops. Thus, 2 minutes may remain following pupil dilatation during which the patient may still be resuscitable. So pupil size does not help one to decide whether to initiate CPR.

What about *respiratory effort*? Without circulation, the patient may still make irregular, gasping respiratory efforts produced from the brainstem. The nurse who waits until this respiratory effort ceases has waited too long. In fact, this author is aware of several episodes in which the breathing pattern continued to be normal, despite sustained ventricular fibrillation for 45 seconds. Conversely, the absence of respiration is of no great help either in assessing the circulation, since in approximately half the cases, respiratory arrest is the primary factor for the collapse.

Should one *auscultate* for the *heart beat*? To do so would take precious time, and one may hear regularly occurring heart beats that are pumping little, if any, blood. It is of *no value* in deciding whether to initiate CPR.

To summarize, the following three factors are crucial in determining the appropriateness of beginning CPR: (1) if there is any question as to whether the patient might be resuscitable; (2) if there is an absence of the carotid pulse; and (3) if the level of consciousness is impaired. If these three are positive, begin to resuscitate.

CPR TECHNIQUE

AIRWAY

After the decision to resuscitate the patient is made, what is the first thing to be done? One should quickly *check the mouth for possible obstruction,* such as a piece of meat in the back of the pharynx, a denture turned sideways, or large particles of vomitus. A good way to clear the mouth of vomitus is to make a sweep with the finger to remove the larger pieces and ignore the smaller particles. Do not waste time using a suction apparatus on the smaller pieces and liquid material. The liquid material can be disposed of by turning the head sideways, and the smaller pieces do not significantly obstruct the airway.

Next, the *neck* should be *extended* and the lower jaw pulled forward. Mouth-to-mouth or nose-to-mouth forceful breathing, performed for *four effective breaths,* should be started. The efficacy of this artificial breathing can be assessed by noting the absence of air escaping around the mouth seal and the fact that the patient's chest rises with each inhalation. Also, when the resuscitator removes his or her mouth after each breath, he or she should be able to observe the chest fall and feel a rush of exhaled air.

This relatively simple procedure is effective in as many as 50 percent of those who have sudden arrest or collapse in that immediately after the four breaths a carotid pulse returns. If this is the case, the primary concern from this point is the maintenance of adequate breathing, and endotracheal intubation with maintained ventilatory support should be considered. Conversely, if after the four inhalations a carotid pulse is not present, one must proceed to manual chest compression for circulatory support.

MANUAL CHEST COMPRESSION

Before discussing manual chest compression, a few comments on the *precordial thump* will be made. The importance of the precordial thump is unclear. There are enthusiasts such as Dr. George Griffiths of California and the American Association of Anesthesiology, but their enthusiasm is based on little if any objective data. In the occasional case (perhaps 1 out of 50 or 1 out of 100) a forceful blow with the side of the fist, at the site of hand placement for chest compression, may be effective in delivering a mechanical distention of the ventricle. This blow causes the ventricle to depolarize and then repolarize with a regular rhythm. Logically one would *deliver the blow* and immediately *feel the carotid pulse* to see if the thump was effective in restoring circulation. If ineffective, repeating the blow is not recommended since precious time will be wasted.

Manual chest compression must then be started. One begins the compression by placing the heel of the hand along the length of the sternum on the lower one-third, just above the *xiphoid process*. Pressure must then be delivered truly vertical to the sternum (see Fig. 18-1). If the pressure is applied to either side of the sternum, the resuscitator rolls the heart off the plateau of the vertebrae, does not compress it, and ends up breaking the ribs since the pressure is ap-

Figure 18-1 A cutaway view of the chest. The vertebrae protrude from the back, producing a plateau or ridge several centimeters higher than either side of the chest cavity containing the lungs. The intent of manual compression is to squeeze the ventricles of the heart between the back of the sternum and the vertebrae. *(Adapted from Shapter, R., Clinical Symposia, CIBA, vol. 26, no. 5, New Jersey p. 8.)*

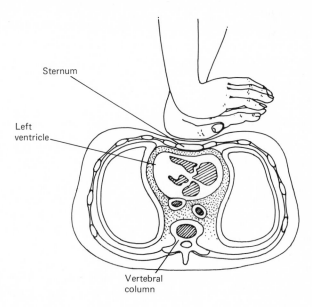

plied against them and not the heart. It is also important for the person compressing the chest to be physically high enough to provide vertical compression and to be able to use the weight of the shoulders with the arms in a stiffened position. A rocking motion of the body should be used to allow the muscles of the abdomen and back to do most of the work rather than the much smaller and easily fatigued arm muscles.

The *rate* and *duration* of compression are also important. The older recommendations were for one compression a second or 60 per minute, which is the minimum rate. The amount of blood being pumped from the heart by chest compression increases in a steady manner between the rates of 50 and 110 per minute. The cardiac output tends to remain stable or actually drop when compression is above that rate. By and large, it is unrealistic to try to compress at a rate of 100 or 110 per minute since it is very fatiguing and much of the necessary coordination is lost. It is better to aim for the middle of this range, that is, 75 or 80 per minute. Then being a few beats per minute off is not critical. It is also important to remember that rapid or jerky movements defeat the purpose of compression, which is to pump blood from the heart. A too-brief application of pressure does not allow the necessary time for the cardiac valve to open and the blood to be ejected. It may transmit an impressive pressure wave, but a pressure wave is not desirable at the cost of effective blood flow. *Steady, even compressions* and *relaxations,* equally timed and rhythmic, are better than spasmodic thrusts with brief rests.

INITIAL DRUG THERAPY

CORRECTION OF ACID-BASE BALANCE

When a patient has a cardiopulmonary arrest, typically two kinds of *acidosis* are present. One is produced by *carbon dioxide* that is not exhaled. The second is produced by *lactic acid* that is formed by the body's attempt to produce adequate energy with inadequate oxygen. Normally, glucose is broken down by the cells to carbon dioxide and water by the addition of oxygen and the release of energy. Without adequate oxygen this process can proceed only partway, and lactic acid rapidly accumulates (see Fig. 5-6). The average amount of acidity or pH of a patient receiving CPR is 7.1, and the normal is 7.4. Correcting this acidosis is critically important since the enzyme systems of the cell and the consequent production and use of energy function best at a pH of 7.4. In addition, epinephrine produces only a small fraction of its usual effect at a pH of 7.1. To correct this acidosis, one must administer approximately *100 meq sodium bicarbonate immediately* and *50 meq every 10 minutes* to keep up with the continued production of lactic acid. Since this requires administering 100 cc fluid immediately, an intravenous route is needed.

INTRAVENOUS INSERTION

This intravenous route is usually provided by a large plastic cannula in the *anticubital fossa* vein. Alternate sites might be the external or the internal jugular vein or a cutdown on the ankle.

A brief discussion of the procedure for a cutdown is necessary. The cutdown is being performed in an emergency where every second counts, and it is nonsensible to waste time with gloves, draping, skin preparation, or even local analgesic. One should make a very rapid 1-inch horizontal incision just above and anterior to the medial malleolus (inside knob of the ankle). Any sizable structure external to the heavy fascia covering the muscle and the bone is a vein that can be opened quickly with the same scalpel, and a polyethylene tube can be inserted rapidly for IV access. The suturing, antiseptic ointment, and sterile dressing can be attended to later.

EPINEPHRINE ADMINISTRATION

In addition to the bicarbonate, one usually administers *epinephrine*. With the alpha- and beta-mimetic effects of this drug, an increase in blood pressure and blood flow should occur. One could use other medications to produce these effects independently, but since both are desired, epinephrine seems to be the preferred drug. Many ask, If the patient has ventricular fibrillation, why make the heart beat faster? If epinephrine is given prior to defibrillation, there is a greater chance of sustaining normal sinus rhythm because of the increased vigor of contractions and the decreased systemic demands on the weak pump. This enhances blood flow to the coronary arteries and therefore the myocardium as well as other vital areas.

The epinephrine is administered as 0.5 to 1 mg diluted 9 to 1 with normal saline. It is mixed with 9 cc saline primarily for the purpose of ensuring that the volume is large enough to travel through the intravenous tubing and into the patient. If there is a delay in obtaining an IV route, the epinephrine may be given undiluted, *transtracheally.* A needle is inserted between the rings of the trachea below the larynx, in the midline of the neck, and the medication injected directly in the trachea. With a breath, the drug is immediately absorbed. As a general recommendation, epinephrine should be given as 0.5 to 1 mg *every 10 minutes* during the resuscitation effort.

In summary, the treatment to this point has corrected the hypoxia and stimulated the heart to improve a low cardiac output. These measures alone revive the majority of those to be resuscitated. The therapies from this juncture diverge depending upon the rate and rhythm of the heart. Thus, it becomes necessary to know the electrocardiographic pattern of the patient.

DEFINITIVE THERAPY

An *electrocardiographic determination* of rate and rhythm can be obtained from an oscilloscope with needle electrodes or, more commonly, with two leg electrodes and the right arm electrode. If the rate is *too slow,* the general approach is to speed it up by *atropine, Isuprel,* or eventually a *pacemaker.* On the other hand, if the rate is *too fast,* the procedure is to apply *electric shock* and/or decrease the irritability with drugs. The third possibility is pump failure with a ventricular rate between 60 and 150. In this situation, one needs to increase the vigor of contraction of the heart.

BRADYARRHYTHMIAS

For slow rates, 1 mg *atropine* given intravenously causes the heart rate to increase by reducing vagal tone. Giving more than 3 mg atropine is rarely effective if the drug has not produced the desired change up to that point. This treatment would be particularly beneficial for a patient with an acute diaphragmatic myocardial infarction who develops complete heart block (see Fig. 18-2a and b).

If the atropine is ineffective in increasing the heart rate, one may give 0.2 mg *Isuprel* (1:5000 dilution) mixed with 9 cc normal saline intravenously. If the emergency is not too great, one may deliver the Isuprel in an intravenous drip, consisting of 500 cc D$_5$W and 2 mg Isuprel (1:5000 dilution). This should be administered at an approximate rate of 1 to 2 cc/min. Finally, if neither of these drugs is effective, an attendant cardiologist may wish to place a pacemaker using a balloon-tipped floating pacemaking catheter through the arm or subclavian vein.

Bradyarrhythmias

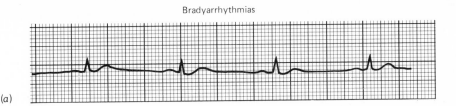

(a)

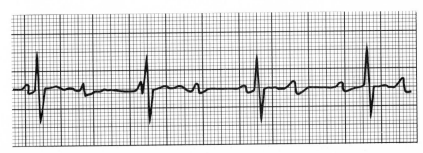

(b)

Figure 18-2 (a) Sinus bradycardia at ventricular rate of **34.** *(Taken from Conover, M., Cardiac Arrhythmias: Exercises in Pattern Interpretation, Mosby, St. Louis, 1974, p. 13.)* (b) **Third-degree heart block with a ventricular rate of 33.**

TACHYARRHYTHMIAS

The electrocardiogram will determine whether a rapid heart rate is a ventricular tachycardia, ventricular fibrillation, atrial fibrillation with a rapid ventricular response, or an atrial flutter with a 1:1 or 2:1 response (see Fig. 18-3a to d). If any of these is associated with *cardiovascular collapse,* electric countershock is indicated.

COUNTERSHOCK   Generally, the equipment needed for countershock is a DC defibrillator with two large paddles that are to be applied with pressure on either side of the heart, that is, beneath the right clavicle and the apex of the heart. The amount of energy delivered is considerable, and it is important to distribute that energy over a large area. The paddles are of substantial size, approximately 4 cm in diameter. This size helps to avoid burning the skin, as would occur if the energy were delivered through a smaller electrode.

To distribute the energy from the paddle to the skin, one must have a *good conductor* of electricity. ECG paste or gauze pads

Tachyarrhythmias

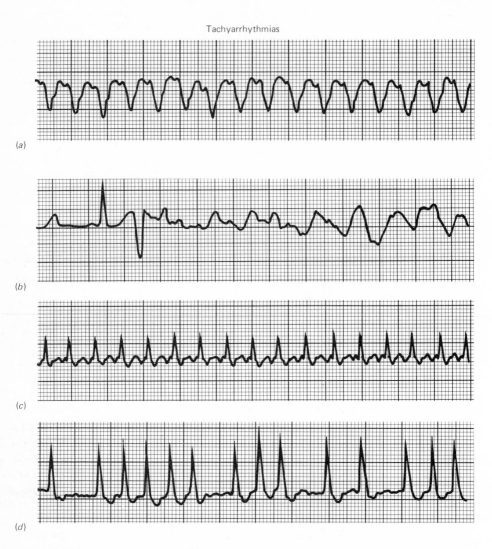

(a)

(b)

(c)

(d)

Figure 18-3 (a) Ventricular tachycardia at a rate of 16.0 *(Taken from Conover, M.,*
Cardiac Arrhythmias: Exercises in Pattern Interpretation, Mosby, St. Louis, 1974, p. 53.)
(b) **Ventricular fibrillation caused by an R-on-T premature ventricular contraction.**
(Taken from Conover, M., Cardiac Arrhythmias: Exercises in Pattern Interpretation, Mosby,
St. Louis, 1974, p. 57.) (c) **Atrial flutter with 2:1 conduction; ventricular rate is 150.**
(d) **Atrial fibrillation with a rapid ventricular response of 140.** *(Taken from Conover, M.,*
Cardiac Arrhythmias: Exercises in Pattern Interpretation, Mosby, St. Louis, 1974, p. 21.)

soaked in saline provide good electrical contact. The saline-soaked pads are preferred because, following countershock, one must return to manual compression, and the ECG paste leaves the skin very slippery and difficult to compress. Another disadvantage to the paste is that if it spreads between the two paddles, the electricity may go along the paste rather than into the skin and the heart. One should never use alcohol pads because the electricity can set them on fire and they are also a poor conductor of electricity. The saline pads have to be separated by a distance of 2 to 3 inches to prevent arcing of the electricity.

To aid in better electrical contact, one should exert about 25 lb pressure on the paddles when delivering the shock. Since the amount of electricity that should be delivered to the heart is directly proportional to the size of the body, a general recommendation for setting the amount is *200 watt-seconds* for *small persons* and *400 watt-seconds* for *large persons*.

It is of prime importance to *resume CPR* after the delivery of a countershock because results may take up to 1 minute to be observed correctly due to monitor recovery and dissipation of the initial parasympathetic effect.

DRUGS   If electric countershock fails to convert the tachyrrhythmia, one would want to give a drug to decrease the irritability of the heart. For example, if the patient has *ventricular fibrillation* and the shock is delivered but the rhythm is not altered, 100 mg *Xylocaine* may be given intravenously. This drug decreases PVCs and at the same time does not significantly decrease the strength of contractions. Usually up to 400 mg can be given immediately, assuming an average size adult.

An alternative drug would be *procainamide;* this is usually given in a 250-mg dosage as a slow IV injection rather than as a bolus as with Xylocaine. The reason for this slowness is that this drug decreases the vigor of contractility; generally up to 1 gm can be given without a marked decrease. These two drugs are best for ventricular irritability. Atrial irritability and sometimes ventricular irritability can be decreased by *propranolol* 0.5 mg IV.

PUMP FAILURE

In the third category, pump failure with a ventricular rate between 60 and 150 per minute, one may wish to increase the vigor of contraction. The three drugs commonly used are *digoxin, Cedilanid,* and *calcium chloride.* Cedilanid is preferred because of the slightly faster onset of action. One-half of a digitalizing dose would be 0.8 mg IV, and one must be sure that the patient has not received a digitalis preparation previously. The preferred calcium preparation is calcium chloride given intravenously as 10 cc of a 10% solution which equals 1 gm. The calcium is doubly effective after a countershock in decreasing ventricular irritability and increasing the vigor of contraction. One must be very careful when giving the calcium if the patient has *received digitalis* because it can increase the chances of digitalis toxicity. There are numerous other drugs that one may wish to use in specific situations, but the attempt here is to provide simplified guidelines for general situations.

ENDOTRACHEAL INTUBATION

The approach to CPR described above is one that can be applied by every ED nurse. A large number of techniques have not been commented on, the most significant being *endotracheal intubation.* If one has the capability for it, endotracheal intubation is highly desirable very early in the process of resuscitation because the cuffed tube gives greater control of ventilation and prevention of aspiration of stomach contents. It is important, however, that one deliver mouth-to-mouth or mouth-to-nose ventilation as soon as possible to provide at least partial ventilation before taking time to perform endotracheal intubation. Even with the most experienced person doing the intubation, the patient is frequently vomiting and struggling. Altogether too much time is devoted to individual unsuccessful attempts at endotracheal intubation. One should allow only 15 to 30 seconds for each attempt and make perhaps only a total of three attempts separated by periods of vigorous ventilation by other means. Mouth-to-mouth or mouth-to-nose is the most reliable. Using a bag with a mask requires some experience to prevent escape of air around the mouth. The Elder valve-to-mask technique is somewhat easier, freeing both hands to attain and maintain a good seal. If the patient is not being adequately ventilated and endotracheal intubation is difficult, one should consider an emergency tracheostomy.

BLOOD GASES

A brief discussion of aterial blood gases is warranted. The recommendations on ventilation and treatment of acidosis usually produce a pH between 7.2 and 7.6, but occasionally this is not so. One good check is to obtain an arterial BGA as soon as possible to make sure that one is neither undertreating nor overtreating the acidosis. A large error in either direction contributes to ventricular irritability.

One final point should be made regarding the treatment of cardiac arrest. The general recommendations of treating precipitating causes leading to the arrest, such as hypoxia and acidosis, may not be the most logical approach in a few clinical situations. An example of this is the patient with an acute myocardial infarction and primary ventricular fibrillation where no time has elapsed since the collapse. This patient is best treated with immediate delivery of countershock.

BIBLIOGRAPHY

Braunwald, E., "Control of Myocardial Oxygen Consumption: Physiologic and Clinical Consideration," *American Journal of Cardiology,* vol. 27, 1971, pp. 416–432.

Committee on Emergency Cardiac Care, "Statement on First Aid for Foreign Body Obstruction of the Airway," American Heart Association, January 1976.

———, "Standards for CPR and ECC," suppl. to *JAMA,* vol. 227, no. 7, February 18, 1974.

Dahl, C. F., et al., "Myocardial Necrosis from DC Countershock," *Journal of Circulation,* vol. 50, November 1974, pp. 956–961.

Maroko, P. R., et al., "Factors Influencing Infarct Size Following Experimental Coronary Artery Occlusion," *Journal of Circulation,* vol. 53, January 1971, pp. 67–82.

Marriott, H. J. L., *Practical Electrocardiography,* 5th ed., Williams & Wilkins, Baltimore, 1972.

CHAPTER 19
MULTIPLE TRAUMA
CAPT. CAROL ANN ISAAC, ANC, R.N., M.Ed.

TRAUMA AS AN EPIDEMIC

TRAUMA as a human event is ubiquitous. It recognizes no boundaries of time, place, age, sex, or economic status. A consideration of some statistics regarding trauma as an epidemic in the American population is important before studying its effects on the individual:

1. For the population as a whole, accidents rank only behind cardiovascular disease, cancer, and strokes as a leading cause of death.

2. During the decade 1964 to 1974, 450,000 persons died from accidents on the highways.[1] Health care professionals have been led to a growing awareness that trauma as a human event has reached epidemic proportions. As a result, ED practitioners have developed an *emergency consciousness.*

In the past decade a marked improvement in the care of the severely injured has been seen. The following are four areas in which progress has been made:

1. First aid care has improved through the use of more highly trained ambulance personnel and through the evacuation of the injured even in sparsely populated areas.

2. Radio communication between ambulances and hospital emergency departments has helped to prepare for the arrival of injured individuals and has allowed for care to begin in the ambulance itself, under the guidance of a physician.

3. Complete furnishing of equipment and skilled staff in hospital EDs has provided improved service to those needing immediate care. [2]

4. Intensive care units have been developed and staffed with experienced and interested personnel to provide extended emergency care to the severely traumatized patient.

Trauma units have been organized as a subspecialty of emergency care for two reasons:

1. Because of vehicular and industrial accidents, many people are being injured in such a way as to involve multiple organ systems.

2. Trauma management is not merely resuscitation. It also involves:
a. Stabilization of all organ systems
b. Establishment of monitoring parameters
c. Performance of diagnostic procedures
d. Preparation of the patient for surgery, if indicated
e. Prevention of complications not directly related to the injury

The management of patients with multiple trauma is a complex task. It is one which can be best facilitated by nurses and physicians who have a thorough knowledge of the priorities of emergency management as well as an ability to safely and quickly care for the patient who has been traumatized. An important aspect of trauma care is that the treatment chosen must not be detrimental to one organ system while intending to remedy the insult that has been made to another.

The epidemic is here. Treatment must be immediate, appropriate, and complete. No information is available as to the number of deaths which would be prevented annually if treatment were ideal, but it certainly seems reasonable to assume that a significant percentage of these patients might be saved if circumstances were optimal.

PHYSICAL PREPARATION OF THE TRAUMA UNIT AND ITS PERSONNEL

It has been said that when an emergency has been prepared for, the emergency ceases to exist. The physical preparation of the trauma unit and the readiness of its personnel are important factors determining the final outcome of the traumatized individual.

After the alert call has been received, the following activities should take place:

1. *Gather equipment.* Clear the unit of excess equipment or supplies which may have been stored there. Ensure the readiness of this equipment:

a. Airway, tracheostomy tray, endotracheal tubes, oxygen mask and oxygen supply, bag mask, and thoractomy tray
b. Defibrillator and ECG monitor
c. IV fluids and tubing on mobile IV cart
d. Fully stocked dressing cart
e. Chest tubes and suction machine, with water seal drainage bottles and tubing
f. Resuscitation cart with emergency drugs
g. Foley catheter tray
h. Chart with forms needed by physicians
i. Nurses' flow chart, lab slips, and nurses' notes
j. Arterial blood-gas analysis equipment
k. Restraints and safety straps on mobile stretcher
l. Plastic bag for bloody clothing

2. *Alert others.* Call these people and alert them for the arrival:
a. Physician
b. Respiratory therapy group
c. X-ray department
d. Blood bank
e. Department of anesthesia and the operating room
f. Intensive care unit

3. Clear the hallway for the arrival.

4. *Direct traffic.* Direct police and curious on-lookers to an area where they will not impede the passage of the victim into the trauma unit.

5. *Assign staff.* This function is a broad one encompassing many factors which will be discussed separately in the following section. Generally, this function involves the nurse in charge assigning the roles of runner, recorder, and vital signs monitor.

ORGANIZATION OF THE TEAM APPROACH TO TRAUMA CARE

It is essential that each person involved in administering initial emergency care to a traumatized victim be assigned a functional role. Assignment of functional roles serves three purposes:

1. It ensures continuity of care. Each team member can be free to do his or her assigned job thoroughly without interruption for other tasks.

2. It provides for an orderly system of operation in a typically small working area.

3. It organizes communication channels for providing and recording data. The nurse in charge should make assignments before the arrival of the patient. The following is a sample list of essential team members and their respective functions.

Runner: The runner ensures delivery of all specimens to the laboratory, procures blood from the blood bank, serves as messenger, and disseminates information regarding the results of laboratory data.

Recorder: The recorder, usually the nurse in charge, initiates and maintains the flow sheet and nurse's notes. This person provides the physicians with the necessary forms for obtaining a history and physical. The recorder charts procedures and their results and medications administered and the times; keeps track of time elapsed since admission or arrest; and is responsible for administrative tasks related to the care of the patient, including admission procedures to the hospital.

Vital signs monitor: This person stays close to the bedside and keeps close observation on vital signs and neurological checks. The monitor records all intake and output; assists physicians with procedures; and may assist in the placement of the Foley catheter, IVs, nasogastric tube, and the ECG hook-up.

Other roles may be assumed if more than three people are available for assistance. These may include:

Family liaison: This person can explain the injury and the immediate treatment required and may take a nursing history from an available family member on behalf of the patient.

Surgical preparation team: If surgery is indicated, this team may specifically prepare the patient by shaving and cleansing the proposed operative sites, having the permit signed, and making arrangements with the department of anesthesia and the operating room.

Procedure assistant: This person sets up equipment for diagnostic procedures and prepares the patient for the procedure. The assistant is responsible for communicating to the recorder all results of diagnostic tests and therapeutic interventions.

Complete and accurate channels of communication must be established among all health care team personnel in the trauma unit. Each member must be aware of all role expectations and limitations. The task to be accomplished is the optimum care of the patient. It necessitates a team approach, wherein each member plays a specific, vital role in the patient's first step toward rehabilitation.

TRAUMA AS A REAL LIFE EXPERIENCE— A SIMULATED SITUATION

A young woman was admitted to the ED with multiple injuries suffered in an automobile accident. Her injuries were those of impact; that is, she presented with a crushed chest, multiple fractures, abdominal trauma, and a head injury.

On admission, her vital signs were as follows: BP 60/30, P 144, and R 28. She presented with the following signs and symptoms:

1. Unconsciousness, with a fixed, dilated left pupil

2. Left scalp laceration

3. Rapid, labored, noisy, paradoxical respirations

4. Cool, pale, cyanotic, and diaphoretic skin

5. Distended abdomen with no bowel sounds auscultated; hematuria

6. Open fracture of the left femur and fibula

Admission laboratory data revealed an elevated white blood cell count and a hematocrit of 26 percent.

This experience in the life of a young woman became the beginning of a long rehabilitation period. She, like many others, was injured in such a way as to need extended emergency care. The system of *assessment and action* was utilized in the early stages of her emergency maintenance. It is this system that will now be discussed.

TRAUMA AND PROPERTIES OF CARE

As the patient with multiple trauma arrives in the ED, two simultaneous interventions must occur. These are:

1. Assessment and maintenance of vital body functions (respirations and heartbeat)

2. Assessment of injuries with necessary action taken once the assessment has been made

AIRWAY

It is imperative to establish an airway first. This may include suctioning the pharynx for blood, vomitus, or secretions, the performance of a tracheostomy in the event of wet-lung syndrome or profuse neck swelling, or the insertion of an endotracheal tube.

BREATHING

Once an airway has been established, ventilation must take place. This may be accomplished through the use of an Ambu bag to provide a few deep breaths to revive the patient, or a volume-cycled respirator to provide extended respiratory support. If the patient has spontaneous respirations, oxygen may be administered 3 to 5 liters/minute by mask.

Auscultation of breath sounds provides information about adequacy of ventilation. It is possible that an endotracheal tube may have passed into the right main-stem bronchus and only one side may be aerated. This would also be obvious by observing the chest during inspiration for symmetry.

Periodic *arterial blood-gas* determinations are needed to assess the effectiveness of respiratory-support interventions and acid-base balance. The severely traumatized patient is likely to hyperventilate because of pain, anxiety, metabolic acidosis, and probable hypoxemia.

Once an airway has been established and breathing is taking

place, either mechanically or spontaneously, the second priority demands action.

CIRCULATION

The second priority in the management of the patient with multiple trauma is to *control bleeding*. This may be done with pressure to the area which is bleeding, or it may take the form of more sophisticated treatment for shock. Once bleeding has been controlled, circulation may have to be supported. Circulatory support may take the form of closed-chest cardiac compression. This must be done in conjunction with ventilation support. The administration of intravenous fluids and the necessary blood products and vasopressors must be carried out as ordered.

Airway—breathing—circulation: These are the top three priorities in trauma management. A thorough assessment of injuries—from head to toe—must also be carried out, but not until the basic life functions, breathing and circulation, have been reestablished. Injuries involving any of the organ systems must be assessed in terms of their effect on the respiration and circulation. *If there is no breath, there can be no life.* Ventilation must not be carried out without perfusion support. That is, merely providing oxygen to the patient's lungs is not enough—it must be assisted in its transfer to the tissues.

TRAUMA AS IT AFFECTS MAJOR ORGAN SYSTEMS

An important priority in caring for the multiple-trauma patient is to obtain a past and present history from a family member or from someone who may have been with the patient at the time of the injury. The history facilitates the diagnosis of the nature of the injury and helps to rule out various causes. In addition, the whole physical and emotional organism must be quickly assessed but only after the airway—breathing—circulation interventions have been made.

INJURIES TO THE CENTRAL NERVOUS SYSTEM

HEAD INJURY A head injury results from the sudden application of force to the *head* and thus to the *scalp, skull,* and *brain.* These three structures are often but not always injured together. The semisolid brain is free-floating in cerebrospinal fluid. At the time of impact, the brain swirls in proportion to the force of the external blow. Mild blows to the head result in little more than a headache. A moderate blow causes clinical neurologic symptoms. As the brain swirls more forcefully, it tends to twist the upper brainstem, a structure which is not free to move. This results in temporary impairment of the function of the reticular activating system, and thus a loss of consciousness. Severe blows result in severe brainstem twisting and hemorrhage from which the brainstem may not recover; prolonged loss of consciousness is the result. This loss of consciousness results from not only brainstem injury but also damage to other loci in the brain, most likely the *medial temporal structures* (Fig. 19-1).[3]

Head injuries may be classified as *open* or *closed*. With open head injuries there is communication between the cranial contents

Figure 19-1 **Mechanisms of head injury.** *(Taken from Smith, R., Head Injuries, in Sproul, C. W., and Mullanney, P. (eds.), Emergency Care: Assessment and Intervention, Mosby, St. Louis, 1974, p. 225.)*

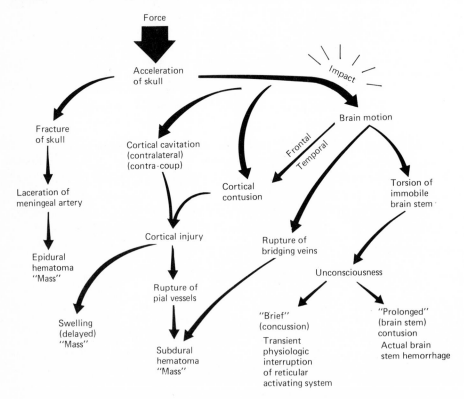

and the air. In addition, the integrity of the scalp or skull has been damaged. With closed head injuries there is also damage to the brain. Although there may be no outward indication of this injury, a thorough neurological examination will reveal this damage. In open or closed head injuries, brain damage, associated hemorrhage, and increased intracranial pressure are the most important aspects for the nurse to consider.

Emergency management of the patient with a head injury involves a system of rapid assessment and action. The principles of treatment outlined below apply to any type of head injury. They are especially applicable for brainstem contusions, cerebral contusions, and hematomas.

1. Determine the state of vital functions of respiration and heartbeat; maintain as necessary. *Suspect accompanying cervical neck injury in all head-injured patients until proved otherwise.*

2. Conduct an immediate minineurological examination. Reassess at frequent intervals, watching for symptoms of increased intracranial pressure (Fig. 19-2):
a. Level of consciousness: orientation to person, place, and time
b. Pupil size and reactivity to light
c. Bilateral movement and sensation of extremities

3. Determine the presence of other injuries and assess for evidence of shock. If any symptoms of shock are present, assess for other organ damage.

4. Determine the nature and extent of the head injury.
a. Obtain a *history* immediately: Note the time that has elapsed since the injury, any loss of consciousness, and any suspicion of drug ingestion.
b. Assess *scalp* injuries: These fall into the categories of contusions, hematomas, abrasions, and lacerations. Stop any bleeding on or about the head. Apply ice to contusions and hematomas and thoroughly cleanse abrasions and lacerations.
c. Assess *skull* injuries: These are classified as *basilar, depressed,* or *linear* fractures. Basilar skull fractures frequently produce hemorrhage from the nose, pharynx, or ears, and blood may appear under the conjunctiva. The escape of cerebrospinal fluid from the ears and the nose is a diagnostic sign of importance. Bloody spinal fluid, if present, suggests brain laceration or contusion.[4] These fractures are best treated with antibiotics to prevent meningitis. A nonemergency operation is the treatment for a depressed skull fracture. However,

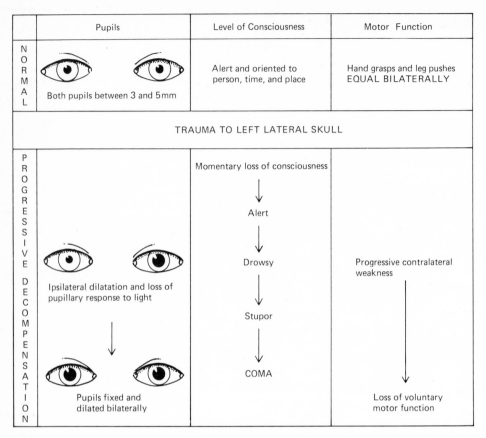

	Pupils	Level of Consciousness	Motor Function
N O R M A L	Both pupils between 3 and 5mm	Alert and oriented to person, time, and place	Hand grasps and leg pushes EQUAL BILATERALLY
	TRAUMA TO LEFT LATERAL SKULL		
P R O G R E S S I V E D E C O M P E N S A T I O N	Ipsilateral dilatation and loss of pupillary response to light Pupils fixed and dilated bilaterally	Momentary loss of consciousness ↓ Alert ↓ Drowsy ↓ Stupor ↓ COMA	Progressive contralateral weakness Loss of voluntary motor function

Figure 19-2 Neurological signs of increased intracranial pressure for the head-injured patient. The ipsilateral pupil dilatation occurs in 90 percent of the head-injured population and is caused by compression of cranial nerve III.

these patients must be closely assessed for *increased intracranial pressure.* Linear skull fractures require no treatment except for observation.

d. Assess brain injuries (see Table 19-1). These fall into four categories:

(1) Concussion. The natural history of brain concussion is one of rapid improvement to an alert level of consciousness. No treatment is indicated.

(2) Brainstem contusion. This is caused by a hemorrhage into and damage to the upper brainstem.

Table 19-1   Assessment of brain injuries.

	Epidural hematoma	Subdural hematoma	Intracerebral hematoma
Cause	Rupture of the middle meningeal artery	Venous hemorrhage underneath the dura	After a fall, most frequently in the elderly
Location	Most frequently in the temporal lobe	Since it is venous in origin, the blood spreads over the entire surface of the brain	Within the cerebrum
Signs and symptoms	Momentary loss of consciousness at the time of the injury, followed by an interval of apparent recovery, then sudden manifestation of muscle twitching due to pressure on the motor cortex	Coma Rising blood pressure with slowing of pulse and respirations	Scattered petechial hemorrhages Coma Confusion
Treatment	Burr holes	Surgical evacuation by suction	Evacuation of clot via craniotomy
Onset	Rapid	Slow, insidious	

(3) Cerebral contusion. This causes lack of nerve function of the bruised portion of the cerebral hemispheres.

(4) Hematomas. *Lateralized neurologic responses usually mean hematoma.* This condition is a neurosurgical emergency.

5. Start an IV line with fluids TKO unless otherwise ordered. Administer fluids with care to prevent fluid overload. *Keep accurate intake and output records.*

6. Protect the patient from self-injury during any period of restlessness or seizures. Orient the patient to three spheres (person, place, and time) in an effort to bring him or her back to the realm of the familiar which may be comforting.

Increased Intracranial Pressure: Every effort must be taken to prevent or to decrease the brain damage that can be caused by increased intracranial pressure. While surgical intervention will most probably be mandatory, the following intermediate treatment may be instituted to prevent further deterioration until the neurosurgical team is mobilized:

1. Artificial hyperventilation. This lowers the patient's *carbon dioxide* levels and causes *cerebral vasoconstriction.* Intravascular blood volume within the brain is reduced, thus providing more space for the expanding hematoma. There is less shift of the brain and a temporary reduction in brainstem compression.

2. Steroids and diuretics. Steroids such as dexamathasone are used to reduce cerebral edema. While many authorities question the effectiveness of this drug, steroids are believed to protect cerebral blood vessels and reduce subsequent cerebral compression during edema.[5] Osmotic diuretics such as mannitol or urea promote water loss from the interstitial space, reduce brain bulk, and allow more room for the expanding hematoma.

Since increased intracranial pressure and its accompanying cerebral damage can occur in minutes, *the sine qua non of emergency management of the head-injured patient is careful, repetitive observation* and *rapid intervention when necessary.*

SPINAL FRACTURES AND DISLOCATIONS   Fractures and dislocations of the spine are serious because of the danger of injury to the *spinal cord* (see Fig. 22-1). They appear most frequently in the Vth, VIth, and VIIth cervical, the XIIth thoracic, and the Ist lumbar vertebrae because there is a greater range of mobility of the vertebral column in these areas.[4]

In effecting immediate treatment, the emergency staff should place the patient in a *neutral position,* that is, with the head, back, legs, knees, and arms straight. The patient must be evaluated for *motor* and *sensory changes.* X-rays must be taken to determine the presence and level of the fracture. Moving the patient onto a Foster or Stryker frame must be done, keeping the head immobilized in a neutral position and with sandbags and a cervical collar. The body must not twist. *The emergency nurse must suspect any multiple trauma patient of having a spinal injury until proved otherwise.*

It is imperative to watch these patients for signs and symptoms of spinal shock, although it rarely occurs. In this complicating syndrome, there is a depression of all reflexes. The blood pressure falls and there may be an abrupt onset of fever. Since sympathetic activity has been blocked to any paralyzed limbs, the patient will not perspire in these areas; hence there is less opportunity for him or her to lose heat in this manner.[4]

If it is necessary to establish an airway in a patient with suspected spinal fracture, the use of the *modified jaw thrust* is suggested. This involves "jutting" the lower jaw forward to open the airway. It would be dangerous to utilize the technique of hyperextension of the head with these patients.

INJURIES TO THE RESPIRATORY SYSTEM

In vehicular accidents, the chest is particularly vulnerable to trauma. Many kinds of injuries occur when a blow to the chest is experienced.

FLAIL CHEST   When the chest is crushed between two objects, multiple rib fractures may occur so that one portion of the chest wall no longer has a bony connection with the rest of the rib cage. This is called a *flail chest* (Fig. 19-3). These injuries are commonly accompanied by the collection of blood in the chest cavity (*hemothorax*) or the escape of air from the injured lung into the pleural cavity (*pneumothorax*). Needle aspirations or chest tube drainage of the blood and/or air allows the lung to reexpand. Intubation with mechanical ventilation is often instituted until the flail chest has resolved.

TENSION PNEUMOTHORAX   Air may be drawn into the pleural space from the injured lung or through a small hole in the chest wall. In either case, the air that enters the chest cavity with each inspiration is trapped there; it cannot be expelled through the air passage or small hole in the chest wall. A tension builds within the chest, which produces a collapse of the lung and may even push the heart and the great vessels toward the normal side of the chest (*mediastinal shift*).

It is important to:

1. *Look* at the patient's color and observe the quality of the respiration; note the position of the trachea.

2. *Listen* with stethescope for decreased breath sounds.

3. *Feel* with the hands, by palpating, for crepitus and deviation of trachea.

A tension pneumothorax is a life-threatening chest injury, requiring immediate intervention. If a chest tube cannot be inserted *stat,* an 18-gauge needle can be inserted in the *second intercostal* space on the injured side at the *midclavicular line,* thus relieving tension. A chest tube to suction can then be inserted in the pleural space.

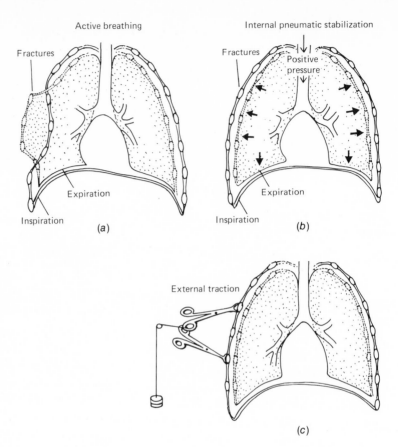

Figure 19-3 Stabilization of the flail chest. (*a*) The paradoxical motion associated with active breathing. (*b*) Stabilization of the fractured segment in the "out" position throughout the respiratory cycle by controlled positive pressure respiration. (*c*) Stabilization of the fractured segment in the "out" position by external traction, using towel clips and orthopedic weight suspension. (*Taken from Ballinger, W., Rutherford, R., and Zuidema, G., The Management of Trauma, Saunders, Philadelphia, 1968, p. 300.*)

SUCKING CHEST WOUNDS An open pneumothorax may occur when there is an opening in the chest large enough for air to pass freely in and out of the thoracic cavity with each attempted respiration. This rush of air produces a sucking sound. The lung is collapsed, and the heart and great vessels are pushed toward the uninjured side with each inspiration and toward the injured side with expiration. This embarrasses circulatory function. *It is lifesaving to stop the flow of air through the* *opening in the chest.* A gauze soaked with petrolatum jelly can seal the hole and prevent respiratory distress.

WET LUNG SYNDROME   Any substance which serves to interfere with the normal passage of air into the lungs can cause the "wet lung syndrome." Increased secretions and blood in the tracheobronchial tree and inability to cough due to pain can cause these symptoms: cyanosis, shallow, labored respirations, and noisy breath sounds. One must institute remedial measures even before central cyanosis appears. *Central cyanosis is one of the last overt signs to occur in respiratory distress and indicates that oxygen saturation is 85 percent or less.*

Trachestomy is almost always necessary. It is important to suction the secretions and keep the patient in high Fowler's position, if possible, to facilitate respiration. Hyperextension of the neck may be necessary to ensure adequate air exchange. (This is done only if cervical neck injury has been ruled out.)

PULMONARY AND CARDIAC CONTUSIONS   Two other manifestations of chest trauma are pulmonary and cardiac contusions.

When the patient has sustained a blow on the anterior chest or a crush injury, there may be bleeding into the pericardial sac. This may result in compression of the heart—a life-threatening condition. The myocardium may be contused, and the patient may exhibit signs and symptoms of myocardial infarction. When the heart has been damaged in this manner, the patient exhibits *symptoms of pericardial tamponade:*

1. Cyanosis

2. Dyspnea

3. Weak, thready pulse

4. Paradoxical pulse

5. Narrow pulse pressure

6. Falling blood pressure

7. Loss of consciousness

8. Distended neck veins

9. Increased central venous pressure

Immediate decompression of the pericardial sac is indicated and can be accomplished by needle aspiration through the left parasternal fifth or sixth interspace. Serial enzymes, daily ECGs, and bed rest must also be ordered.

The patient with pulmonary contusions manifests with deteriorating arterial blood gases and often requires ventilatory support because of a tendency to breathe shallowly. There is a radiodensity in parts of the lung field upon x-ray which must be observed daily for changes in characteristics and size. [4]

It is important to note that even if the patient has not suffered direct trauma to the chest, there may be life-threatening pulmonary complications from injuries to other organ systems. For example, an injury to the brainstem may cause depressed respirations and hence atelectasis secondary to shallow respiratory excursions. Abdominal trauma may cause damage to the diaphragm which will also hamper breathing effectiveness.

Oxygen administration is helpful for these patients as it facilitates effective tissue nourishment. The oxygen must be warmed and humidified if administered through a tracheostomy or endotracheal tube, as it bypasses the normal respiratory tract.

INJURY TO THE CIRCULATORY SYSTEM

Trauma to the circulatory system implies an injury to a vascular structure or to the heart itself. Since injury to the heart was discussed briefly in the section on chest trauma, bleeding injuries will be discussed here.

The first priority is to control accessible bleeding by a pressure dressing. Accessible bleeders can be clamped with hemostats to control hemorrhaging. Secondly, the patient must be assessed for signs of shock. Since blood volume may be reduced by more than 10 percent before any signs of shock develop, it is critical to *assume shock initially until proved otherwise.*

Circulatory shock is defined as an abnormal state of circulation in which the cardiac output is so reduced that the tissues of the body are inadequately perfused. Shock may be divided into three states: mild, moderate, and severe.

Signs and symptoms: Respirations in mild shock are rapid and deep; as shock becomes more severe, respirations become rapid and shallow. The skin is cool and pale, unless there is a high fever as may occur with severe head injuries. As shock deepens, skin changes continue to occur. Skin temperature becomes cold and the extremities become moist and cyanotic. The blood pressure in early shock may be normal or slightly elevated owing to the action of epinephrine and norepinephrine. But as shock continues and loss of circulating volume increases, the blood pressure starts to drop.

As the shock state worsens, the level of consciousness changes from alertness and apprehension to mental cloudiness and coma due to *cerebral hypoxia* and an increasing level of *lactic acid.* Urine output is decreased in moderate shock and may be absent in severe shock. As the circulation deteriorates, the pulse becomes rapid, weak, and easily collapsible. The patient's complaints, if he or she is awake, can include thirst, pain, or fear.

INJURY TO THE SKELETAL SYSTEM

The skeletal system assessment includes observation of all extremities for *pain, swelling,* obvious *deformity,* and *movement.* An injured extremity should be immobilized. There are four categories of acute orthopedic emergencies: (1) vascular injury; (2) bony or soft tissue injury; (3) open fractures; and (4) dislocations. In each of the above injuries, one should observe for the following five signs and symptoms: *pain, pulse, paresthesia, paralysis, and pallor.*[6]

Fat embolism is a constant danger after multiple fractures. The theory is that fractures, particularly of the long bones, allow fat droplets to be released from the marrow into the general circulation. From there, they lodge in the lungs or brain. Most frequently, fat emboli occur within the first 24 hours after trauma. Signs and symptoms of fat emboli are listed in Table 19-2.

INJURY TO THE ABDOMEN

The abdomen should be closely inspected for signs of abdominal trauma: *contusions, abrasions,* or *wounds.* It should also be inspected for distention or rigidity, indicating possible internal injury. Increasing distention can be detected by taking frequent girth measurements. The patient, if conscious, should be questioned about the presence of any abdominal pain. If the abdomen is rigid, the physician may want to do a paracentesis to confirm the presence

Table 19-2	**Signs and symptoms of fat emboli.**
	Apprehension
	Mild agitation
	Shortness of breath
	Diaphoresis
	Tachycardia, pallor, and cyanosis
	Classic sign: Petechial hemorrhages of the chest and shoulders, which may extend to the axillae, flanks, and conjunctivae
	Decreased PaO_2

of blood. If present, this would be an indication for exploratory surgery.

A nasogastric tube should be inserted to detect the presence of upper gastrointestinal bleeding. A rectal examination should be performed also to detect lower gastrointestinal bleeding. Vital signs must be monitored closely, and *recorded,* as they may be the only indication of internal injury in the early stages.

In the case of protrusion of any of the abdominal organs, cover them with a sterile saline dressing to prevent drying of the viscera. Do not try to manipulate the organs back into the abdomen. Doing so may cause shock and peritonitis. Flex the knees of the victim— this prevents further protrusion.[4] Tetanus toxoid should be administered in an effort to prevent infection by the clostridium bacilli.

TRAUMA ON A CONTINUUM—MONITORING PARAMETERS

Throughout the descriptions of the myriad signs and symptoms of multiple trauma, various monitoring parameters have been mentioned. It is critical that measurements of the patient's condition be made accurately and completely. These measurements must also be recorded completely and correctly, as the patient's record is an extension of that person while in the hospital. It must be given as much care as the patient is given! Data recording is also of legal and medical importance and must be carried out to its full extent. It is important to note a *pattern of changes* with regard to these parameters and not their mere absolute values. The use of a flow sheet greatly facilitates the recording of these data (see Table 19-3a and b).

EMOTIONAL REACTIONS TO TRAUMA

The patient and family can be conceptualized as going through four stages in their emotional reaction to the traumatic event. These are the stages of impact, retreat, acknowledgement, and reconstruction.

The stage of impact is the patient's initial encounter with the critical situation. The patient enters a state of shock and exhibits much automatic and poorly controlled behavior. It is a stage of depersonalization and numbness.[7]

Table 19-3a   Comprehensive flow sheet to be used for all critically ill or injured patients. *(Adapted from Medical Programs. Inc.: Emergency Department Nursing Student Workbook, American Journal of Nursing Co., New York, 1973, p. 19.)*

NAME: _Mary Phillips_   AGE: _42_   DATE: _____

PROBLEM: _Head Injury: Possible Epidural Hematoma_
Fractured ® Femur
Multiple Lacerations + Abrasions
Old Anteroseptal MI 6/72   TETANUS TOXOID: _IMAT0645_

TIME	PUPILS L	PUPILS R	LOC	BP	P/R	CVP	Hb/Hct	ARTERIAL BLOOD pH/HCO₃⁻	pO₂/PCO₂	1 IV FLUID cc/Tot.	2 IV FLUID cc/Tot.	BLOOD cc/Tot.	IN cc/Tot.	URINE cc/Tot.	OTHER OUTPUT cc/Tot.	REMARKS
0600	•	•	4	130/80	96/22	3.5	12.5/34	7.46/24	80/34	periph. 50/50	↑UP 50/50	NONE	100/100	Foley 200/200	N.G. 20/20	skull films
																family here

Table 19-3b	This neurological chart describes four levels of consciousness. It should be attached to the flow sheet (Table 19-3a) for easy reference.

Levels of consciousness

1. *Alert:* The patient responds immediately, fully, and appropriately to visual, auditory, and other stimuli.

2. *Lethargic:* Responses to stimulation are delayed or incomplete, and increased stimulation is necessary to get the patient to respond. Patient may be delirious and restless, or quiet, falling asleep again when left alone.

3. *Stuporous:* The patient can be aroused only by vigorous and continuous stimulation. Such stimulation may arouse the patient enough to answer simple questions with one or two words, or responses may be only restless motor activity or purposeful behavior directed to avoiding further stimulation.

4. *Semicomatose:* The patient is unresponsive except to superficial, relatively mild painful stimulation to which he or she makes some purposeful avoiding motor response. Spontaneous motion is uncommon, but the patient may groan or mutter.

5. *Comatose:* The patient is unresponsive to all but very painful stimuli to which he or she may make fragmentary, delayed reflex withdrawal. In deeper stages, all responsiveness may be lost. There is no spontaneous movement and respirations may be irregular.

The stage of *retreat* is a time of great anxiety. The numbness brought on by the impact causes the patient to retreat in an attempt to return to what existed before the critical event occurred. The emotional reactions of the patient indicate not so much a refusal to face the trauma as an *inability* to do so at the given time. The patient may demonstrate behavior ranging from indifference to euphoria.[7]

The *acknowledgement* stage brings the patient to the realization that loss has occurred. The patient enters the process of grieving, starting with shock and disbelief. It is important in this stage to be available to the patient to help him or her verbalize recollections of the events which have transpired.[7]

In dealing with the physically traumatized patient and family members, it is best to give short, simple, truthful answers to their questions. These people are very anxious! Giving false reassurance is poor nursing care and makes their grief more bitter in the long term, as they then have not been prepared to cope with possible loss.

Table 19-4 Nursing care plan for the patient with multiple trauma.

Date	Potential problems	Nursing interventions	Goal to be achieved	Deadline

	1. Respiratory distress due to:
	 a. Chest trauma
	 b. Central nervous system trauma (cerebral edema)
		At least q. 5 minutes observe:
		 Character and rate of respiration
		 color (pale, cyanotic)
		 lung sounds
		 pulse rate and quality
		 signs of hyperventilation
		 anxiety level
		 level of consciousness
		 symmetry of respiratory excursions
		 If in distress:
		   Insert airway
		   Suction p.r.n.
		   Administer O_2
		   Tracheostomy tray on stand-by
			No cyanosis
			 Adequate blood gases
			 Clear breath sounds
			 Slow, regular respirations
				By time of transfer

	2. Hypotension and shock due to:
	 a. Volume loss
	 b. Infection
	 c. Pump failure
		At least q. 5 minutes observe:
		 Signs and symptoms of shock
		 BP
		 Pulse rate and quality
		 Skin temperature, color
		 Monitor CVP
		 Respiratory rate
		 Draw blood for CBC
		 Insert foley catheter
		 Elevate feet
		 Allay patient's apprehension
		 Prevent massive circulatory overload
		 Apply pressure dressing to any wounds
		 Keep patient warm
		 Administer O_2, if ordered
		 Start an intravenous route
		 Administer blood and blood products, as ordered
			Stable vital signs
			 Stable hematocrit
			 Adequate replacement with fluids or blood products
			 Adequate perfusion to:
			   CNS
			   Renal arteries
			   Periphery
				By time of transfer

(continued)

Table 19.4 (continued)

Date	Potential problems	Nursing interventions	Goal to be achieved	Deadline

	3. Potential neurological damage	At least q. 5 minutes, observe:
		Level of Consciousness and VS
		Pupils: fixed, reactive, dilated, constricted, equal
		Presence and nature of seizures
		Obtain history from attendants
		Elevate head of bed
		Keep IV TKO
		Place sandbag to immobilize head and neck
		Protect from self-injury due to restlessness
		Watch for signs of increasing intracranial pressure:
		  Increase in temperature
		  Slowing of pulse
		  Slowing of respirations
		  Widening pulse pressure
		  Change in behavior
			Stable neurological vital signs including reactive pupils, level of consciousness, sensation, and movement of extremities.	By time of transfer

	4. Abdominal trauma	Observe abdomen for wounds, rigidity, distention Check for hematuria Observe for respiratory impairment Listen for bowel sounds Assist with diagnostic procedures	Stable vital signs Completion of paracentesis and abdominal x-rays	By time of transfer
	5. Fractures	Observe for pain, pulselessness, pallor, paralysis, paresthesia, swelling, open wounds Immobilize an extremity with a suspected fracture Assist with x-rays	Immobilization of fractured extremity Stable vital signs	By time of transfer

6. Pain	Obtain analgesia order from medical department Make positive statement regarding effectiveness of medications Ice towels for thirst	Verbalizes less pain Lies quietly for short intervals (several minutes)	By time of transfer
7. Anxiety due to: a. Abrupt injury b. Extremely upsetting or unknown diagnosis, or prognosis c. Stress factors: Pain Embarrassment Legal/financial concerns Patient's perception of situation Lack of control over situation Family demands	Observe emotional response Explain all procedures Answer all patient's questions Talk with patient Listen and reassure as needed If a family member is fairly calm, allow to stay with the patient at intervals Actively listen	Understands procedures deemed necessary for diagnosis and treatment Aware of plan of treatment Verbalizes anxieties Calm effect	By time of transfer

The final stage, that of *reconstruction,* is one of reintegration of the new body image. The patient is reorganizing social values and making adjustments to new technical devices which help in the activities of daily living. A renewed sense of self-worth should come over the patient. It is important for caring personnel to be emphathetic to the patient's anxieties. This is a time which may be awkward for the patient, and much encouragement is needed.

Finally, nurses need to review their basic beliefs concerning the person who becomes a patient. A nurse's feelings regarding the traumatic event which brought this patient to the hospital must be examined. Judgments of those persons involved in the injury or a repugnance of the patient's physical appearance should not be communicated to the patient or family. Facial expressions and attitudes easily communicate feelings of acceptance or rejection.

Trauma as a human experience demands that ED practitioners provide skilled and concerned care. The care provided must involve an orderly system of prompt assessment and immediate initiation of treatment. A comprehensive summary of problem-oriented assessment and intervention is included in Table 19-4 which appears on pp. 293–295. This system of *assessment* and *action* can save the lives of patients—all of whom have a *right* to high-level emergency care.

REFERENCES

1. Stephenson, H., *Immediate Care of the Acutely Ill and Injured,* Mosby, St. Louis, 1974, p. xiii.

2. Baker, Robert J., et al., "Priority of Management of Patients with Multiple Injuries," *Surgical Clinics of North America,* February 1970, pp. 3–10.

3. Youmans, J., *Neurological Surgery,* vol. II, Saunders, Philadelphia, 1973, pp. 947–948.

4. Brunner, L. S., et al., *Textbook of Medical-Surgical Nursing,* 2d ed., Lippincott, Philadelphia, 1970, pp. 384, 815–954.

5. Smith, R., "Head Injuries," in Sproul, C. W., and Mullaney, P., *Emergency Care: Assessment and Intervention,* Mosby, St. Louis, 1974, p. 238.

6. Webb, K. J., "Early Assessment of Orthopedic Injuries," *American Journal of Nursing,* June 1974, pp. 1048–52.

7. Lee, J. M., "Emotional Reactions to Trauma," *Nursing Clinics of North America,* December 1970, pp. 577–587.

BIBLIOGRAPHY

Bouterie, Ronald L., "STAT! How Would You Manage This Patient," *Journal of Emergency Nursing,* September–October 1975, pp. 41–44.

Northfield, D. W. C., *The Surgery of the Central Nervous System,* Blackwell Scientific Publications, Ltd., London, 1973.

Stein, Alice, et al., "Multiple Fractures," *Nursing '74,* November 1974, pp. 26–32.

Tharp, Gerald D., "SHOCK: The Overall Mechanisms," *American Journal of Nursing,* December 1974, p. 2208.

Wagner, Mary, "Assessment of Patients with Multiple Injuries," *American Journal of Nursing,* October 1972, pp. 1822–1827.

CHAPTER 20
ABDOMINAL EMERGENCIES
J. B. GREENWELL, JR., M.D.

A CUTE abdominal disease and trauma, which have many common diagnostic and therapeutic aspects, are discussed in this chapter. This presentation will outline the general nature of the acute abdomen with emphasis on the initial clinical and laboratory evaluation. While specific examples of abdominal diseases will be provided to illustrate key concepts, primary emphasis will be placed on abdominal trauma. It is not possible to discuss every surgical disease separately and fully. Correlative reading in surgical and nursing texts will be helpful.

ABDOMINAL ANATOMY

The abdomen is the cavity lying below the muscular diaphragm which separates it from the thoracic cavity. It includes the hollow pelvis below, the spinal column at the back, and the abdominal muscular wall in front. Part of this space is bounded by the ribs above and the pelvic girdle below. The peritoneum, a thin glistening membrane, lines this space and also the outside surface of most of the organs.

The abdominal organs either lie in a *retroperitoneal* position or are held in place by the *mesentery,* a thin suspending membrane which contains the blood, nerve, and lymphatic supplies. The abdomen is divided into a number of reference areas which are summarized in Fig. 20-1. With these reference areas the position of organs and pathologic findings can be described accurately. The locations of the abdominal organs, with few exceptions, are quite regular, as illustrated in Fig. 20-2.

THE ACUTE ABDOMEN

The acute abdomen is a general term which includes diverse conditions, both traumatic and nontraumatic, requiring urgent care. These conditions include infection, hemorrhage, peritonitis caused by perforations of various organs, vascular problems, inflammatory conditions without infection, space-occupying masses, and various mechanical problems, including torsion or obstruction of the gut or other

Figure 20-1 Abdominal areas. Dotted lines divide the abdomen into its four major quadrants: left and right upper and lower quadrants. The numbers mark the following areas: 1,3, right and left hypochondrium; 2, epigastrium; 4,6, right and left flanks; 5, periumbilical area; 7,9, right and left iliac areas; 8, hypogastrium or suprapubic area.

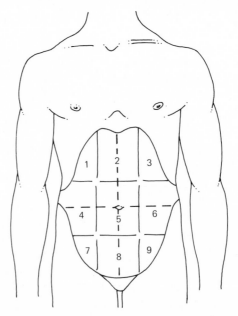

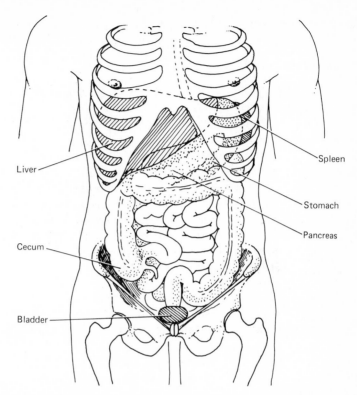

Figure 20-2 Normal location of the abdominal viscrea. *(Taken from Dunphy, J., and Botoford, T., Physical Examination of the Surgical Patient, Saunders, Philadelphia, 1958, p. 103.)*

organs. Some of these problems are obvious, others are more subtle. They may range from an acute gastric perforation in the newborn baby, presenting mainly as respiratory distress, to appendicitis in a 90-year-old patient, which may have none of the expected hallmarks of that disease. While there are many conditions which cause an acute abdomen, a few basic principles in *examination, diagnosis,* and *treatment* are common to all.

EXAMINATION

Examination of the abdomen for disease or injury is only a part of the total assessment of a patient. Examination of other systems may also help in the recognition of abdominal disease. For example, vital signs may indicate that shock is present in the case of a ruptured spleen, and the pale color of the mucous membranes can attest to a low hemoglobin from the blood loss. Jaundice may point to liver dysfunction or biliary obstruction. There are four essential maneuvers in examining the abdomen: *inspection, palpation, auscultation,* and *percussion.*

INSPECTION Inspection of the abdomen may indicate signs of trauma or disease. Normally the abdomen is described as flat or *scaphoid.* Abrasions contusions, lacerations, or distention of the abdomen with blood may be seen with blunt trauma. Discoloration of the umbilicus (*Cullen's sign*) can indicate intraperitoneal bleeding, while ecchymosis in the flanks is seen occasionally with hemorrhagic pancreatitis (*Grey Turner's sign*). Specific organs may occasionally be enlarged and visible, such as a liver involved with tumor, distended loops of bowel with intestinal obstruction, or an incarcerated hernia. One may look for distended collateral veins on the abdominal wall in advanced cirrhosis with portal hypertension.

AUSCULTATION Generally auscultation is carried out next as it is a gentle maneuver. The stethoscope is placed in the different quadrants of the abdomen to listen to the bowel activity. Bowel sounds are normally *active* and *intermittent.* In the case of bowel obstruction, they may become high pitched or tinkling, while in severe injury or peritonitis they become *hypoactive* or absent. A special maneuver is to listen for the *succussion splash* of fluid in a distended or obstructed stomach. Vascular sounds or bruits may accompany blood vessel disease.

PALPATION The third step in examining the abdomen is palpation, that is, examining with the hand. One first determines if the abdominal wall is tense or soft. In the healthy, relaxed patient, the abdomen is soft; with gentle examination there is no tenderness. It may become tense from distention of the bowel with fluid or gas, ascitic fluid from liver disease, or advanced cancer. Tenseness may also be produced by muscle contraction of the abdominal wall. This is described as *spasm,* which may be *voluntary* (guarding) or *involuntary.* Severe generalized spasm is known as *rigidity.* It is important to determine and describe the location of tenderness (direct and rebound), spasm, and the presence of masses. Any enlargement of the various organs is also important to note.

PERCUSSION Finally, one performs percussion. This consists of gentle tapping of one finger with another over the entire abdomen, listening to the note produced, and again observing for tenderness (*direct* and *rebound*). One may also determine the size and position of solid organs and ascertain the presence of gas, either free or in the bowel.

ETIOLOGY OF THE ACUTE ABDOMEN

When considering the etiology of an acute abdomen, one may conveniently think in terms of several major subdivisions.

INFLAMMATION   Inflammatory disease is one of the commonest causes of the acute abdomen. *Appendicitis* is the most common surgical abdominal disease and occurs in all age groups. The diagnosis may be difficult at both extremes of age. It is well treated by appendectomy. *Cholecystitis* with inflammation of the gallbladder is also a very common disease; some episodes resolve, while others demand urgent surgery. *Diverticulitis* is a serious disease due to inflammation of a diverticulum, a small out-pocketing of the colon, which usually occurs in the middle and later years of life. Again, this disease may resolve spontaneously or go on to produce complications such as local abscess, perforation, or obstruction, all of which require surgery. *Pancreatitis* varies from a very mild to life-threatening disease. The most common causes are alcoholism and gallstones. Ulcerative colitis, regional enteritis, primary pediatric peritonitis, and Meckel's diverticulitis are examples of other inflammatory diseases causing an acute abdomen. *Viral gastroenteritis,* a common self-limited disease, can sometimes cause diagnostic concern as it may appear as acute inflammatory abdominal disease. Recognizing it is important because surgery is obviously not indicated.

PERFORATION   The most common spontaneous perforations include duodenal and gastric ulcers, appendicitis, diverticulitis and cancer of the colon, ovarian cysts, ectopic tubal pregnancies, and, much less commonly, perforation of an organ like the gallbladder. Surgical anastomoses may occasionally leak, producing an acute abdomen. Foreign bodies that are swallowed or introduced into the rectum or endoscopic procedures on the gastrointestinal tract may cause perforations which result in serious acute abdominal disease. Trauma may cause perforations of any of the hollow organs.

OBSTRUCTIONS   The third major subdivision is obstruction, and the gastrointestinal tract is mainly involved. Obstructions are classified as (1) *complete,* when no further gas and fluid will pass the point of obstruction, or (2) *partial,* when some gas and fluid are passed. Partial obstructions sometimes resolve spontaneously with conservative treatment, while most complete obstructions will require surgery.

Obstruction of the bowel or other organs may be caused by tumor, inflammations, a torsion (volvulus), adhesions, or hernias. *Intussusception* of the bowel occurs when a portion of the bowel telescopes into the distal part causing obstruction; this condition is most common in childhood. Foreign bodies may obstruct the intestine. For example, bezoars are concretions of material, usually plant fiber, which may collect in the stomach over many years to create gastric obstruction. Gallstones may erode from the gallbladder into the gut and result in an obstruction called gallstone ileus. The biliary tract can be obstructed by tumor or stone to create acute abdominal disease. On rare occasions, severe constipation in a bedridden patient may pose as an obstruction, which does not need surgical relief. Again, this is only a partial list of examples of this category of disease.

VASCULAR PROBLEMS   A fourth category of acute abdominal disease, vascular problems, includes both *venous* and *arterial* events. Mesenteric vascular occlusions can occur in the artery owing to emboli from the heart or to closing off of vessels from arteriosclerotic disease. Venous mesenteric occlusion usually occurs in elderly patients with cardiac disease and congestive heart failure. Loss of circulation to a portion of the bowel with resulting necrosis may occur when the bowel is strangulated in a hernia or when a volvulus of the intestine occurs. Abdominal aortic aneurysms may rupture with pain, bleeding, and shock. Dissecting aortic aneurysms usually develop in the thoracic aorta, proceeding downward to the abdominal vessels, and create acute pain and problems secondary to the obstruction of various branch vessels.

TRAUMA   Another large subsection of acute abdominal disease, trauma, is discussed later in this chapter.

BLEEDING   Bleeding may occur in the general abdominal cavity or into the lumen of the intestine. Aside from trauma, the common causes of bleeding are ulcers of the upper gastrointestinal tract, tumors of the stomach and colon, congenital anomalies such as a Meckel's diverticulum of the ileum, and inflammatory disease such as ulcerative colitis and Crohn's disease. Bleeding from the upper gastrointestinal tract may result in either hematemesis or melena; bleeding from the lower bowel results in dark melena or passage of bright blood (hematochezia). Bleeding may or may not be accompanied by inflammation and pain. It often appears simply as shock.

Table 20-1	A partial list of clinical conditions which may mimic acute abdominal disease.	
1. Coronary thrombosis		8. Renal and prostatic infections
2. Pneumonia		9. Sickle-cell anemia
3. Malaria		10. Tabetic crisis
4. Typhoid		11. Lead poisoning
5. Herpes zoster		12. Severe constipation
6. Acute hepatic congestion in heart failure		13. Ingestion of toxins
7. Diabetic ketoacidosis		14. Bite of black widow spider

OTHER CONDITIONS   There is a large group of conditions which are *mimics* of the acute abdomen. In the pediatric patient, infections of the ear, nose, and chest are often accompanied by abdominal complaints. These conditions are important to mention since it is necessary to exclude them in the differential diagnosis (see Table 20-1).

INTERIM CARE OF THE PATIENT

The patient with abdominal disease or injury requires general observation, diagnostic maneuvers, and treatment. The goal is to provide comprehensive care while evaluating the abdominal problem.

Maintenance of the *airway* is the first consideration. A patient who is vomiting or comatose is in danger of aspirating stomach contents into the lungs. Suctioning the oral cavity, providing supplementary oxygen, positioning the patient appropriately, using oral airways or endotracheal intubation as required, and providing artificial support of ventilation are of the first importance.

The control of *bleeding* is also of primary importance. Sometimes it can be controlled with pressure, particularly in the extremities and in lacerations. Internal hemorrhage, if massive, will, of course, require urgent surgery. Vital signs need to be recorded and watched closely since shock may develop rapidly or insidiously. The urine output and central venous pressure (CVP) may also need to be monitored as indicators of circulatory status. Early treatment for shock or shock prevention will consist of administering intravenous fluids or blood as the situation dictates.

Transportation without delay is essential, both outside and within the hospital. Position of the patient is determined by the problem. Usually, the patient is placed flat on the back. The head may be lowered if the patient is vomiting or in shock. Nothing should be given by mouth.

If the patient's abdomen is *impaled* by an object, this should not be removed, but simply stabilized with dressings and removed later in the operating room. In the event that abdominal viscera are protruding through wounds, these are best covered with *sterile saline dressings.* No attempt is made to replace organs in the abdomen until later in the operating room.

Medications may need to be started early in the treatment of abdominal problems. However, one usually avoids using narcotics during the evaluation of abdominal trauma, especially in the unstable patient. These may obscure pain, hinder the diagnosis, and also potentiate shock. Antibiotics and other drugs should not be given until the provisional diagnosis is made and treatment plans are established.

HISTORY

Important points in history-taking must always be sought when evaluating the patient with an abdominal crisis since the history may give as important clues as the physical examination. The frequency of a disease relates to *age.* While intussusception might be the commonest cause of melena in a 2-year-old, colon carcinoma becomes important in the older patient. The patient's *sex* is obviously important in evaluating pelvic symptoms, and a menstrual history must always be taken.

The *course of onset* of the disease may provide important data. Chronic pain, bleeding, weight loss, change in bowel or digestive habits, jaundice, and other signs are most significant. In addition, one must always know the *past history* of operations and illnesses.

The history from relatives or paramedical personnel may add much to what one hears from a desperately ill patient. Other significant data includes a *history of exposures,* such as to hepatitis, *geographic factors* such as recent visits to tropic areas, *drugs* that may cause surgical disease, such as aspirin, alcohol, or steroids. One should always elicit a history of *allergies* and *bleeding tendencies.*

SIGNS AND SYMPTOMS

Having taken the history and performed a total examination of the patient, one may then focus on the specific abdominal findings. The principal symptoms and signs to consider in acute abdominal disease are four: *pain and tenderness, distention, rigidity,* and *vomiting.*

These signs and symptoms can often lead the examiner to a specific diagnosis or, if that is not possible, to general judgments about therapy. Sometimes surgery is required without a diagnosis. At other times, repeated observation and further diagnostic maneuvers are best.

PAIN AND TENDERNESS

In the majority of cases of acute abdominal disease, pain is the main symptom and must be carefully evaluated. As a general rule, in a previously healthy patient, severe pain of over *6 hours duration* is most often of surgical importance. Pain may be very sudden in onset, as in a perforated ulcer, or more gradual over a period of a day or so, as in appendicitis. The *location* and *character* of pain are very important. Gastric and biliary colic are in the upper abdomen; small bowel pain is felt in the periumbilical area and the large bowel in the lower abdominal region. It may be localized, for example, in early appendicitis, or generalized, if the appendix has perforated and peritonitis has occurred. One must also ask, is the pain steady as in diverticulitis or cholecystitis, or is it colicky (crampy and intermittent) as in gastroenteritis or intestinal obstructions? A patient with peritonitis will lie still, avoiding movement, while one with colic may writhe about in agony.

Referred pain must be considered. A ruptured spleen or ectopic pregnancy may cause shoulder pain in the phrenic nerve distribution (c. 3 to 5 dermatone) due to irritation of the undersurface of the diaphragm by blood. Pneumonia or pleurisy are, in contrast, intrathoracic conditions which could produce the same symptoms. A fractured lumbar vertebra can also cause abdominal pain and findings to suggest an acute abdomen.

Tenderness often goes along with pain but must be distinguished from it. Pain is a feeling which the patient complains of and which is subjective, while tenderness is an objective finding which the examiner elicits. Carefully map the area of tenderness with one finger and by light percussion of the abdomen first. Then check for *cough tenderness,* having the patient indicate the area which hurts. *Rebound tenderness* is a test for peritoneal irritation; after pressing on the abdomen slowly, one removes the hand quickly and may elicit tenderness in another inflamed area. One must not omit examination of the *flank,* the *costovertebral angles* over the kidneys, the *lower costal area,* or the *rectum* and *pelvis.* Always ask if a patient has been given narcotic drugs or antibiotics which might obscure the present findings.

DISTENTION AND PERISTALSIS

Distention and peristalsis are important to assess by visual, palpatory, and auscultatory means. Bowel sounds may be increased (hyperactive) as in gastroenteritis, or characteristically high-pitched with quiet intervals as in intestinal obstruction. They may be diminished or absent in severe inflammation as in generalized peritonitis. Paralytic ileus is usually on a reflex basis, suggesting some intraabdominal problem. It will occur in advanced appendicitis, cholecystitis, toxic megacolon, and many other diseases and trauma.

Many abdominal problems can cause distention, for example, ascites due to liver disease, intestinal obstruction, or masses such as the bladder or an enlarged organ. Percussion is done to determine whether the distention is due to a solid organ or gas. It may be helpful to elicit a succussion splash in the obstructed and distended stomach. Always carefully palpate all hernial areas for sites of obstruction.

RIGIDITY

Rigidity or spasm of the abdominal wall is carefully noted. It may be the *voluntary spasm* due to early appendicitis or an uncooperative patient or a true *involuntary spasm* of serious advanced abdominal disease. Severity can range from a localized spasm over the right rectus muscle in moderately advanced appendicitis to a board-like rigidity of the abdomen in diffuse peritonitis caused by a perforated ulcer. Some abdominal crises, of course, may not be accompanied by rigidity. For example, early intestinal obstruction or massive gastrointestinal bleeding may be accompanied by a soft abdomen. Furthermore, inflammation in the so-called *nondemonstrative* areas of the abdomen, particularly the deep pelvis and the subdiaphragmatic areas, may show relatively little on abdominal examination. Always beware of the very *obese patients* in whom findings may be less clear.

In the pediatric patient, examination may be made easier after an appropriate dose of sedative since this will not abolish the true spasm or tenderness. A simple sugar nipple or pacifier in an infant may assist in the examination; the frightened child may need to be examined while being held in its mother's arms.

VOMITING

Vomiting occurs with many abdominal catastrophies as well as with a variety of medical conditions. While often nonspecific, it is a classic finding in the well-developed *obstructions* of the intestine. The higher the obstruction, the earlier the vomiting will occur. Its projectile character in *pyloric stenosis* is so characteristic that it may often be diagnosed by telephone. *What* is vomited may be revealing. Is it bile or blood? Does it smell like feces as with lower intestinal obstruction? A gastric outlet obstruction will result in vomitus containing only old food or gastric fluid which does not contain bile since it cannot reflux from the duodenum. Because vomiting empties the upper intestine, higher obstructions may not be clinically evident without further studies, since distention is not present.

PELVIC AND RECTAL EXAMINATIONS

The pelvic and rectal examinations, though generally done last, must never be omitted. They are best done in the *lithotomy position* and both may be done bimanually. If the patient has a colostomy, digital examination through this orifice may be useful. Signs and symptoms may be elicited from these examinations that might be missed otherwise with conditions like pelvic appendicitis, an ovarian cyst or torsion, acute prostatitis, gonorrheal pelvic inflammatory disease, a pelvic abscess, or rectal tumor. One might find the signs of abortion, which might require surgical intervention. As with the abdominal examination, the pelvic and rectal examinations are sometimes best repeated under anesthesia prior to making an incision.

In summary, the first step in the care of the patient with acute abdominal disease is a thorough assessment through history-taking and physical examination. Therapy may then be instituted early. With the aid of laboratory and radiologic studies, a specific diagnosis will be made on which further treatment is based. Complete descriptions of any given disease process can be found in surgical textbooks. The remainder of this chapter will deal specifically with abdominal trauma.

ABDOMINAL TRAUMA

Trauma is the primary cause of death in the United States in the age group under 35 years and is fourth among all causes of death. Abdominal trauma constitutes only a small percentage of this total, but the mortality and morbidity of abdominal trauma are relatively high compared with other sites of injury. With the increase in automobile traffic and industrialization, trauma has increased. However, due to improvement in emergency services, including rapid transportation, the health team now has an opportunity to see and treat cases earlier and save more lives. Having trained personnel and equipment at the scene of the accident, en route to the hospital, and at the receiving hospital are keys to greater success. During this early phase of care the basic principles of attention to the airway, hemorrhage, suctioning, oxygen, and rapid transportation are essential.

BLUNT VS. PENETRATING INJURIES

Abdominal injury is sometimes conveniently divided for purposes of discussion into *blunt* trauma and *penetrating* (open) injuries, though these may often be concomitant. Examples of the open injury are stab or gunshot wounds. These injuries are usually obvious, and evisceration of bowel or mesentery may be present, clearly indicating the need for operative treatment. It is the blunt nonpenetrating injuries that are more easily and frequently overlooked. The basic principles involved in care of both these forms of injury are the same.

The frequency of injuries to abdominal organs indicates that for *blunt* trauma, the spleen, liver, vascular structures, small bowel, kidneys, and bladder are the most commonly injured structures in descending order. In children, the order may be slightly altered with spleen, liver, urologic injuries, intestinal injuries, and retroperitoneal injuries heading the list. In the case of *penetrating* abdominal injuries, the most commonly injured viscera are the liver, vascular structures, small bowel, colon, stomach, spleen, and duodenum in descending order. The two commonest injuries will be described further.

SPLEEN The spleen is the organ commonly injured with *blunt* abdominal trauma. It is friable and has a thin capsule, and injury to it is often one of several concomitant injuries. Usual findings include left upper quadrant pain, tenderness, and moderate rigidity. There may be left shoulder pain (Kehr's sign), and signs of hemorrhage are common. X-rays often reveal fractures of the left lower ribs. The diagnosis may be obvious, but it may be more subtle if bleeding is slow. Late or delayed rupture of the spleen may occur up to a month later, when the *subcapsular hematoma* which formed at the time of injury breaks and bleading starts again. The treatment of splenic rupture is splenectomy. The mortality is low unless there are multiple injuries.

LIVER The liver is also frequently injured by blunt and penetrating trauma, most commonly the result of automobile accidents. These injuries vary from small lacerations which are easily sutured, debrided, and drained to major lacerations and fractures of the liver which may require partial hepatectomy. *Massive hemorrhage* is a common operative and postoperative problem. Other associated injuries, particularly open injuries to the colon, are associated with a higher mortality.

GENERAL RESUSCITATION

General resuscitative measures have first priority and include (1) the maintenance of the airway and proper ventilation, (2) treatment of hypovolemic shock by insertion of large-bore needles and catheters and the infusion of balanced salt solutions and blood, (3) preparation for monitoring both arterial and central venous pressure, and (4) placement of a urinary catheter for diagnostic and monitoring purposes.

HISTORY

Conventionally, the history of illness is taken first, but in trauma cases it may become secondary. The history of injury is usually clear, but on occasion may be vague as in the case of a battered child or in the intoxicated patient. Occasionally after trauma, the appearance of the problem may be delayed for hours, days, or even occasionally weeks as with delayed splenic rupture or the development of pancreatic pseudocyst.

EXAMINATION

Physical examination, all acute abdominal problems, is of critical importance. A main point to remember is that the clinical course following severe trauma is seldom static. Continuing clinical observation by a responsible surgeon and the members of the health team is the most valuable diagnostic tool of all. Physical signs are an accurate guide in the alert patient but may be lost in the unconscious patient in whom additional diagnostic maneuvers become mandatory. Just as minimal or early acute abdominal disease may be overlooked, so may patients with seemingly minor abdominal trauma be released by a hospital, only to develop serious complications later.

When examining the traumatized patient, *muscle wall* tenderness must be distinguished from *intraabdominal* tenderness. A useful maneuver is to have the patient contract the abdominal muscles during palpation. Tenderness of the intraabdominal structures is notably reduced in contrast to abdominal wall tenderness, which is more marked during palpation with the muscles contracted.

Rigidity may range from the voluntary spasm of the mildly contused abdominal wall to the true involuntary spasm which accompanies the traumatic ruptured viscus with peritonitis. Rigidity, however, may be absent in the presence of shock. *Distention* is less often important diagnostically in early abdominal trauma, but intraabdominal bleeding may result in visible distention after a period of time. The absence of *bowel sounds* should always be sought as a sign of intraabdominal injury. It is important to listen to the abdomen long enough (several minutes) to obtain a representative sampling of the sounds.

A nasogastric tube is usually passed into the stomach to check for *bleeding.* The swallowing of blood from nasal injuries must be considered as a source. *Vomiting* is quite nonspecific and can occur with any abdominal problem. Decompression of the stomach helps avoid aspiration.

COMPLICATIONS

Multiple injuries exist in many cases of trauma. One has to guard against missing some injuries or missing the significance of abdominal injury because of more pressing problems, such as severe head injury or a flail chest. Multiple injuries increase the risk of mortality.

Shock may be grave and sometimes the only important sign of intraabdominal injury. The patient with a traumatic rupture of the spleen is the most common classic example. Shock may be neurogenic or cardiogenic in origin, but is most often *hypovolemic.* Obvious shock always requires rapid and vigorous treatment, sometimes with little delay before transporting the patient to the operating room. The health team must be suspicious of the patient who has transient hypotension, then seems to compensate with the early resuscitative measures. These individuals may have further internal bleeding.

Since early surgical intervention is usually required, prepare for transfusion soon after the patient enters the ED. A tube of blood should be drawn and sent for type and cross match along with any other necessary studies. Blood-gas analyses are also essential in monitoring shock patients.

DIAGNOSTIC TESTS

LABORATORY AIDS   There are several laboratory aids commonly used in cases of abdominal trauma. A *complete blood count* is always obtained early for reference. In the case of bleeding, the hematocrit level drops as the body equilibrates by transcapillary refill and by dilution from intravenous infusions. The *white blood count* is usually increased following trauma but is nonspecific. An important indicator of injury to the pancreas is the *amylase* level. It should be drawn in all cases of abdominal trauma, particularly when there is upper abdominal pain or tenderness, since pancreatic injuries produce considerable mortality and morbidity. The *urinalysis* gives important information. Gross hematuria may indicate injury to any portion of the genitourinary tract while gross blood at the urethral orifice can signify urethral transection.

X-RAYS   X-rays are important in most injuries; in skeletal trauma they are diagnostic. *Pelvic, spine,* or *lower rib* fractures may be found in association with abdominal injuries. With a pelvic fracture, one is alerted to the possibility of *bladder* injury, while with left lower rib fractures, *splenic* injury may have occurred. Likewise, right lower rib fractures may be associated with *liver lacerations.* Plain x-rays of the abdomen (abdominal series) have limited value in trauma but on occasion may indicate (1) perforation by the presence of free air, (2) splenic rupture by an enlarged splenic shadow with associated rib fractures and stomach compression, or possibly (3) the obliteration of fat planes suggesting intraabdominal fluid such as blood. Chest x-rays are indicated if there is any thoracoabdominal injury and as a base-line study for any seriously ill surgical patient.

CONTRAST STUDIES   X-ray contrast studies are occasionally useful in abdominal trauma. An *upper gastrointestinal* series is not often indicated but might be diagnostic of a duodenal hematoma with obstruction. Barium enemas are not often required. Intravenous *pyelograms* are commonly indicated in the patient with hematuria to locate and assess the degree of injuries. *Cystograms* are also commonly done in the patient with pelvic trauma in order to rule out bladder rupture, which will require surgical attention. A *retrograde urethrogram* may be indicated if there is inability to pass a catheter and one suspects urethral transection.

ARTERIOGRAPHY   Arteriography and selected vessel study can be utilized in certain instances of abdominal injury. These techniques do not supplant the history and physical examination in ruling out visceral injury. However, when organ injuries are suspected but the physical examination and other studies are equivocal, these studies may be indicated. For example, with a left upper quadrant injury and fractured ribs, pain, but no evidence of major blood loss and a negative abdominal tap, one might utilize a splenic angiogram to assist in determining whether there is significant splenic injury. *Scanning techniques* are also growing in importance and can be used to study the spleen and other organs after trauma.

In recent years attempts have been made to limit routine laparotomy for all cases of abdominal injuries because of the high incidence of negative exploration. *Sinograms* (injection of dye into wound tract) has had limited success in the diagnostic management of stab wounds. Other approaches include local wound exploration, peritoneal *aspiration* by four-quadrant tap (see below), and peritoneal *lavage.*

PARACENTESIS   Paracentesis is a very important diagnostic tool in the evaluation of abdominal trauma as well as other abdominal crises. Some medical centers recommend it routinely for patients admitted for observation of abdominal trauma. There are two commonly used methods. The *four-quadrant tap* has been utilized for a number of years. A spinal needle attached to a saline-filled syringe is inserted into each of the four quadrants with gentle aspiration. A positive tap produces nonclotting blood and can be a very meaningful diagnostic finding.

The second procedure is *diagnostic peritoneal lavage.* This is a fairly simple and quite accurate procedure done under local anesthesia. A dialysis catheter is introduced into the abdomen through a trochar or small peritoneal incision. Saline or another balanced salt solution can be infused, and following a period of distribution, the fluid is allowed to return through the catheter for study. Gross appearance is checked, and microscopic examination for red and white blood cells, amylase, bacteria (Gram's stain), and enteric contents (Wright's stain) is performed. The test is interpreted as *positive* if gross blood, bloody fluid or many RBCs (greater than 100,000 per cubic millimeter), bile, bacteria, or a high amylase level is present. Clear or very light pink fluid may be considered negative pending the other laboratory studies. Obviously there are occasional false positive and false negative tests. Continuing frequent clinical examination of the patient with abdominal trauma is one's major tool.

SURGICAL INTERVENTION

Following the World War II experience, an approach had developed where routine laparotomy for abdominal trauma cases was considered best. In recent years, alternative approaches have been offered. Selective conservative management with surgical exploration, when there is evidence or suggestion of peritonitis or hemorrhage, has been used in many centers with consequent reduction in the number of required operations. However, if there is serious doubt about the clinical signs in abdominal trauma, although the other studies are negative, it is probably best to operate.

Gunshot wounds provide a different situation. Clinical signs are generally more obvious than with stab wounds. These patients should undergo laparotomy in almost all cases, unless it can be demonstrated that the shell did not enter the peritoneal space. High-velocity missiles can produce intraabdominal injury through concussive force alone.

Improved patient management has done the most to increase the survival rate in patients with abdominal trauma in recent years. Good anesthesia, aggressive treatment of shock, antibiotics, availability of blood-gas studies and other monitoring functions, and earlier surgery have all contributed.

BIBLIOGRAPHY

Altman, P. P., et al., "Abdominal Emergencies in Infants," *Advances in Surgery,* vol. 9, Year Book, Chicago, 1975, pp. 305–364.

Botoford, T., and Wilson, R., "The Acute Abdomen," *Major Problems in Clinical Surgery,* vol. X, Saunders, Philadelphia, 1969.

Bouterie, R., "The Acute Abdomen," in Sproul, C., and Mullanney, P., *Emergency Care: Assessment and Intervention,* Mosby, St. Louis, 1974, pp. 332–348.

Clain, A., *Hamilton Bailey's Demonstrations of Physical Signs in Clinical Surgery,* Chaps. 22 and 23, Williams & Wilkins, Baltimore, 1972.

Cope, Z., *The Early Diagnosis of the Acute Abdomen,* 14th ed., Oxford, London, 1972.

Dunphy, J., and Botoford, T., *Physical Examination of the Surgical Patient,* Saunders, Philadelphia, 1975.

Jordan, G., and Beall, A. C., "Diagnosis and Management of Abdominal Trauma," *Current Problems in Surgery,* 1971.

Kraft, J., "The Acute Abdomen," *Emergency Medicine,* vol. 5, 1973, pp. 145–151.

"Patient Assessment: Examination of the Abdomen (Programmed Instruction)," *American Journal of Nursing,* vol. 74, 1974, pp. 1679–1702.

Raffensperger, J. G., et al., *The Acute Abdomen in Infancy and Childhood,* Lippincott, Philadelphia, 1970.

Shepherd, J. A., *A Concise Surgery of the Acute Abdomen,* Churchill Livingstone, Edinburgh, 1975.

CHAPTER 21
EMERGENCY CARE OF ORTHOPEDIC INJURIES

VIRGINIA R. DODS, R.N.

THE care of orthopedic injuries is an everday problem confronting the ED nurse and requires a thorough working knowledge of various types of injuries. The purpose of this chapter is to familiarize nurses with the physiology and process of bone repair and some common orthopedic injuries and to discuss practical aspects of care such as splinting, positioning, and emotional support.

PHYSIOLOGY OF BONE

Bone is a specialized connective tissue with a calcified collagenous intercellular substance made up of *33 percent organic* and *67 percent inorganic* material. Bone is either cancellous (spongy spaces filled with bone marrow) or compact (a continuous, hard mass). Cartilege is specialized connective tissue which forms a temporary skeleton for the embryo and persists in the adult in joints, respiratory passages, ribs, and ears. It has no nerves or blood vessels.

The mineral content of bone is a mixture of tricalcium phosphate and calcium carbonate. Calcium content is dependent upon many factors, such as parathyroid hormone and estrogens, dietary intake, stress, and acid-base balance. A slight decrease in pH increases the solubility of calcium carbonate and causes bone demineralization.

A typical long bone, such as the femur, is made up of three main parts: the *diaphysis, epiphysis,* and *metaphysis.* The diaphysis is the shaft and consists of a wall of compact bone enclosing a large cylindrical bone marrow cavity. The epiphysis is the end of the bone and consists of cancellous bone with a thin outer wall of compact bone. The metaphysis is the spongy bone directly beneath the epipyseal plate. The growth plate lies between the epiphysis and the diaphysis. The importance of this is seen in children when the growth plate may slip and cause impaired bone growth. Periosteum is modified connective tissue which covers bone and is a supporting structure through which blood vessels and nerves reach the bone.

TYPES OF FRACTURES

A fracture is defined as any break in continuity of bone or cartilege and may be complete or incomplete, these terms referring to the line of fracture through the bone. A *closed fracture* has no opening through the skin, while an *open fracture* has a communication or tract between the site of the fracture and the outside air.

The general pattern of a fracture is usually determined by the direction and intensity of force and the resiliency of bone. Types of fractures are illustrated in Fig. 21-1.

REPAIR OF FRACTURES

The moment a fracture occurs the stage is set for repair. The biochemical process begins with a local inflammatory response; there is marked increased vascularity which initiates resorption of bone ends and the freeing of calcium.

There are three main stages of repair. In the *first stage* a hematoma forms within the first 48 hours. The *second stage* is marked by consolidation or callus formation, which restores continuity between fragments. After about six weeks cartilege is replaced by bone, and

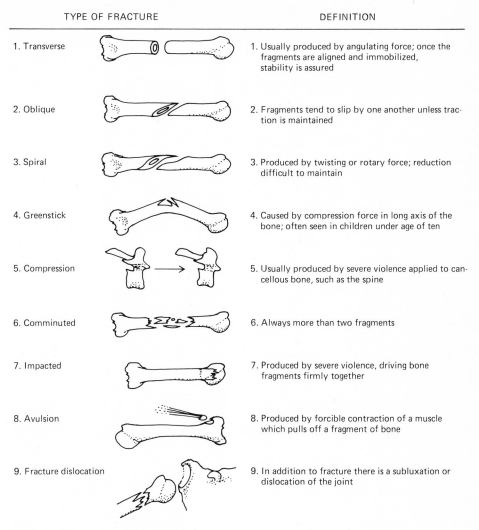

TYPE OF FRACTURE	DEFINITION
1. Transverse	1. Usually produced by angulating force; once the fragments are aligned and immobilized, stability is assured
2. Oblique	2. Fragments tend to slip by one another unless traction is maintained
3. Spiral	3. Produced by twisting or rotary force; reduction difficult to maintain
4. Greenstick	4. Caused by compression force in long axis of the bone; often seen in children under age of ten
5. Compression	5. Usually produced by severe violence applied to cancellous bone, such as the spine
6. Comminuted	6. Always more than two fragments
7. Impacted	7. Produced by severe violence, driving bone fragments firmly together
8. Avulsion	8. Produced by forcible contraction of a muscle which pulls off a fragment of bone
9. Fracture dislocation	9. In addition to fracture there is a subluxation or dislocation of the joint

Figure 21-1 Types of fractures.

at completion of this stage the fragments are united. At this point the cast may usually be removed. *Stage three* is remodeling. The dead ends of fragments are resorbed, cancellous bone is replaced by compact bone, and the union is completed. The rate of union varies from bone to bone and is dependent upon many factors.

Conditions influencing rate of healing include:

1. Age of patient

2. Blood supply to both fragments

3. Proximity of fractured surfaces

4. Stresses at the fracture site

5. Systemic disorders such as malnutrition and local or generalized bone disease

ASSESSMENT OF THE ORTHOPEDIC INJURY

In order to institute proper care and management of the patient with an orthopedic injury, the ED nurse must first recognize and assess the extent of the injury. Clinically, suspect a fracture when there is *history* of injury and *pain* localized to an area of bone. The concept that there is complete loss of function is erroneous since the patient with a fractured forearm can move the finger and the patient with a fractured leg can move the ankle and wiggle the toes. If nerves are intact, motor function will be present, although often painful.[1] The patient should be assessed for the following local and systemic signs of fracture:

1. Deformity

2. Local pain and tenderness

3. Grating, crepitation

4. Swelling

5. Discoloration (eccymosis)

6. Loss of function or abnormal mobility

7. Appearance of fragments

8. Shock

A careful history will assist the health team in determining the type of fracture by knowing the amount of trauma involved, the direction of force, and other possible injuries which may have occurred.

FRACTURE MANAGEMENT

Careless handling of a patient with a fracture of a major bone may convert a simple problem to a serious one. The closed wound may be converted to an open; a clean wound grossly contaminated; an intact spinal cord severed, or major blood vessels and nerves seriously injured. Table 21-1 lists the principles in fracture management.

It is also a good rule to keep any orthopedic injury NPO until thoroughly evaluated by the physician as this person may need surgery to reduce a fracture, repair a tendon, or for other injuries associated with the traumatic event.

METHODS OF REDUCTION AND IMMOBILIZATION

Initial emergency care begins at the scene with proper *assessment* and *immobilization*. Further treatment is generally carried out under the care of the physician in one of the following ways:

1. Closed reduction with external fixation (cast)

2. Balanced traction suspension—pin through bone or skin traction

3. Open reduction and internal fixation—generally agreed upon in the following cases:

a. Displaced and separated fractures of the olecranon

b. Displaced and separated fractures of the patella

c. Displaced fracture of the neck of the femur

d. Small fragments in the joint

e. Fractures that cannot be reduced by any other method

Table 21-1   **Fracture management: general principles of care.**

---

1. Avoid unnecessary handling
2. Immobilize
3. Apply clean dressings to wounds
4. Control hemorrhage with direct pressure (tourniquets are a last resort in hemorrhage control and may lead to loss of the involved limb)
5. Check for the "5 P's" of vascular occlusion distal to injury
   a. Pain
   b. Pulselessness
   c. Paresthesia
   d. Pallor
   e. Paralysis

COMPLICATIONS OF FRACTURES

Hemorrhage, shock, nerve and tendon damage, and infection are all possible complications of fractures. The patient should be watched carefully for signs of *shock* as discussed in Chap. 14. *Fat embolism* is another grave complication, especially in long bone fractures, and is also discussed in Chap. 19. *Prevention of infection* of open fractures by immediate IV administration of broad-spectrum antibiotics and tetanus prophylaxis is essential. A search for *nerve, tendon,* and *circulatory damage* is mandatory in all injuries and can be a part of the initial nursing assessment by using the "5 P's" outlined in Table 21-1.

SPLINTING

It is often difficult to assess initially the extent of an orthopedic injury. Types of injury may include *fracture* (a break in the bone); *sprain* (a partial tear of a ligament); *strain* (overstretching of a muscle); *dislocation* (displacement of a bone end from a joint); or *subluxation* (incomplete separation of the joint surfaces). It is best to assume the worst and treat all these injuries as fractures and immobilize them until further evaluation through x-ray and the physician's examination.

Basically splints are of four types: rigid, inflatable, traction, and spine boards. It is possible to improvise any of these types from materials at hand such as rolled newspapers, boards, cardboard, or pillows. Even a door may be used as a backboard. The primary objective of splinting is to prevent motion of fragments; properly applied, splints can help prevent the following complications:

1. Damage to muscles, nerves, or blood vessels caused by broken ends of the bone

2. Laceration of the skin by broken bones

3. Interruption of blood flow to an area as a result of pressure of bone ends on blood vessels

4. Restriction of sensation or function due to nerve damage

5. Excessive bleeding into the surrounding tissue as a result of unstable bone ends

6. Increased pain associated with movement of bone ends

7. Paralysis of extremities due to fractured or dislocated vertebrae

GENERAL CONSIDERATIONS IN SPLINT APPLICATION

These guidelines represent basic principles of management for any type of orthopedic injury:

1. Immobilize before moving the patient or applying traction—"splint 'em where they lie."

2. Do *not* straighten dislocations.

3. If an open fracture, stop bleeding and dress wound before splinting; do *not* push protruding bone back inside.

4. Immobilize broken bone or dislocated joint one joint above and one joint below point of injury.

5. Apply slight traction (steady downward pull) while splinting and maintain until splint is in place.

6. Splint tightly, but do not interfere with circulation.

7. *Check pulse, color, pain, and sensation distal to injury before and after splinting.*

8. Suspect injury to neck or spine in any accident which could cause fracture or dislocation.

9. Pad the splint carefully to prevent pressure points and discomfort to the area.

SOME COMMON ORTHOPEDIC INJURIES

CLAVICLE

One of the most frequently fractured bones in the body is the clavicle since this area is easily exposed to severe forces. The fracture can be either seen or felt as a lump over the area of pain. Treatment is generally a figure-of-eight splint for 3 to 6 weeks. Open reduction is very rarely indicated (see Fig. 21-2).

SHOULDER DISLOCATIONS

The clinical picture of a shoulder dislocation includes the history of a fall and immediate disability. The patient holds the arm rigidly immobile in abduction and avoids any movement which is extremely painful. The normal rounded appearance of the shoulder is replaced by a flattening (see Fig. 21-2).

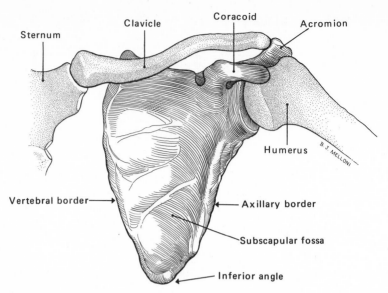

Figure 21-2 The scapula, anterior view, joined to the humerus and the clavicle. The head of the humerus articulates in the glenoid cavity. *(Taken from Langley, L., Telford, I., and Christensen, J., Dynamic Anatomy and Physiology, McGraw-Hill, New York, 1974, p. 104.)*

The head of the humerus may slip out of the glenoid fossa either *anteriorly* or *posteriorly*. The most common type of shoulder dislocation is the anterior. The patient should be placed in a position of comfort while awaiting x-ray to rule out a fracture before the shoulder is manipulated and reduced. Generally a semisitting position is preferred with pillows used to splint the arm as it lies. This is a very painful injury due to the severe muscle spasm, and no attempt at manipulation should be made. Closed reduction of these dislocations may be done in the ED with the patient well sedated and the arm then manipulated, placed in a shoulder immobilizer (for 3 to 6 weeks), and a postreduction film taken.

Posterior dislocation is very rare (it constitutes about 4 percent of all types of dislocations); however it may occur during a seizure or in patients undergoing electric shock therapy. Again, the clinical picture is history of trauma, abduction of the shoulder, internally rotated arm, and decreased prominence of the humeral head. Treatment is usually reduction under general anesthesia.

In young people (dislocations usually appear between the ages of 20 and 45 years) dislocations are prone to recur, particularly if the first episode is not followed by immobilization. De Palma advocates an immobilization period of 3 weeks to allow firm tissue healing.[2] Each subsequent dislocation occurs with greater ease and less pain, indicating that stretching and laxity of soft tissues have occurred.

In all shoulder dislocations it is important to check for *circumflex nerve injury by* pin prick over the deltoid. Watch for numbness and stiffness of fingers. Check for pulses distal to the injury and note the color of the extremity.

RIB

The most commonly fractured ribs are the *seventh* and *eighth,* usually laterally. As a general rule, one rib fracture presents little problem as far as complications are involved. The patient will present with much pain after a history of trauma to the area. Treatment after x-ray is usually pain medication. Rib belts and taping are sometimes ordered for immobilization. The danger of *atelectasis* in this treatment must be considered, especially in the elderly patient. Simultaneous fractures of three or more ribs will generally find the patient admitted to the hospital under the care of the chest surgeon. The possible complications of tension pneumothorax, heart contusion, and hemothorax must be ruled out.

ELBOW

The elbow is formed by the articulation of three bones, the radius, ulna, and humerus (see Fig. 21-3). Besides flexion and extension at the elbow, there is rotary motion of the radius which makes movement of the forearm possible. Numerous ligamentous and bone injuries can occur in and around the elbow joint.

Elbow fractures are often associated with severe soft tissue damage. Extreme swelling may result in a deformity known as *Volkmann's contracture.* This is a claw-hand deformity caused by constriction of the brachial artery resulting in ischemia, pain, swelling, cyanosis, and loss of movement of the fingers. Any delay in treatment of this condition is disastrous since 3 to 4 hours of ischemia may cause irreversible damage. It is extremely important to check the radial pulse and circulation and to test for motor and sensory function as soon as this patient arrives in the ED (see Table 21-2). This author feels an air splint should not be used on this type of fracture because it may add pressure to an already compromised area. Other complications of elbow fractures include myositis ossificans, a calcium deposit in soft tissues with resultant limited joint movement and nerve damage.

Figure 21-3 Bones of the upper extremity. (a) Anterior view. (b) Posterior view. *(Taken from Langley, L., Telford, I., and Christensen, J., Dynamic Anatomy and Physiology, McGraw-Hill, New York, 1974, p. 105.)*

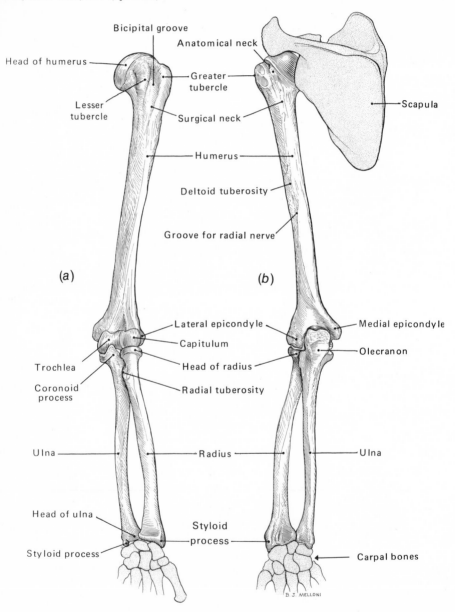

Table 21-2	An abbreviated sensory and motor nerve assessment for the upper extremity.	
	Sensory	*Motor*
	Median nerve	
	Pin prick index or middle finger on flexor surface	Oppose thumb to tip of little finger
	Ulnar nerve	
	Pin prick ulnar side of little finger	Spread fingers apart
	Radial nerve	
	Pin prick web space of thumb and index finger	Extend wrist

WRIST

The term *colles fracture* describes a fracture of the distal end of the radius within 1 inch of the wrist joint (see Fig. 21-4). It is usually caused by a fall on an outstretched hand and may result in a characteristic dinner-fork deformity. Splint this fracture as it lies, including the hand and forearm up to the elbow. Check for pulse, color, and sensation before and after splinting.

Another type of fracture caused by a fall on an outstretched hand is the *scaphoid* or *navicular fracture* of the wrist. X-ray often does not show this fracture immediately; it may be diagnosed

Figure 21-4 **Bones of the wrist and hand.** *(Adapted from Langley, L., Telford, I., and Christensen, J., Dynamic Anatomy and Physiology, McGraw-Hill, New York, 1974, p. 106.)*

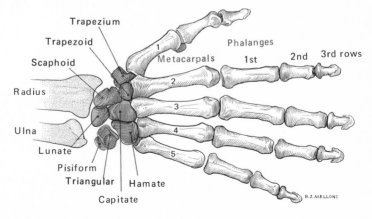

clinically by history and by pain in the "snuffbox"—the indented area visible at the base of the thumb where the sensory branches of the radial nerve are located. Healing time is prolonged in this area because the bones of the wrist are variable in their blood supply, and a fracture may leave one fragment of the bone with no blood supply. Interruption of circulation results in disintegration or death of bone called *aseptic necrosis*. Treatment of this fracture is usually immobilization with a short arm cast or splint for 8 to 10 weeks.

PHALANX

A chip fracture of the posterior surface of the distal portion of the distal phalanx results in a "baseball finger" fracture (see Fig. 21-5a). The injury results from the tearing of the extensor tendon in this area which pulls the chip of bone into the joint. This injury can result in inability to extend the distal phalanx with loss of function; it must be splinted in a special manner. The treatment is exaggerated and prolonged (4 to 6 weeks) hyperextension of the distal joint of the finger to allow sufficient time for reattachment of the tendon (see Fig. 21-5b). In most other types of fractures of the fingers, the general principles are to splint in a position of function with the joints slightly flexed and immobilize *only the affected fin-*

Figure 21-5a "Baseball finger" fracture. (*b*) Splinting the "baseball finger" fracture. Note that (1) proximal interphalangeal joint is flexed at 90°; (2) distal joint is hyperextended.

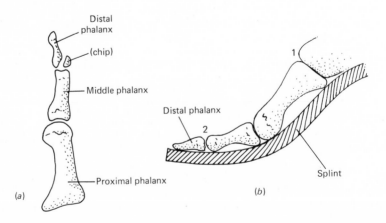

ger to allow free, active use of the uninvolved fingers and avoid stiffness and loss of joint function.

HIP

The term "broken hip" includes injuries ranging from the very upper end of the femur to the region at the base of the neck of the femur. The upper end of the femur is called *intracapsular* and farther out in the neck, *extracapsular*. The region of femur at the base of the neck is called the *trochanter*.

Fractures of the hip are divided into two major groups:

1. Fractures within the joint capsule

2. Fractures at the base of the neck with involvement of one or both trochanters (see Fig. 21-6)

Prognosis for union and restoration of normal function varies considerably in the two groups, because the blood vessels which supply nutrition enter the neck of the femur and reach the head inside the bone.

In intracapsular fractures with displacement, the neck vessels will be torn, blood supply may not be sufficient to nourish the entire femoral head, and aseptic necrosis may result. This is the chief cause of nonunion which can occur even with perfect reduction. These fractures are treated with open reduction and internal fixation connecting a fair amount of neck with the head fragment.

Intertrochanteric fractures occur distal to the hip joint capsule, rarely sever important arteries, and almost invariably heal although there may be some loss of normal angulation between shaft and neck due to the strong pull of the muscles. Treatment may be traction or open reduction with internal fixation.

Clinically the patient with a hip fracture tends to be in the older age group with a history of a fall and pain in the hip area. If this is an impacted fracture, the leg may be in normal position, and the hip can be moved, although painfully. A leg in *marked external rotation* with no movement possible generally suggests a complete fracture of the neck of the femur with separation. The leg in internal rotation with the hip flexed and the knee toward midline usually indicates dislocation.[3]

In the ED, allow this patient to find and maintain a position of comfort, in a supine position, and place a pillow or soft roll between the legs so that skin surfaces do not touch. *Do not attempt traction* as this may fragment the fracture in the joint or cause tearing of blood vessels to the area. The patient should be kept NPO

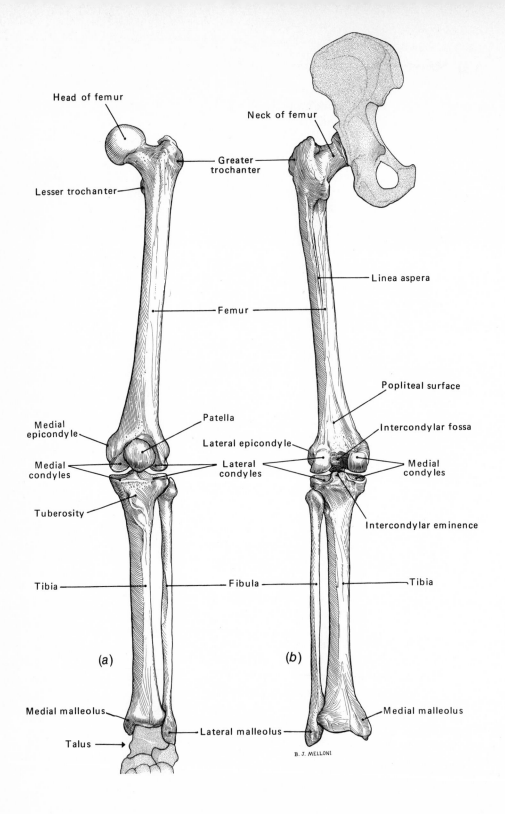

Head of femur

Lesser trochanter

Medial
epicondyle

Medial
condyles

Tuberosity

Tibia

Medial malleolus

Talus

Patella

Lateral epicondyle

Lateral
condyles

(a)

Lateral malleolus

Neck of femur

Greater
trochanter

Linea aspera

Femur

Popliteal surface

Intercondylar fossa

Medial
condyles

Intercondylar eminence

Fibula

Tibia

(b)

Medial malleolus

B. J. MELLONI

and an IV started in readiness for surgery. It is possible for the patient to lose 300 to 500 cc blood into the area, and routine blood work should include a stat CBC and type and cross match for whole blood. The x-ray order should include an anteroposterior view of the pelvis with a lateral view of the affected hip, and, if fracture is fairly certain, a *chest film* should also be taken at this time. Trauma to the hip may also have included trauma to the pelvis and bladder, so a urine sample is also needed.

These patients who undergo open reduction with internal fixation may be greatly reassured by the knowledge that, barring complications, they will not be bedridden for months, but instead be up and ambulating with a walker within a few days and possibly weight-bearing in a very short time.

FEMUR

A fracture of the femur just below the trochanter (see Fig. 21-6) is one of the most difficult to treat as it tends to project forward at right angles to the body, abduct, and rotate outward due to the strong muscle pull of the iliopsoas and gluteus medius. Treatment is traction and reduction.

With a fracture of the shaft of the femur there is strong action of the gluteus medius muscle which has the tendency to pull the upper fragment of the femur outward, and the adduction group causes bowing at the fracture point. This fracture should be reduced immediately. A *Thomas* or *Hare traction splint* should be applied. This type of splint decreases the pain by reducing muscle spasm, prevents overriding of the bones, and lessens the chance of hemorrhage. A patient may lose up to *2000 cc blood* into the thigh with this injury, and an IV should be started upon arrival in the ED. Once the traction splint is applied, the patient thoroughly assessed for any other injuries, an IV started, and pain medication administered, she or he may proceed to x-ray, where vital signs should continue to be monitored closely.

KNEE INJURIES

The knee is a hinge and pivot joint dependent upon the quadriceps and collateral ligaments for stability in extension and guarded by the semilunar cartilages (menisci) which act as shock absorbers

Figure 21-6 Bones of the lower extremity. (a) Anterior view. (b) Posterior view. *(Taken from Langley, L., Telford, I., and Christensen, J., Dynamic Anatomy and Physiology, McGraw-Hill, New York, 1974, p. 110.)*

(see Fig. 21-7). Patients with knee injuries are evaluated for patellar fractures, sprains or tears of the ligaments, meniscus tears, or fractures into the joint.

MENISCUS TEARS A rupture of the internal cartilege is a common athletic-type injury and may be called a "bucket handle" tear because of its shape. A history of twisting while the knee is flexed and the leg fixed firmly to the ground (as with cletted shoes on soft turf) while the thigh is violently rotated is common. The cartilege is split, and part enters the central compartment of the knee, while the other part remains in a normal position. Repeated locking of the knee is indicative of this condition. Meniscus tears do not show up on ordinary x-ray. The tear is outlined by *arthrography* which involves injecting dye into the joint space prior to x-ray. Treatment of this tear is usually surgical removal of the meniscus. Dense collagenous tissue which is rarely torn replaces the cartilege after a period of time.

When locking of the knee joint occurs from a tear in the meniscus or other injury, treatment should not be delayed as the tension may fray and stretch other ligaments and cause serious damage to the joint structure. The knee may be locked in either flexion or extension and the patient unable to move from that position. *Do not* attempt to straighten or reposition. Rather place a pillow under the flexed knee. Treatment is generally surgery.

FRACTURE Patellar fractures are usually repaired surgically because the action of the quadriceps muscle may separate the fragments several inches at the time of injury, and they must be wired back together or, in badly comminuted fractures, all the fragments removed.

SYNOVITIS Swelling in varying degrees accompanies most knee injuries and is due to either synovial fluid or blood in the joint. This is called *effusion.* Synovial membrane lines joint cavities, tendon sheaths, and bursae, and its smooth moist surfaces protect against friction from the moving parts.

Acute synovitis may result from a tearing of the synovium or ligamentous attachments. Synovial fluid accumulates slowly over 12 to 24 hours and results in a very swollen knee, although seldom tense or severly painful. *Traumatic hemarthrosis* refers to blood in the joint and is a sequel to all types of intraarticular fractures, tears in the menisci, and rupture of ligaments. There is a farily rapid onset of symptoms associated with much pain.

The treatment for either of these effusions is usually joint aspiration. This is a *sterile procedure*. Xylocaine is first injected into the area for local anesthesia. A large (50 cc) syringe with a large bore (usually 18 gauge) needle is used to aspirate the fluid. The area should be prepared with a 10-minute scrub and the patient given much reassurance.

Figure 21-7 The knee joint. (*a*) Articular surfaces and ligaments, anterior view. (*b*) Sagittal section through the joint to expose muscles, tendons, ligaments, and bursae. (*c*) Articular surface of the tibia in cross section through the knee joint. (*Taken from Langley, L., Telford, I., and Christensen, J., Dynamic Anatomy and Physiology, McGraw-Hill, New York, 1974, p. 115.*)

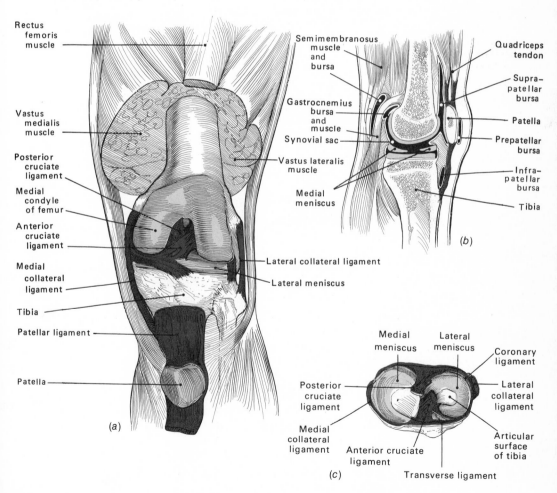

SPRAINS Sprains of the knee ligaments are generally treated with ice, a bulky supportive wrap, and activity as tolerated by the patient. Do not apply heat over the joint area as it will result in more swelling. Start the knee wrap at midcalf and terminate it at midthigh, beginning at the most distal portion and wrapping upward. Some type of cotton padding (cast padding is fine) followed by a large Ace bandage will provide good support. The Ace wrap should not be pulled tight as the elasticity of the bandage itself will provide adequate support.

LOWER LEG

The tibia is the main weight-bearing bone of the leg and is well covered with muscle in the upper and middle portions except at the shin (see Fig. 21-6). The lower one-third of the tibia is one of the most frequent sites of nonunion because of the sparse covering of subcutaneous tissue and poorer circulation to this area. Injuries to this area are quite painful as there is little protection to the sensitive periosteum. Immobilization can be obtained by the use of either the traction splint, a long-leg air splint, or well-padded cardboard splint.

ANKLE

Ankle fractures may be *medial malleolar* (tibia), *lateral malleolar* (fibula), or *bimalleolar,* where both sides are fractured. A *trimalleolar,* or Pott's, fracture is a serious injury involving fracture of the internal malleolus, posterior end of the tibia, and lateral malleolus (see Fig. 21-6). Treatment is open reduction and internal fixation.

Sprains of ankle ligaments are common (see Fig. 21-8). A sprain is a partial or complete rupture of the fibers and is often accompanied by effusion into the joint. Sometimes a strong ligament will take a piece of bone with it—an *avulsion fracture.* Treatment is generally a padded wrap, such as a cast padding under an Ace bandage, ice, elevation, and crutches to prevent weight-bearing. After a few days, when swelling has subsided, a short leg walking cast may be applied if needed for the patient's comfort.

Because it is often difficult to differentiate clinically between a sprain and a fracture, owing to the amount of swelling in the area, these injuries should be splinted and treated as a fracture until x-ray can confirm the diagnosis. A boot-type air splint, cardboard splint, well padded, or even a pillow may be used to immobilize

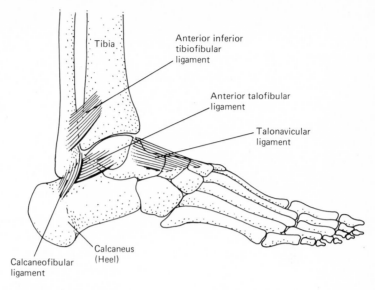

Figure 21-8 Ligaments of the ankle.

the ankle. The patient should lie down with the injured ankle elevated while awaiting treatment.

FOOT

Fractures of the *heel* (calcaneous bone) are usually caused by direct violence from a fall with the victim landing on his or her heels. This is often associated with a compression fracture of the spine, usually T12 or L1, as the force is transmitted upward. Initial treatment for this patient should include a good history and assessment for back injury. The patient should be positioned on a firm surface, on the back, and not be allowed to move around until back injury is ruled out. The foot may be elevated on a pillow and ice packs applied. Place the pillows so that there is no pressure on the heel area.

The main problems with fractures of the *metatarsal bones* and *toes* are restoration of length and alignment. Improper healing could result in a deformity that leads to irritation from shoes and weight-bearing. Initial splinting can be done with a boot-type air splint, padded cardboard splint, or pillow splint. Treatment consists of immobilization by splint or cast, ice packs, elevation, and crutches. These fractures usually heal in about 4 weeks. Toes may be splinted by placing cotton padding between the web spaces and then taping them together.

PEDIATRIC FRACTURES

Most fractures in children seem to heal fairly well even with almost indifferent treatment, *proper alignment* being the chief requirement. Injuries to the growth plate account for about one-third of skeletal trauma in children; possible complications include progressive angular deformity, a discrepancy in limb length, and joint incongruity.[3] Although growth plate damage has potential for causing many problems, the area usually repairs well, and these complications are rare. The diagnosis by *x-ray* is very important and often confusing because of epiphysial and growth lines which must be differentiated from the actual fracture line. X-rays of both right and left parts in similar position and in two projections should be taken for comparison.

SUBLUXATION

One of the most common orthopedic injuries seen in the ED is *subluxation*. The patient is usually a child between 1 and 4 years of age who has suddenly refused to move an arm and holds it slightly flexed and pronated. Parents often think the arm is paralyzed or the clavicle is fractured and seldom mention that the problem began as the child was being pulled along by the wrist, the usual cause.[4] A sudden jerk on the child's hand subluxes the radial head, and for this reason the injury has sometimes been referred to as "curbstone dislocation" or simply a pulled elbow. This dislocation is easily reduced by supination and flexion of the elbow with no local anesthetic needed. There should be an audible click, and the child will begin to use this arm at once. Many times this maneuver occurs inadvertently as the child is positioned by the radiologist for x-ray, and findings are negative, which makes a good history invaluable. Authorities differ over the importance of immobilizing these injuries after treatment.

The general principles of fracture management are the same as those applied for an adult, with much reassurance for both the child and his parents.

EMOTIONAL SUPPORT

Orthopedic patients are a nursing challenge as they involve a full spectrum of emotions including anxiety and fear, compounded by the pain of the injury. To the apprehensive patient and family orthopedics may appear at times very brutal as it involves strange-looking devices (splints, tractions apparatus, finger traps), and teaching must begin immediately to allay anxiety. It is important to establish a quick rapport which allows enough confidence on the patient's part to allow the nurse to touch the injury and assess the situation. Gentle but firm handling, splinting to reduce some of the pain, and explanation as the nurse is doing these things are important. Positive, firm handling instills confidence in the frightened patient. The nurse must give as much information as possible about what to expect—i.e., the splint, the cast, the x-ray (*check with females for possible pregnancy*), and other treatment. If there is an obvious deformity and possibility of surgery, keep the patient NPO and explain why. If the patient is going home, let him or her know how much pain to expect, what the danger signals are, and the importance of not hesitating to call or return if any problems develop.

CAST CARE

The cast material is plaster of paris imbedded in a fine mesh. It is dipped in lukewarm water and then applied wet over a stockinetted and padded area. It begins to set almost immediately and gives off *heat* as it dries. The patient will experience this heat and needs to know that it only lasts for a few minutes. The cast itself takes from 24 to 48 hours to dry completely, although it may appear so on the outside an hour after application.

Points to cover with the cast patient include the importance of keeping the cast dry as water will revert it to its former soggy state. Also instruct the patient that no autographs are allowed for 24 hours until the cast is completely dry—then caution not to paint the entire area since this may clog the porous material and prohibit circulation of air through the cast. The patient must also be given a return appointment for a circulation check the next day.

The role of the ED nurse is expanding to include first-line care of many types of orthopedic injuries. Nurses need a practical working knowledge of initial assessment, splinting, and wrapping as well as knowledge of the possible complications as they function as pivotal members of the health care team.

REFERENCES

1. Schneider, F. R., *Handbook for the Orthopedic Assistant,* Mosby, St. Louis, 1972, p. 25.

2. DePalma, A., *Management of Fractures and Dislocations,* Saunders, Philadelphia, 1970, p. 361.

3. Cole, J., et al., "Injuries of the Bones, Joints and Related Soft-Tissue Structures," in Cosgriff, J., and Anderson, D. L., *The Practice of Emergency Nursing,* Lippincott, Philadelphia, 1975, p. 408.

4. Rang, M., *Children's Fractures,* Lippincott, Philadelphia, 1974, pp. 1–9, p. 361.

BIBLIOGRAPHY

Anthony, C. P., and Koltnoff, N. J., *Textbook of Anatomy and Physiology,* Mosby, St. Louis, 1974.

Committee on Trauma: American College of Surgeons, *Early Care of the Injured Patient,* Saunders, Philadelphia, 1972.

Crenshaw, A. H. (ed.), *Campbell's Operative Orthopaedics,* vols. 1 and 2, Mosby, St. Louis, 1971.

DePalma, A., *Surgery of the Shoulder,* Lippincott, Philadelphia, 1973.

Goldstein, L., and Dickerson, R., *Atlas of Orthopaedic Surgery,* vols. 1 and 2, Mosby, St. Louis, 1974.

Helfet, A. J., *Disorders of the Knee,* Lippincott, Philadelphia, 1974.

Larson, C., and Gould, M., *Calderwodd's Orthopedic Nursing,* Mosby, St. Louis, 1974.

Riehl, C. L., *Emergency Nursing,* Bennett, Peoria, Ill., 1970.

Rockwood, C. A., Jr. and Green, D. (eds.), *Fractures,* Lippincott, Philadelphia, 1975.

Sproul, C., and Mullanney, P., *Emergency Care,* Mosby, St. Louis, 1974.

Turek, S. L., *Orthopaedic Principles and Their Application,* Lippincott, Philadelphia, 1967.

CHAPTER 22
INJURIES OF THE SPINE
MAURICE W. NICHOLSON, M.D.

THE ED nurse is seeing more patients with spinal injuries because of the increased number of automobile accidents and the increased amount of time people spend in recreational activity.

Injuries in the area of the spine may damage a variety of structures and may occur singly or in combination. Injuries may affect (1) muscles and ligaments, (2) bone, (3) spinal nerve roots, and (4) spinal cord. Severity can vary from a very mild flexion-extension injury, the so-called "whiplash," to a very severe cord damage with quadriplegia.

The *cervical spine* is the most commonly injured area, followed by the lumbar spine, then the thoracic spine. The most common level of injury is *C5-6* and *C6-7*.

ED personnel must always think of possible spinal injuries in any patient with *multiple trauma* following motor vehicle accident, any patient with a *head injury,* and any patient who has sustained a *fall* from a height greater than several feet. In addition, in coastal areas, *surfing* and *swimming accidents* are a frequent cause of cervical spine injuries.

CLASSIFICATION OF INJURIES

BONE INJURIES

SUBLUXATION   With this condition, one vertebra slides forward or backward out of line with the adjoining vertebra. A fracture of one of the articulating facets is usually present to allow this dislocation to occur. However, this fracture may not be visualized. Subluxation may or may not be associated with neurological abnormalities (see Fig. 22-1a).

COMPRESSION FRACTURES   These usually occur without subluxation and usually involve only one vertebra. These fractures are often stable as posterior bony elements are intact. The variant of a compression fracture which is very unstable is a comminuted or bursting fracture of the vertebral body (see Fig. 22-1b).

FRACTURE DISLOCATIONS   In these cases the facets or intraarticular joints are subluxated, and usually the pedicles or other bony elements are fractured, allowing the vertebral bodies to slide forward. These may be associated with a severe neurological deficit (see Fig. 22-1c).

CORD AND ROOT INJURIES

CONCUSSION   These patients may present with complete loss of sensory and motor function. However, they recover rapidly within a few hours and are left with no neurological deficits.

CONTUSION   This is a more advanced stage from the concussion, and usually the neurological deficit lasts for days or weeks. Usually, there is almost complete recovery of neurological function.

LACERATION   This is self-explanatory and is usually associated with compound wounds such as bullet or knife injuries to the spine.

COMPRESSION   A variety of injuries may cause compression of the spinal cord. It is usually found in fracture dislocations but may be secondary to epidural or subdural hematomas or to an acute rupture of the intervertebral disk.

HEMATOMYELIA   This is a hemorrhage into a substance of the spinal cord.

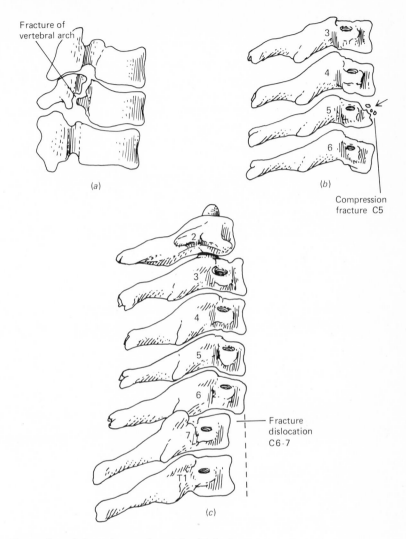

Figure 22-1 Examples of three types of vertebral injuries.

SPINAL ROOT DAMAGE   A spinal root may suffer a concussion, a contusion, a transection, an avulsion, or a compression. The *compression* may be from bone or disk impingement. *Transection* may occur from a missile or knife wound. *Avulsion* of the nerve roots occurs most frequently with automobile accidents where the patient is forcibly twisted or thrown with the arm outstretched. This causes the nerve root to be pulled completely out of the spinal cord. This injury has no cure.

ED MANAGEMENT

Persons suspected of having a spine injury must be treated as though they had one. The following is an explanation of the emergency management.

RESPIRATION

Adequacy of respiratory function must be determined immediately. If the patient is alert, as many of these patients are, ask him or her to take a deep breath. Check to see if the chest and diaphragm are moving in a normal manner. If the patient is not responsive, observe the thoracic and abdominal movements. If there is increased motion of the abdomen, this is suggestive of *diaphragmatic breathing*. One should be alert to a possible lower cervical cord injury with paralysis of the thoracic muscles. Check the color of the nail beds and skin. Arterial blood should be obtained at an early time if there is any question of inadequate pulmonary function.

IMMOBILIZATION

Patients with spinal injuries must be immobilized. It is especially important that no flexion or extension of the spine be allowed. If a patient is having respiratory distress and needs intubation, nasotracheal intubation or tracheostomy should be considered to avoid the hyperextension that occurs with the routine endotracheal intubation.

BLOOD PRESSURE AND PULSE

If the patient is in shock, the nurse should suspect some other injury since neurological injuries rarely produce more than a mild hypotension and bradycardia. Severe shock usually indicates hemorrhage from other injury. Blood pressure must be stabilized.

NEUROLOGICAL EXAMINATION

If the patient is alert, his or her cooperation can be elicited to perform a brief neurological examination (see Fig. 22-2). The examination can be performed in a few minutes by the ED nurse.

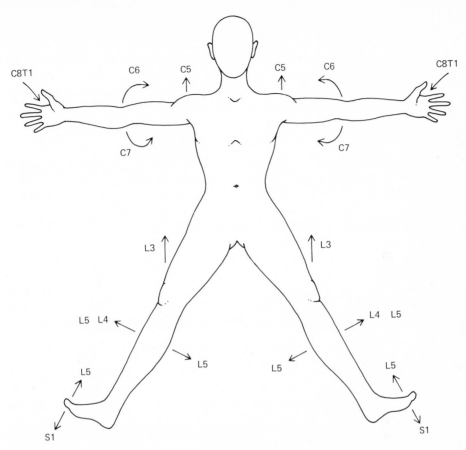

Figure 22-2. Summary chart for brief neurological examination. The patient must be checked bilaterally. See text for explanation.

EXAMINATION SUMMARY   Starting at the cervical area, ask the patient to do the following: (1) *Lift* the elbows up to shoulder height—C5; *bend* the elbow—C6; *straighten* the elbow from a flexed position—C7; *grip* —C8 and T1. (2) *Lift* the leg off the bed or flex the hips—L3; *extend* the knee—L4 and L5; *wiggle* the toes backwards—L5; *push* the toes downward—S1. If the patient can do all these, a severe cord injury is not present. If he or she is able to bend the elbows but not extend the elbows, then one has to suspect a lesion between C6 and C7. If the arm function is intact and the chest is moving, but the patient is unable to move the legs, then the site of concern is in the upper lumbar area. If the examination

shows that one arm moves well but the other arm does not, suspect a *nerve root injury* on the nonfunctioning side. This brief
examination can help the ED nurse to assess the severity of the
injury quickly.

If the patient is comatose the nurse can do the following tests:
(1) Rub the sternum with the knuckles to see if the arms or legs
move. If all move, then there is little chance of a severe injury. If
one side moves and the other side does not, the nurse has to be
concerned with a *hemiplegia*. If the arms move and the legs do
not, a lower spinal cord injury has to be considered. (2) Squeeze
the muscles in the axillary fold on each side to allow comparison
of movement of one arm with the other arm. Squeezing the Achilles
tendons allows assessment of leg motion.

SPECIFIC TREATMENT

If a cord injury is present, intravenous *dexamethasone* 10 to 20
mg should be given. There is some controversy about the use of
this drug. However, many neurosurgeons, including the author feel
that it is of value.

Oxygen by nasal catheter or mask should be given if there is inadequate respiratory function. Damaged nerve tissue becomes
more severely damaged by low PaO_2 or high $PaCO_2$.

Skeletal traction (skull tongs) for fracture dislocation of the cervical spine is often inserted in the ED. There are two main types of
tongs: *Vincke tongs,* which are inserted into the skull in the temporal area in front of the ears, and *Crutchfield tongs,* which are
put in the parietal skull closer to the vertex. Traction of 12 to 15
pounds is usually instituted to stabilize the fracture.

SUPPORTIVE THERAPY

The nurse should start intravenous fluids with a catheter and at the
same time may draw blood for blood grouping, hematocrit, blood
sugar, electrolytes, barbiturates, and alcohol. A foley catheter must
be used in any patient with paraplegia or quadriplegia. A nasal
gastric tube should be introduced in all serious cervical cord injuries to alleviate vomiting and possible aspiration. Open wounds
must be covered with sterile bandages.

DIAGNOSTIC PROCEDURES

In addition to the neurological examination, the patient with a
spinal injury must have *x-rays.* These are necessary for a diagnosis

of a fracture or fracture subluxation. The x-ray technicians must be advised that there is a possible spine injury so they will use a minimum of motion in obtaining their films.

A lumbar puncture is rarely of diagnostic value in these patients and, if performed, should be done by a neurological surgeon.

Details of sensory neurological examination have not been included as ED nurses are too busy to perform these tests and they are not really their function. The emergency nurse who is alert to the possibility of a spinal cord injury can often prevent further injury by proper assessment and care for the patient. Spinal cord injuries can be devastating to the patient, and it is tragic to see a young, healthy individual suddenly changed from an active person to a paralyzed, bedridden patient for the rest of his or her life. Good care by the ambulance attendant at the scene of an accident and by the ED personnel can prevent any further damage to the nervous tissue in spinal injuries.

BIBLIOGRAPHY

Croff, L., et al., *Traumatic Cervical Syndrome and Whiplash*, Lippincott, Philadelphia, 1967.

DeJong, R. N., *The Neurological Exam*, Harper & Row, New York, 1976.

Hardy, A., and Rossier, A., *Spinal Cord Injuries*, Publishing Sciences Group, Acton, Mass., 1975.

Nicholson, M. W., "Whiplash: Fact, Fantasy or Fallacy," *Journal Hawaii Medical Association*, vol. 33, no. 5, May 1974.

CHAPTER 23
THE EMERGENCY TREATMENT OF BURNS

JAMES PENOFF, M.D., F.A.C.S.

THE treatment of burns has several critical and unique characteristics but overall is quite similar to all other pathological situations. Sound observation, understanding of the pathophysiology, and good judgment in selecting the treatment mode set a sound course for proper management. There are many acceptable approaches in the treatment of burns—the methods mentioned here represent one of several.

Burns can be classified in several ways. The extent of the burn as well as the characteristics of the burning agent and depth must be considered.

AGENT

The burning agent should be determined as soon as possible since it slants the treatment.

1. Burns caused by *heat* (e.g., scalding with hot liquids or flame) have surface involvement almost exclusively.

2. Burns caused by *chemicals* (acids or bases) continue to cause damage for quite some time and should be noted so that a program of multiple and prolonged showers can be started.

3. *Electrical* burns are characterized by many hidden problems since the passage of the current can cause cardiac arrhythmias, hemoglobinurias, aneurysms, or late cataracts.

DEPTH

Burns are classified in degrees which denote the depth of burn. The degrees are not always immediately distinguishable but are important to assess since second- and even more so third-degree burns are accompanied by fluid loss from the vascular system.

1. *First degree.* These burns are characterized by erythema and tenderness. The best example is the well-known sunburn.

2. *Second degree.* These burns have the erythema of the first-degree burn plus the formation of *blebs* or blisters. They represent deeper injury to the skin but heal unless an infection destroys the epithelial remnants.

3. *Third degree.* These represent injury through all the layers of the skin and appendages and cannot be healed without the formation of heavy scar. They are characterized by open raw areas or *escars* (crusts) and are classically considered insensitive to pain (but this is not always true). *Skin grafting* is the usual treatment. The appearance can vary anywhere from a pale white skin to a charred crust.

SURFACE AREA

The amount of body burn is important since this determines the seriousness just as much as the depth. The "rule of nines" is a frequently used method of evaluation (see Fig. 23-1).

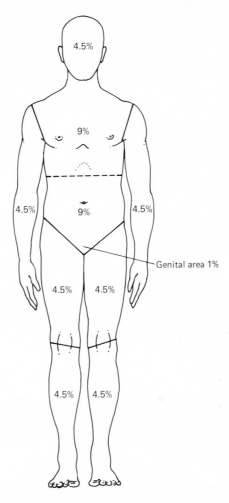

Figure 23-1 Percentage of body burns by "rule of nines." Anterior aspect shown. The percentages are the same for the posterior aspect.

BURNS TO HOSPITALIZE

A *20 percent second-* or *third*-degree burn in an adult or a *15 percent* similar burn in a child is usually considered of sufficient magnitude to warrant hospitalization. The fluid losses are such that they should be closely monitored in a hospital setting. Burns of critical areas (e.g., face, ears, perineum, hands, and feet) may also warrant hospitalization despite the fact that they may cover less than 20 percent of the surface area.

TREATMENT

FIRST-DEGREE BURNS

Pain is the hallmark of these, but fortunately it is usually greatly diminished in 12 to 24 hours. A cold wet towel is probably the most comfortable bandage. This need be applied only as long as the area is uncomfortable. The pain is due to exposure of the burn to air, and a moist towel protects it. Greasy dressings also do this but are not recommended since they are difficult to remove and retain moisture and may, therefore, encourage bacterial growth.

SECOND-DEGREE BURNS

Whether to leave or remove the blisters has been a subject of debate. Since the blebs usually burst anyway, it is best to carefully remove them and wash the area with saline. A dressing of *Xeroform* gauze (or similar nonadhering dressing) in a single layer with a layer of absorbent gauze (e.g., Kerlix) is placed over this. The outer dressing is removed in 24 to 48 hours, and the Xeroform allowed to dry and separate spontaneously. It should be checked approximately two to three days later to make sure that the area is dry. If there is moisture, a secondary infection or perhaps a misdiagnosed third-degree burn should be suspected.

THIRD-DEGREE BURNS

These burns have no epithelial remnants beneath and require skin grafting unless they are quite small. The burned tissue and escar need to be treated and removed before grafting. This is done during hospitalization.

TREATMENT OF HOSPITALIZED BURNS

Upon entrance to the ED, the *tetanus immunization status* should be determined. If there is no past history of immunization, *hyperimmune human serum* should be used and tetanus immunization begun. Otherwise, updating the tetanus toxoid is done when indicated.

History determination of the burn is important. If the burn occurred in an enclosed area, the patient should be carefully watched for respiratory difficulties as either steroids or tracheostomy may be indicated. (Overall, the use of tracheostomy in burns is not common.) All large burns should have blood-gas and pH determinations since this is a sensitive index of the lung status. If an acid or other chemical was the burning agent, repeated flushing with showers is indicated for the first 12 hours after admission as these agents continue to chemically destroy tissue even after the initial first-aid flushing and irrigation. An electrical burn should have cardiac evaluation in the ED with an ECG since cardiac arrhythmias are not uncommon and must be noted.

INTRAVENOUS AND ORAL FLUIDS

The morbidity of burns in the first week almost always is caused by *fluid* and *electrolyte imbalance.* The sequestration of fluid in extravascular areas is significant, and there is often marked hypotension. This begins at the time of the burn and is most marked in the first 24 hours. Several elaborate formulas have been devised where replacement of the fluid is based upon the weight of the patient and percent of total body burn. The aim of all these formulas is to replace the lost fluids to a sufficient degree to maintain circulating blood volume. However, this author believes that the best index of adequate blood volume and blood flow is shown by *urinary output.*

As a result, a good replacement can be achieved by placing an indwelling urinary catheter and giving intravenous normal saline with 1 ampule bicarbonate per liter at a sufficient rate to cause a urinary flow of 50 to 60 cc per hour in the adult or 30 to 40 cc per hour in the child. An IV rate of 250 to 300 cc per hour may be required to do this. The IV should be with a large-bore catheter that is a *central venous line.* A *cutdown* (directly through the burn if necessary) is usually indicated. At the time of cutdown an initial CBC, BUN, electrolytes, and creatinine should be done to establish base-line levels. *The prompt replacement of intravenous fluids in the ED is the most important function of the emergency team.*

Large burns raise the possibility of an accompanying *ileus,* and upon admission the patient should be placed NPO and serious consideration given for a *nasogastric tube.*

LOCAL TREATMENT

The burn should be washed with a mild soap solution or saline and dressed appropriately. If the type of dressing has not been determined, a sterile sheet is adequate.

At present treatment with *silver sulfadiazine* ointment (Silvadene) either open or with dressings is probably the most popular. It gives good antibacterial protection of the burn without the hyponatremia of silver nitrate solution or the carbonic anhydrase inhibition action of Sulfamylon. Topical gentamicin has been used, but this is considered not to be as acceptable a method of treatment as Silvadene at the present.

SYSTEMIC ANTIBIOTICS

The use of systemic antibiotics is becoming less and less popular. The most common approach is to use either no antibiotics or aqueous penicillin (or its equivalent) for 5 days to protect from a streptococcal infection.

SPECIAL TREATMENT (EARS, HANDS)

Burns of the *ears* can easily result in chondritis and complete loss of an ear, so special care must be taken to carefully cleanse and apply the ointment as indicated.

Because *hands* are so important and can easily stiffen beyond a useful level, all efforts must be directed toward their proper care. The correct method of treatment is to place them in the most useful position (the position of function). This is accomplished by *dorsiflexing the wrist* and allowing the MP and IP joints of the fingers to flex in their position of rest. This position is easily obtained with the wrist in dorsiflexion and can be achieved by a splint that extends from the forearm into the palm or by resting the relaxed hands on folded towels.

ANCILLARY TREATMENT OF BURNS

The use of *porcine skin* (pig skin) is one of the newer methods of treating burns. This is a biological dressing and should not be considered as a true skin graft. Its use is best confined to either the second-degree burn from which the blebs have been removed and is painful on exposure to air or to a third-degree burn that is an open, clean wound. The porcine skin acts as a biological covering and, therefore, decreases fluid and electrolyte loss as well as provides comfort.

There has been some recent work showing that the use of *heparin* in burns for 7 days results in a quicker healing of the burn since the vascular sludging and thromboses that occur in small vessels adjacent to burns can be decreased significantly. This has been advocated only recently, and its true value has not been ascertained.

EXPECTED COURSE

The most important role of the ED is the *evaluation* of the burn and *stabilization* of problems (primarily the hydration and replacement of hypovolemia with intravenous solutions). The start of an overall definitive plan of therapy is in the ED.

In the first 4 to 5 days, the problems of fluid and electrolyte imbalance must be carefully monitored by hemoglobin, electrolyte, blood-gas, and pH determinations. After the first week, the plan is to prepare the burn for grafting with debridement and topical antibacterials. This lasts until 3 to 4 weeks after the initial burn. Coverage with split-thickness skin grafts follows, and the most significant burns are ready for discharge in 1 to 3 months after admission.

After this come the long-term problems of scar contracture and cosmesis. The total rehabilitation may take 2 to 3 years. At present, the best results are only satisfactory.

Table 23-1	Summary chart for the emergency care of burns

1. Classification of burns
   a. Agent: Thermal, electrical, chemical
   b. Depth: First degree: red skin
      Second degree: red skin plus blisters
      Third degree: red skin plus blisters plus crust or pure white skin or loss of all skin
   c. Surface area: rule of nines

2. ED treatment
   a. First degree: Cold towels
   b. Second degree: Remove blebs and dress with Xeroform and Kerlix
   c. Third degree: Hospitalize

3. Treatment of hospitalized burns
   a. Tetanus immunization
   b. Tracheostomy evaluation
   c. Evaluation of burning agent
      (1) If chemical, flush well
      (2) If electrical, get ECG
   d. IVs: Normal saline solution and indwelling catheter; run IV at rate to get urinary output of 30 to 50 cc hour
   e. Local treatment: Cleanse the burn with saline and dress with appropriate dressing (probably Silvadene for all large burns)
   f. Systemic antibiotics: None or penicillin for 5 days
   g. Special treatment (ears, hands): Close attention to problems of ears, and hands in position of function
   h. Oral intake: All large burns NPO; consider nasogastric tube

BIBLIOGRAPHY

American College of Surgeons, *Early Care of the Injured Patient,* Saunders, Philadelphia, 1972.

Artz, C. P., "Burns: From First Aid to Skin Graft," *Drug Therapy,* vol. 5, no. 4, April 1975, pp. 127–135.

Baxter, C. P., "Concepts in Management of Major Electrical Burns," *The Surgical Clinics of North America,* vol. 50, December 1970, pp. 1401–1418.

Larson, D. L., et al., "The Burned Child," *Texas Medicine,* vol. 67, April 1971, pp. 58–67.

CHAPTER 24
TETANUS PROPHYLAXIS—THEN AND NOW

LIZABETH LOVE RYAN, R. N.

IN 1909 there were 1373 deaths from tetanus recorded in only 18 states of North America.[1] Grandma had more familiarity with the disease than most doctors today. She may have seen at least one case, and the source of her academic knowledge would have been her home medical volume, perhaps the venerable *Dr. Chase's Recipes* or *Information for Everybody* revised and enlarged in 1900 to include:

> *Locked Jaw Tetanus:* A disease in which the muscles of the body are in a state of rigidity with occasional spasms and excruciating pain. The cause of this disease is injury to the extremities of the nerves, punctured or lacerated wounds of the hands or feet, surgical operations, or the use of narcotic poisons.[2]

Dr. Chase's treatments included "drachm doses of laudanum" to reduce spasms, turpentine enemas, hot baths, wound debridement, and poultices of "slippery elm and lye."

Tetanus has been almost eradicated since Dr. Chase wrote that recipe at the turn of the century. During the first 2 months of World War I, deaths from tetanus among the wounded were legion. In the middle of October 1914, tetanus antitoxin was administered to the wounded and the rate dropped dramatically in only 2 weeks. After the war the use of the new medication dropped civilian deaths from tetanus below prewar levels. With the introduction of *tetanus toxoid* in 1924 and with an improved preparation with alum in 1934 and aluminum phosphate in 1952, the disease has become rare in the United States. In 1970 fewer than 200 cases were reported. Today's statistics show a rise in the disease among drug abusers and that fatality is largely confined to individuals over 35 years of age. An understanding of the organism and the disease process can quickly explain these statistics, and will help ED nurses give better care and education to these potential victims of what Dr. Chase terms "that dread convulsive disease."

PATHOPHYSIOLOGY

Considering the wide distribution of the bacillus, the disease is infrequent. The anaerobic *Clostridium tetani* is found in the intestines of grass-eating animals and in human intestine, and then through elimination is transferred to the soil.

Anytime the skin's protection is compromised, the bacilli can enter the body. Few emergency nurses would neglect to administer tetanus protection for the classic puncture wound, deep lacerations, crushing wounds with much tissue destruction, burns, compound fractures, gunshot wounds, or those containing splinters. But tetanus can also occur after frostbite, oral lacerations, fractures of the maxilla or the mandible affecting dental sockets, dental surgery, induced abortion, childbirth, and intestinal operations. In addition it can occur in the newborn and even develop after a wound revision. Tetanus is rising among *drug users,* especially those who "pop" drugs directly under the skin where blood supply and oxygenation are poor—perfect conditions for the anaerobic growth of this bacillus. The majority of cases occur with wounds that go unnoticed or are considered too minor for treatment.

No matter what the injury, the deposited bacilli multiply and produce toxins for an *incubation period* of 3 to 14 days in acute tetanus or 4 to 5 weeks in so-called chronic tetanus. The organism usually stays at the site of injury, but the toxins are distributed to local and/

or systemic nerves. Two *toxins* are produced: *tetanolysin* that produces some lysis of erythrocytes, and *tetanospasmin* that joins with the nerve cell to cause the characteristic spasms of tetanus. Once the tetanospasmin joins the nerve cell, it is impossible for any presently known therapy to neutralize it. The earliest symptoms are evidence of this union.

SIGNS AND SYMPTOMS

The onset of the disease is usually gradual, with *stiffness of the jaw* and of the *muscles* of the *esophagus and neck* the first symptoms. Soon the jaws are rigidly fixed, and the facial muscles contract giving the patient a wild, excited expression. *Spasms* produce a blend of laughter and crying. Tetany spreads to the muscles of the back and penis. The spasms are reflex and are brought on by the slightest irritation. The patient has a high *fever* and great *pain,* yet the mind remains clear as he or she suffers from hunger, thirst, and fatigue. The illness may be swift or linger for weeks with death usually the result of exhaustion or asphyxia. The *chronic form* of tetanus, with slower onset and less severe symptoms, is an infection in a healed wound that is reopened by accident or surgery. Local tetanus affects only the limb or area of the wound.

Fatality varies with age, treatment, length of incubation, and geographical location. Tetanus today has special significance for one age group: 90 percent of fatalities occur in people over 35 years of age. Surveys show that a high percentage of the middle aged and elderly do not have protection against tetanus. Because tetanus toxoid was not introduced until 1924, and childhood immunization programs started even later, these people have missed the series of immunizations. It is important to notice that routine immunization of infants and schoolchildren against tetanus has reduced the mortality in people under 35 to about 1/300 the rate at the beginning of the century.

Emergency nurses are rarely involved in the care of the actuely ill tetanic patient. For further coverage of this topic, please check the bibliography. Their primary role is in the prevention of the disease. Therefore all emergency personnel should understand the basics of active and passive immunization so they can give the best protection to each patient. The basic points about immunization are listed in the following sections.

ACTIVE IMMUNIZATION

Active immunity is produced by stimulating the production of antitoxin by the patient's own immune system.

FLUID (UNMODIFIED) TOXOID

Preparation: Tetanus toxin modified with formaldehyde and heat so
it does not have toxic effects.

Basic immunization: Three subcutaneous injections at least 3 weeks
apart. Adequate circulating antitoxin present 2 weeks after last injection. Fortifying booster may be given at 1 year, then every 5 to 10
years. Neonatal tetanus is prevented by boosting during pregnancy.

Untoward effects: Redness, swelling, itching, regional lymphade-
nopathy.

Appearance: Clear, colorless to brownish-yellow.

Expiration: Two years after date of manufacture or issue.

Storage: Two to ten degrees Celsius.

ADSORBED TETANUS TOXOID

Preparation: Four different preparations of the active part of the
fluid, the actual toxoid, modified with alum, aluminum hydroxide,
or aluminum phosphate, and then suspended in saline.

Basic immunization: Requires only two doses 4 weeks apart.

Advantages: Slower absorption from the site of injection than fluid,
thus providing higher levels of antitoxin. Now recommended for both
active immunization and boosters because of higher level of longer-
lasting immunity.

Untoward effects: Local reactions more common because of slow
absorption.

Appearance: Turbid as a white, grayish, or pinkish suspension.

Storage and expiration: Same as fluid toxoid.

Nursing implications: Give deeply IM in lateral upper arm to avoid sterile abcess formation. Shake well as active toxoid is in the precipitate at the bottom of vial or prefilled syringe.

PASSIVE IMMUNIZATION

Passive immunity is produced by the injection of tetanus antitoxin actively produced by another source. *Tetanus antitoxin,* in theory, neutralizes the toxins produced by the bacillus.

ANTITOXIN OF EQUINE OR BOVINE ORIGIN

Preparation: Extracted from the blood of horses or cattle hyperimmunized with tetanus toxoid.

Disadvantages: Of those receiving this antitoxin, 5 to 30 percent have *allergic reactions.* Authorities feel that it should no longer be used unless the tetanus immune globulin is not available within 24 hours.

TETANUS IMMUNE GLOBULIN

Preparation: From the blood of adults who were hyperimmunized with tetanus toxoid.

Advantages: Does not produce the serious reactions of the former. The protective levels of antitoxin last 3 to 4 weeks.

Untoward effects: Soreness at injection site, urticaria, angioedema.

Appearance: Transparent or slightly opalescent. May develop harmless granular deposit.

Storage: Two to eight degrees Celsius. Do not freeze.

Expiration: Two years after date of manufacture or issue.

Nursing implications: Must be given IM in the gluteus; it is important to draw back on the plunger to be sure a blood vessel has not been entered. No gamma globulin preparation should be given IV because of the danger of a hypersensitivity reaction. Theoretically the same amount of toxin is produced and must be neutralized in both adult and child. May also be given to unimmunized patient for surgical wound revision.

ACTIVE AND PASSIVE IMMUNIZATION CONCURRENTLY

By giving the adsorbed toxoid in the ED along with the immune globulin, levels of the antitoxin that last several weeks can be developed.

When a patient comes to the ED for treatment of any wound, a standard procedure for giving tetanus prophylaxis is necessary. Table 24-1 lists the widely accepted recommendations of the American College of Surgeons.[3]

One final point in the emergency prevention of tetanus is the *immunization history.* Note in the guide the phrases "documented previous immunization" and "unimmunized or without good evidence of it." Never assume that anyone has been immunized. Legal decisions on this point give the physician the right to rely on the patient's statement, but many times the nurse takes the tetanus history. The patient who says he or she had a tetanus shot 2 years before may only have been given immune globulin with no instruction for follow-up. For the current injury the patient may have no level of circulating antitoxin to boost with an injection of toxoid. The ED nurse can assist in determining this person's status by getting records of previous visits and calling private physicians' offices. Documentation of the present injection helps ensure the patient's future safety from tetanus.

A *written record of immunization* should be given to each patient. A printed card enables emergency personnel to record the information quickly and easily and gives the patient a durable record. If the patient has never been immunized and the first toxoid is given in the ED, the card can carry the dates on which he or she should receive the remaining injections. These could be checked off by the private physician as they are given and the card would then give a complete tetanus history. By encouraging all patients to know their own status and giving special scrutiny to patients over 35 years of age and to drug abusers, many cases of tetanus, especially those that occur after injuries that seem too small to warrant medical attention, could be prevented.

In his campaign against tetanus, Dr. Chase used everything from slippery elm and milk to hot bricks and vinegar. Seventy-five years of research and development have given all some advantages; many have never seen a single case of tetanus. To keep it this way, all nurses must take reliable tetanus histories and then return to "Grandma's ice box" for the appropriate drug to prevent the disease in every patient.

Table 24-1   Standard procedure for tetanus prophylaxis. *(Adapted from the Committee on Trauma: "Guide to Tetanus Prophylaxis," The Bulletin of the American College of Surgeons, vol. 56, no. 6, June 1971, pp. 22–23.)*

History	Intervention
1. Documented previous immunization a. Booster within 12 months b. Completed series within 12 months	Meticulous surgical care
2. Immunization 1 to 10 years ago in wounds that do not seem tetanus-prone	0.5 cc of adsorbed toxoid
3. Previous immunization took place from 6 months to 1 year ago and wound is severe, neglected, and more than 24 hours old	0.5 cc adsorbed toxoid
4. Immunization 1 to 10 years ago and wound seems especially tetanus-prone	0.5 cc adsorbed toxoid 250 units human tetanus immune globulin Prophylactic antibiotics
5. Unimmunized or *without good evidence of immunization:* a. With clean minor wounds in which tetanus is most unlikely	0.5 cc adsorbed toxoid
b. With any but a very minor wound	0.5 cc adsorbed toxoid 250 units human tetanus immune globulin Possibly prophylactic antibiotics
c. With severe, neglected, or old wounds	0.5 cc adsorbed toxoid 500 units human tetanus immune globulin Prophylactic antibiotics

REFERENCES

1. Osler, W., *The Principles and Practices of Medicine,* 9th ed., E. N. Appleton, New York, 1920.

2. Beal, J. B. (ed.), *Dr. Chase's Recipes or Information for Everybody,* University of Michigan Press, Ann Arbor, Mich., 1907, p. 237.

3. Committee on Trauma, "Guide to Tetanus Prophlaxis," *The Bulletin of the American College of Surgeons,* vol. 56, no. 6, June 1971, pp. 22–23.

BIBLIOGRAPHY

Benenson, Abram S. (ed.), *Control of Communicable Diseases in Man,* 11th ed., The American Public Health Association, New York, 1970.

Eckert, K., *Emergency Room Care,* 2d ed., Little Brown, Boston, 1970.

"Growing Old Without Tetanus," *Emergency Medicine,* Fischer-Murray, New York, July 1971.

Hummel, R. P., "Too Many Tetanus Boosters?" *Consultant,* February 1975, pp. 45–47.

Muller, J., Marshall, F. N., Davison, K. J., and Lepreau, F. J., "Tetanus in Haiti," *The Lancet,* Feb. 15, 1975, p. 383.

"Tetanus Umbilicus," *Emergency Medicine,* vol. 7, no. 11, November 1975, p. 134.

"Tetanus When It Really Happens," *Emergency Medicine,* Fischer-Murray, New York, January 1974, p. 46.

CHAPTER 25
EMERGENCY CARE OF THE COMATOSE PATIENT

ROBERT C. HINMAN, B.S., M.D.

COMA results from conditions that widely and directly depress (destroy) the functions of the cerebral hemispheres or the brainstem with its integral alerting mechanisms (*reticular activating system*) for the maintenance of consciousness. The causes of coma can be placed into three categories:

1. *Supratentorial mass lesions* as intracerebral hemorrhages, subdural hematomas, and epidural hematomas that bilaterally depress hemispheric function or unilaterally depress one hemisphere with attendant medial displacement of the temporal lobe with secondary brainstem compression.

2. *Subtentorial mass* or destructive lesions that compromise the brainstem such as cerebellar and pontine hemorrhages.

3. *Metabolic disturbances* which are naturally occurring as in hepatic failure and those due to the ingestion of a central nervous system depressant such as barbiturates.

CLINICAL ASSESSMENT

The most important aspect in evaluating the comatose patient is an adequate *history* obtained from friends or relatives. Information thus gained that a patient ingested barbiturates will prevent much fruitless searching for the etiology of the patient's coma and more precisely direct the continuing care of the patient.

Observations made during the physical examination (and enumerated below) will help to distinguish structural damage or compressive dysfunction which is usually focal in nature from metabolic disturbances due to endogenous or exogenous toxins (see Table 25-1).

Table 25-1   Final diagnosis in 386 patients with coma of unknown etiology.*
(Modified from Plum, F., and Posner, J. B.: Diagnosis of Stupor and Coma, 2d ed., Davis, Philadelphia, 1972, p. 3.)

I. Supratentorial mass lesions	(18%)
A. Epidural hematoma	
B. Subdural hematoma	
C. Intracerebral hematoma	
II. Subtentorial lesions	(13%)
A. Brainstem infarction	
B. Brainstem hemorrhage	
C. Cerebellar hemorrhage	
III. Metabolic and diffuse cerebral disorders	(68%)
A. Anoxia or ischemia	
B. Concussion and postictal states	
C. Infection (meningitis and encephalitis)	
D. Exogenous toxins, medications, and poisons	D + E (42%)
1. Sedative drugs	
a. Barbiturates	
b. Nonbarbiturate hypnotics (i.e., diazepam)	
c. Ethanol	
d. Opiates	
2. Enzyme inhibitors	
a. Heavy metals	
b. Organic phosphates	
c. Cyanide	
d. Salicylates	
3. Decreased oxygen tension	
a. Carbon monoxide	

Table 25-1 (*continued*)

    E. Endogenous toxins and deficiencies
       1. Decreased cerebral blood flow secondary to increased vascular resistance
         a. Hypertensive encephalopathy
       2. Hypoglycemia
       3. Cofactor deficiency
         a. Thiamine
       4. Diseases of nonendocrine organs
         a. Liver failure
         b. Kidney (uremia)
         c. Lung (CO_2 narcosis)
       5. Hyper- or hypofunction of endocrine organs
         a. Pituitary
         b. Thyroid
       6. Water, pH, and ionic abnormalities (increased or decreased)
         a. H_2O
         b. Na
         c. K
         d. Ca
         e. Magnesium
         f. pH
       7. Other problems:
         a. Sickle-cell anemia
         b. Heat stroke
       8. Central nervous system disease
         a. Creutzfeldt-Jakob disease
         b. Alzheimer's disease
         c. Huntington's chorea

*It should be noted that exogenous or endogenous toxins account for nearly 50 percent of the total number of comatose patients presenting in an ED. Psychologically induced comatose-like states are extremely uncommon.

1. Simple observation of the patient will often reveal the level at which the patient is presently functioning. In *decorticate posturing* (arms flexed at the elbow and legs extended), there is bilateral hemispheric dysfunction, but the brainstem is generally intact. *Decerebrate posturing* (arms and legs extended) implies bilateral dysfunction of the hemispheres and the brainstem to the level of the midpons. Neither of these postures helps to distinguish metabolic from structural dysfunction.

2. Flaccidity (decreased muscle tone) with depressed reflexes and flexor plantar responses on stimulation of the sole of the foot, but without any suggestion of hemiparesis, usually indicates a *metabolic etiology* for the coma. Asymmetrical pupils, reflexes, or tone, especially in association with a unilateral Babinski's response, suggest a focal and structural lesion. Myoclonic jerks (random and irregular rapid movements of a muscle or muscle group) suggest an anoxic etiology for the coma.

3. There are many patterns to patients' respirations that might be noted, but the most helpful fact to remember is that *hyperventilation* frequently indicates a metabolic disturbance, i.e., acidosis as in diabetic ketoacidotic coma.

4. The *pupils* are of great significance in the overall evaluation of the comatose patient. Preserved pupillary responses to light stimulation with the appropriate constriction and equality of the pupils in the absence of other focal signs and the presence of *doll's eye response* (a rolling of the eyes from side to side with lateral and brisk rotation of the head from left to right) suggest a metabolic cause for the coma. *Unreactive pupils* may suggest that atropine has been used or that the patient has ingested a central nervous system depressant such as glutethimide. *Reactive pupils* to light imply an intact upper brainstem. *Pinpoint pupils* which often seem unreactive (except with magnification) to a bright light indicate dysfunction in the pontine area of the brainstem. This is usually secondary to a focal and destructive lesion such as pontine hemorrhage. It is important to note that drugs used in the treatment of glaucoma (pilocarpine) also cause pinpoint pupils, and in elderly patients this should be a primary consideration if the pupillary abnormality is bilateral and the only focal disturbance. A *unilateral markedly dilated* pupil which is fixed to light stimulation, with or without outward deviation to the globe of the eye, implies compression of the third nerve on the same side as the dilated pupil. This is a focal sign and suggestive of a structural lesion in the supratentorial region which is usually due to a hematoma in or about one cerebral hemisphere, inducing medial deviation of the temporal lobe and compression of the third nerve on the same side.

EMERGENCY MANAGEMENT

In all comatose patients it is important to maintain an adequate airway, preserve vital functions, establish an adequate intravenous route, and look carefully for allied conditions. An allied condition in a patient with an epidural hematoma sustained in an automobile accident with head injury might be the rupture of the spleen with intraabdominal hemorrhaging.

In patients in whom the etiology of the coma is not apparent historically or by examination, a number of *laboratory tests* might routinely be obtained, e.g., serum glucose, electrolytes, and BUN. Blood-gas determinations should be obtained if there is any suggestion of respiratory embarrassment. A complete blood count is also of value, especially where infection may be the etiology for the coma. Where the ingestion of a central nervous system depressant may ultimately be the etiology, the drawing and freezing of 20 cc blood will allow *toxicological determinations* to be run at a later and more appropriate time. In conditions where trauma seems to have induced the comatose state, *x-rays* of appropriate bony structures as the skull should be obtained. Other laboratory tests or diagnostic evaluations should be at the discretion of the attending physician or neurological consultant.

All comatose patients should be treated with thoughtful dispatch, but two conditions require rapid intervention to preserve life or central nervous system integrity. They are *epidural hematoma* and *hypoglycemia*.

EPIDURAL HEMATOMA

This condition is suggested by the head-injured patient who was initially rendered unconscious for several minutes, regained consciousness and functioned relatively normally for 1 to 2 hours, only to again become unconscious. The pupil on the side of the epidural hematoma may dilate with attendant lateral deviation to the globe of the eye (see above) with an associated contralateral hemiparesis to that of the dilated pupil. (See Fig. 19-2.) Skull x-rays will often demonstrate a fracture transversely through the lateral skull wall that crosses the *middle meningeal artery* from which bleeding into the epidural space is emanating.

In patients where traumatically induced supratentorial hematomas are producing rapid, progressive neurological deterioration, *hyperventilation* will constrict the intracranial vascular bed sufficiently due to the induced alkalosis so that the mass compressive effect of the hematoma will be temporarily reduced. At that point a definitive neurosurgical procedure may be performed, i.e., burr holes or craniotomy.

HYPOGLYCEMIC COMA

Rapid respirations, decerebrate posturing, preserved pupillary light reactions, and intact eye movements suggest hypoglycemic coma.

Twenty-five to fifty cc of 50% *glucose* given intravenously after a concomitant serum glucose has been drawn will return the patient to immediate consciousness providing the hypoglycemic state has not existed for too long a time. Indeed, in many EDs it is standard procedure to administer this volume of glucose to all comatose patients when the etiology of the coma is not apparent by history or examination. It is important to remember that this amount and concentration of glucose serves as a *hyperosmolar agent* and may transiently lighten or improve the comatose patient's state when this coma is attended by cerebral edema or a mass lesion effect as a hematoma. *Obtaining the concomitant blood sugar determination becomes very important!*

In areas where narcotics are commonly "mainlined," 1 to 4 ampules of *naloxone* (0.4 mg per ampule), a narcotic antagonist, may be given intravenously without detriment to the patient and with rapid return of consciousness if the coma is secondary to narcotic excess.

With a little patience and practice all the above observations and interpretations can be carried out by the emergency nurse. Further information about any of the above statements can be obtained from the books and articles in the bibliography.

BIBLIOGRAPHY

Brendler, S. J., and Selverstone, B., "Recovery from Decerebration," *Brain,* vol. 93, 1970, pp. 301–392.

Fisher, C. M., "The Neurological Examination of the Comatose Patient," *Acta Neurologica Scandinavica 45 (Suppl. 36),* 1969, pp. 1–56.

Plum, F., and Posner J., *Diagnosis of Stupor and Coma,* 2d ed., Davis, Philadelphia, 1972.

Suter, C., "Clinical Advances in the Evaluation of Deep Coma," *Medical College of Virginia Quarterly,* vol. 10, 1974, pp. 152–162.

Zervas, N. T., and Hedley-Whyte, J., "Successful Treatment of Cerebral Herniation in Five Patients," *New England Journal of Medicine,* vol. 286, 1972, pp. 1075–1077.

CHAPTER 26
ENDOCRINE EMERGENCIES
JUDITH RAMSEYER, M.D.

EITHER an excess or the absence of endocrine secretions may produce life-threatening clinical situations. A variety of endocrine emergencies are discussed in this chapter.

DIABETIC COMA

PATHOPHYSIOLOGY

Insulin is a protein hormone produced by the beta cells of the pancreas. Diabetic coma is a manifestation of a lack of insulin and is characterized by *hyperglycemia* and *acidosis*. The insulin deficiency may be absolute, for example, in an insulin-dependent diabetic who does not take insulin for several days. It may also be relative as in the case of a diabetic who takes the usual dose of insulin in the face of an increased requirement such as infection or myocardial infarction.

Hyperglycemia and *dehydration* are found in the absence of insulin because most cells are unable to use glucose as a source of energy. The blood sugar rises, increasing the extracellular osmolality. As the osmolality rises, water is pulled from the cell into the vascular space. The kidney attempts to deal with this hyperosmolality by excreting a large volume of urine. If the patient's fluid intake does not compensate for the increased urine output, dehydration will result.

Acidosis is the result of the cell's use of fat, instead of glucose, as an energy source. The end products of fat metabolism are β-hydroxybutyric acid, acetoacetic acid, and acetone. The blood pH falls in the face of the increased acid production. The respiratory center attempts to compensate for the metabolic acidosis by stimulating long deep breaths, thus blowing off CO_2. If the coma is severe enough, these so-called *Kussmaul respirations* may be replaced by depressed respirations.

Other etiologies of coma must be considered. It is important to remember that profound hypoglycemia may present a similar picture to diabetic coma. To assist in diagnosis, laboratory studies include determining the level of glucose and ketones in blood and urine. Blood gases show a low pH and a low PCO_2, characteristic of *metabolic acidosis*. Serum electrolytes often show a *high potassium,* which may be reflected in peaked T waves on the ECG. The high serum potassium is the result of movement of intracellular potassium to the extracellular space in the presence of acidosis.

EMERGENCY THERAPY

Emergency therapy of diabetic coma is directed toward *correcting dehydration and acidosis* and the *administration of insulin.* The use of a diabetic flowsheet greatly simplifies the future care of the patient. This sheet includes a record of the volume and composition of IV fluids, insulin dose, blood pressure, pulse, urine output, and laboratory findings throughout the course of this episode of coma.

Various factors influence the type and rate of fluid administration. *Normal saline* is used initially if the patient is hypotensive and half-normal saline if the blood pressure is satisfactory. The rate of fluid administration is governed by the state of the patient's hydration. If the pH is less than 7.10 or the bicarbonate is less than 10 meq/liter, *bicarbonate* should be added to the IV fluids. *Insulin* is given either as a continuous drip at 6 units/hour or as intermittent IV boluses of 50 to 100 units.

Blood sugar, pH, and potassium are measured every 2 hours until the situation stabilizes. As the acidosis is corrected and serum potassium falls, potassium may have to be added to the IV fluids to prevent hypokalemia. Glucose may have to be given in the later course of the therapy to prevent the blood sugar falling to less than 200 mg %. Finally, the event which precipitated the diabetic coma, such as infection or myocardial infarction, must be searched for and treated.

HYPOGLYCEMIA

PATHOPHYSIOLOGY

The *brain* is dependent on glucose as a source of energy and is the organ primarily affected in hypoglycemia. Hypoglycemia is defined as a blood sugar of less than 50 mg % associated with specific symptoms—confusion or loss of consciousness. Hypoglycemia may produce permanent brain damage. The degree of damage is related to the level of blood sugar, as well as the duration of hypoglycemia. This is the basis of the argument that every comatose patient should have a bolus of glucose after a blood sugar is drawn. Two forms are found: reactive and fasting hypoglycemia.

Reactive hypoglycemia is defined as a blood sugar of less than 50 mg % within 5 hours of ingesting 100 g glucose. It is never associated with coma. Reactive hypoglycemia is usually the result of a lack of feedback control between blood sugar and insulin levels. *Fasting hypoglycemia* is commonly associated with drug administration (insulin or oral hypoglycemics) and is less frequently seen in patients with insulin-producing tumors of the pancreas, hypothyroidism, or hypoadrenalism.

EMERGENCY THERAPY

Patients with reactive hypoglycemia respond best to frequent, low-carbohydrate-content meals. The emergency therapy of the patient with hypoglycemic coma is to give first a *bolus of 50 percent glucose* and then 10 percent glucose until the blood sugar is maintained at 100 mg %.

ADRENAL CRISIS

PATHOPHYSIOLOGY

The adrenal cortical steroids, *aldosterone and cortisol,* are responsible, in part, for maintaining electrolyte balance, blood glucose level, and blood volume. These steroids also carry out ill-defined but essential functions at times of stress. A lack of cortisol and aldosterone produces an adrenal crisis.

The adrenal cortex, in addition to the testes, ovaries, and thyroid, is controlled by the *pituitary*. An adrenal crisis may be the result of either decreased adrenal or decreased pituitary function. If low pituitary function is the cause, the patient will have low cortisol, thyroxine, and sex steroid levels. In contrast, if adrenal function is absent, the pituitary produces large amounts of *adrenocorticotropic hormone (ACTH),* since cortisol normally suppresses ACTH secretion.

The patient with low pituitary function has a sallow complexion and absent facial, axillary, and pubic hair. The increased secretion of ACTH in patients with absent adrenals produces increased skin pigmentation—particularly seen in the gums, scars, and over the knuckles. The patient with adrenal insufficiency may have a history of prolonged diarrhea and weight loss and there may be marked orthostatic hypotension.

A common cause of adrenal crisis is the sudden cessation of oral steroids which have been given to a patient for asthma or arthritis. Rarely, children will present in adrenal crisis because their adrenals lack the enzymes to synthesize cortisol.

Laboratory values may show a low sodium and a high potassium, but may also be normal. These patients usually have a low fasting blood sugar. They will have a low serum cortisol, but the results of this test cannot be obtained immediately.

EMERGENCY THERAPY

If an adrenal crisis is suspected, blood is drawn for serum cortisol, blood sugar, and electrolyte determinations, and the patient is started immediately on normal saline, glucose, and a water-soluble preparation of cortisol. Eventually, either the adrenal or the pituitary glands will have to be implicated as the cause of the adrenal crisis.

THYROID STORM

PATHOPHYSIOLOGY

Thyroid hormone causes increased heat production and mimics the effects of the sympathetic nervous system. Patients who have high levels of *thyroxine* and are in a stressful situation such as infection, myocardial infarction, or an operation may present in thyroid storm. *Storm* is defined as the condition of hyperthyroid patient who has a temperature greater than 100°F, a pulse greater than 120 per minute, and a confused mental status. The source of excess thyroxine may be a diffusely hyperfunctioning gland (*Graves' disease*), a localized area of hyperfunction ("*hot*" *nodule*), or ingestion of exogenous thyroid hormone. These patients usually have a palpable *goiter,* may have a stare or *exophthalmos,* moist skin, and a fine tremor. The major laboratory abnormality is an elevated free thyroxine.

EMERGENCY THERAPY

The treatment of storm involves supplying the fluid which is being lost by evaporation and supporting the increased energy loss secondary to the hypermetabolic state. The third aspect of therapy is to stop the production of thyroxine and inhibit its peripheral effects. Therefore, these patients require large volumes of glucose but must be watched for signs of congestive heart failure since they have a tachycardia and borderline cardiac function. Cooling blankets and sedation to control shivering are used to lower the core temperature. *Antithyroid drugs* are given by stomach tube since no IV preparation is available. (*Inorganic iodide* can be given intravenously to turn off thyroxine production acutely, but this effect is short-lived, and antithyroid drugs must be given chronically.) *Propranolol* is often given to block the sympathetic effect of thyroxine, and the dose is monitored by its effect on the tachycardia. Long-term treatment involves surgery or radioactive iodine.

MYXEDEMA COMA

PATHOPHYSIOLOGY

Myxedema coma occurs in a patient who is profoundly *hypothyroid.* The hypothyroid state may be on the basis of absent pituitary function or may occur in a patient with an absent thyroid and a normal pituitary. A patient in myxedema coma usually has thick dry skin, a pulse less than 60 per minute, and a temperature of less than 97°F. If low pituitary function is the cause, facial, axillary, and pubic hair will be absent, and the testes will be atrophic. Marked *respiratory depression* is a feature of myxedema coma.

Laboratory findings include a *low free serum thyroxine* and a *low serum sodium.* If the patient's pituitary is normal and his thyroid gland is hypofunctioning, the level of thyroid-stimulating hormone (TSH) which is secreted by the pituitary will be high. (In health, TSH secretion is suppressed by normal thyroxine levels.)

EMERGENCY TREATMENT

If the diagnosis is suspected, blood is drawn for serum-free thyroxine, TSH, and electrolyte determinations, and the patient is given IV thyroxine. The patient should be monitored since a therapeutic dose of thyroxine in a hypothyroid patient may precipitate angina and cardiac arrhythmia.

HYPERCALCEMIA

PATHOPHYSIOLOGY

Calcium and *phosphate metabolism* is regulated by the bone, gut, and kidney. The major hormones responsible for controlling the blood levels of these ions are *parathormone* and *vitamin D*. Parathormone is a protein secreted by the parathyroid glands and acts mainly on the kidney and bone. Vitamin D is a sterol which can be either ingested or made in the skin in the presence of sunlight. It is metabolized into an active form by the liver and kidney. Vitamin D controls calcium and phosphate levels mainly through its action in the gut.

Hypercalcemia may result from bone disease such as bone metastases, enlargement of the parathyroids with hyperparathyroidism, excessive use of vitamin D, or eating large amounts of calcium-containing antacids. High levels of calcium slow muscle depolarization and are a potential reason for *cardiac arrest*. The combination of high levels of calcium and high levels of phosphate precipitates calcium phosphate in tissues and urine. Thus, the symptoms of hypercalcemia include *constipation, confusion,* and *renal colic*. The ECG in hypercalcemia shows a prolonged S-T interval. Normal serum calcium is 8 to 10 mg %; a level greater than 14 mg % is considered a medical emergency.

TREATMENT

The therapy of hypercalcemia is to increase the excretion of calcium by the gut and kidney. The renal excretion is enhanced by using *IV normal saline* and *furosemide* since calcium and sodium are excreted together. Loss of calcium from the gut is promoted by the use of *oral* or *rectal sodium phosphate.* This produces non-absorbable calcium phosphate. *Mithramycin,* a chemotherapeutic agent, which absolutely stops bone reabsorption, can also be used to lower calcium levels.

HYPOCALCEMIA

PATHOPHYSIOLOGY

Calcium is present in serum as free (ionized) calcium and is also bound to *albumin.* The active form is ionized. Muscle contraction is enhanced in the presence of a low ionized serum calcium. The patient with hypocalcemia demonstrates *tetany* (persistent contraction of fingers, wrists, and ankles) and increased muscle excitability. (However, the commonest cause of tetany is hyperventilation and respiratory alkalosis.) Hypocalcemia may produce cardiac arrhythmias, which may be worse if the patient is taking digitalis. The ECG may show a short S-T interval.

Low parathyroid function due to damage in the thyroid operation is the usual etiology of symptomatic hypocalcemia. Asymptomatic hypocalcemia may be seen in renal disease or other diseases with low serum albumin, since the ionized calcium may be normal.

EMERGENCY TREATMENT

If hypocalcemia is suspected, samples for bloodgas, calcium phosphate, albumin, and creatinine tests are drawn. *IV calcium gluconate* is given in an emergency; chronic therapy of hypocalcemia includes oral calcium and vitamin D.

BIBLIOGRAPHY

Himathong Kam, T., Newmark, S. R., Greenfield, M., and Dluhy, R. G., "Acute Adrenal Insufficiency," *JAMA,* vol. 230, 1974, p. 1317.

Newmark, S. R., and Himathong Kam, T., "Hypercalcemic and Hypocalcemic Crises," *JAMA,* vol. 230, 1974, p. 1438.

Newmark, S. R., and Himathong Kam, T., and Shane, J. M., "Hyperglycemic and Hypoglycemic Crises," *JAMA,* vol. 231, 1975, p. 185.

———, "Hyperthyroid Crises," *JAMA,* vol. 230, 1974, p. 293.

———, "Myxedema Coma," *JAMA,* vol. 230, 1974, p. 884.

CHAPTER 27
DROWNING AND NEAR-DROWNING
J. K. SIMS, M.D.

DROWNING and near-drowning are usually associated with aquatic environments, although not always. Drownings have been documented as occurring in large industrial vats of paint or beer, tanks of petroleum products, sewers, cesspools, street gutters, and roadside mud puddles, in addition to the more usual ocean, lake, river, pond, bathtub, and quarry sites.

DIFFERENTIATION OF DROWNING FROM NEAR-DROWNING

Drowning may be defined as death by asphyxiating immersion or submersion in any fluid or liquid medium where the cause of death cannot be fully attributed to other lethal disorders (see Table 27-1). Fluid environments are not respecters of preexisting or acute medical problems; *diabetics* and *epileptics* occasionally drown in their bathtubs at home. For *every* drowning, some

Table 27-1	Variables that may be associated with near-drowning*
	• Preexisting medical problems (epilepsy, diabetes, others) • Presence of intoxicants (e.g., alcohol, heroin, glue) and poisoning • Preimmersion food consumption, causing cramps, vomiting, airway obstruction, aspiration • Panic syndrome, fatigue, submersive entanglement • Hyperventilation before breathhold diving (i.e., shallow-water blackout) • Skin and scuba diving emergencies, including equipment failure • Depression leading to suicide attempt • Hot or cold fluid immersion • Allergic reactions to medications, aquatic organism toxins, adverse effects of medications • Mental retardation, elderly state, inadequately supervised children (resulting in risk-taking) • Swallowing liquid medium or aspirating vomitus/fluid • Intraaquatic trauma (e.g., motorboat propellers, runaway surfboards) • Foul play (e.g., attempted murder) • Aquatic cervical spine injuries • Convulsions, electrocution • Chemical, bacterial, particulate composition of inhaled medium • Duration of immersion/submersion

* Each ED should devise its own near-drowning checklist to provide for comprehensive assessment and diminution of complications while managing the victim.

mechanism will be responsible, and the ED is responsible for contributing to the office of the medical examiner any information (e.g., past medical history, blood alcohol level, record of external marks) that might be helpful in determining the actual cause of death for that "routine" case of "D.O.A. from Drowning."

Near-drowning, in contrast to drowning, represents an asphyxiating or partially asphyxiating immersion (or submersion) in a fluid medium; the victim recovers spontaneously or is successfully resuscitated, at least temporarily. Unfortunately some die minutes to days later from factors generally related to the near-drowning event. A few well-appearing near-drowners have been found dead in bed at home the next day, and several initially alert near-drowning hospital admissions have expired in the hospital after several days from severe *pulmonary infections* and progressive *respiratory insufficiency*. Near-drowning can be quite insidious, and comprehensive ED intervention and evaluation are needed upon first contact with the patient.

STAGES OF DROWNING

Current concepts of drowning and near-drowning have been influenced by attempts to reconstruct the intraaquatic stages of drowning from information obtained from survivors of near-drowning and witnesses to drownings. (Fig. 27-1).

Analysis of the stages of drowning reveals that *panic* is seen as an early manifestation (i.e., aquatic panic or hyperventilation syndrome). The degree of panic can be appreciated by realizing that the near-drowning victim has been in juxtaposition to death. This may be responsible for the victim's manifestations of fear, anxiousness, combativeness, pensiveness, or withdrawal, but these psychological manifestations may also be caused by hypoxemia, hypercarbia, hypocarbia, and acidemia. Restoration of the psyche of the near-drowning victim can be achieved with early psychiatric intervention, but this is to be done *after* life-threatening hypoxemia, acidosis, electrolyte imbalances, airway obstruction, cardiac arrhythmias, body fluid shifts, acute pulmonary insufficiency, and other potentially lethal conditions are relieved.

CLASSIFICATION OF FLUID MEDIA

Classification of drownings or near-drownings according to *saltwater* versus *freshwater* should be made, based on laboratory determination of composition of the fluid. For example, saltwater drowning can occur in the Great Salt Lake, Utah, which is 28 percent sodium chloride, or in ocean water which is 3.3 to 3.5 percent saline (human blood is approximately 0.9 percent saline). Accurate chemical analysis of near-drowning immersion fluid is essential for proper emergency management.

SALINE DROWNING

In seawater, when a near-drowner inhales the saline fluid, excessive *intraalveolar* fluid accumulates by *osmosis*. The osmotic gradient for free-water flow is from the 0.9 percent isotonic saline pulmonary capillary fluid to the 3.5 percent hypertonic saline intraalveolar aspirated seawater. Intraalveolar fluid increases while the intravascular space simultaneously becomes dehydrated by loss of free water to the alveoli (this also causes some erythrocytes to be-

Figure 27-1 Stages of drowning and near-drowning. *(As listed in Modell, J. H., The Pathophysiology and Treatment of Drowning and Near-Drowning, Charles C Thomas, Springfield, Ill., 1971. Art work by Randolph Wong.)*

STAGES OF DROWNING

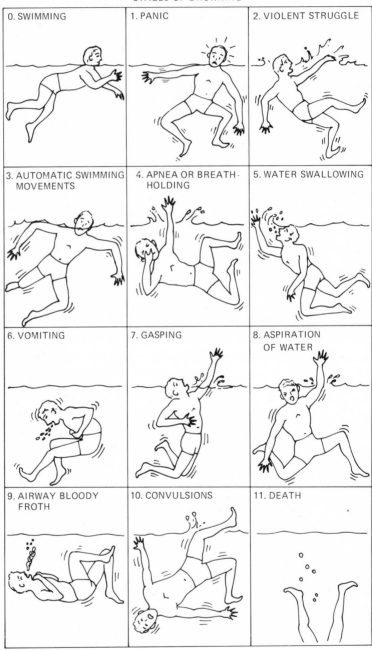

come dehydrated, fragment, and liberate plasma-free hemoglobin, causing *hemoglobinuria*). This excessive intraalveolar fluid can increase to a volume of *1.5* times the original volume aspirated and produce fulminating *pulmonary edema.* Thus, seawater sodium and chloride have a distinct role in producing the increased *intraalveolar fluid accumulation, acidosis,* and *hypoxemia* in the near-drowner (see Table 27-2). *Hypermagnesemia* (from seawater) has been observed in seawater near-drownings; however, the influence of the other electrolytes on the pathophysiology of drowning and near-drowning requires more investigation.

FRESHWATER DROWNING

In the freshwater near-drowning patient, the electrolyte contributions *from the inhaled fluid* have, to date, been relatively inconspicuous and insidious. Distilled water is approximately 0.0 percent saline, but some freshwater sources do contain sodium, chloride, and other electrolytes. Nevertheless, numerous freshwater near-drowners inhale a liquid that is *hypotonic* to the 0.9 percent salinity of pulmonary capillary blood, and this inhaled fluid is rapidly absorbed from the alveoli into the pulmonary capillaries by osmosis. If the victim inhales this hypotonic fluid in significant amounts, then clinical *intravascular fluid overload, hemodilution,* and *hemolysis* (by osmosis) result. Initial difficulties in managing the freshwater near-drowner may be attributed to acute *cardiopulmonary insufficiency* from fluid overload in the presence of pulmonary edema and alveolar collapse. This pulmonary edema and alveolar collapse arise from osmotic fluid damage to the *alveolar-capillary membrane* and *surfactant.* Excessive accumulation of pulmonary interstitial fluid occurs from leaking volume-distended pulmonary capillary endothelial cells and osmotic gradients for free water directed into the pulmonary interstitial spaces.

The hemolysis in near-drowning freshwater is primarily an intravascular osmotic process, with erythrocytes distending by free-water accumulation to the point of rupture. The ruptured red blood cells release hemoglobin as *plasma-free hemoglobin* (i.e., as non-intraerythrocytic hemoglobin). This hemoglobin circulates to the kidney causing *acute tubular necrosis* (producing *acute renal failure* in some patients) and hemoglobinuria when significant hemolysis has occurred. This hemolysis also liberates intraerythrocytic potassium (each erythrocyte in humans contains 120 to 140 meq/liter potassium), which explains why significant hemolysis, in the presence of hypoxemia and acidosis, may predispose the heart

Table 27-2	Factors that can contribute to worsening a near-drowner's acidosis and hypoxia*

- Cardiopulmonary arrest
- Prolonged immersion or submersion
- Convulsions
- Inhalation of the immersion liquid medium with/without incomplete suctioning or incomplete head tilt
- Preoral and/or pre-nasal obstruction to bulk airflow
- Ventricular tachycardia, ventricular fibrillation
- Cardiac electromechanical dissociation or cardiac asystole
- Oral-nasal-pharyngeal airway obstruction or intralaryngeal, tracheal, bronchial, or alveolar obstruction from:
    Tongue (upper airway)
    Vomitus
    Inhaled food
    Blood
    Mud, sand, shell fragments
    Fluid medium
- Laryngospasm or laryngeal edema
- Respiratory muscle dysfunction from
    Traumatic flail chest, rib fractures, sternal fx.
    Open sucking chest wounds
    Neuromuscular toxins from venomous marine organisms
    Aquatic cervical spine injury
- Central nervous system trauma, infarcts, or hemorrhages
- Decompression sickness (i.e., the bends) or air emboli
- Circulatory collapse (e.g., severe hemorrhage) or spinal shock
- Anaphylaxis, poisoning, or drug overdose
- Pneumothorax
    Traumatic
    Spontaneous
    From intracardiac medication injections
    From positive pressure breathing devices (e.g., respirators, Elder-type valves)
    From airway obstruction
- Intratracheal placement of esophageal obturator airway
- Intraesophageal placement of endotracheal tube
- Insufficient rescue breathing or low oxygen percentage administration
- Gastric dilatation by air, fluid, or oxygen; gastric rupture

* These factors should be evaluated and corrected to enhance the near-drowning victim's survival and to decrease the near-drowner's morbidity.

to *ventricular fibrillation, cardiac electrical asystole,* or other electrocardiographic *arrhythmias.*

PREHOSPITAL CARE

Comprehensive clinical assessment of the near-drowning victim in the ED requires a quick reconstruction of the victim's near-drowning event by obtaining a history. Rescue personnel, lifeguards, and ambulance paramedics can particularly assist the ED by obtaining much of the data outlined in Table 27-1 and by (1) carefully documenting in writing all prehospital resuscitation methods used on the near-drowner, (2) properly immobilizing all near-drowners at high risk for *aquatic cervical spine injuries,* (3) collecting an immersion fluid sample (in a sterile container) for subsequent hospital laboratory chemical analysis and microorganism culture, and (4) obtaining an at-scene arterial blood sample for subsequent *arterial blood-gas analysis.*

Particular attention should be paid to prehospital application of a cervical collar and spineboard for possible aquatic cervical spine injury (Table 27-3). Such injuries indicate the need for careful movement of the patient and for cervical spine x-rays (and skull x-rays, in some cases). Should hypoxia be present or develop in the cervical spine-injured near-drowner, hyperextension of the neck and standard endotracheal intubation are contraindicated. Carefully performed nasotracheal intubation, esophageal obturator airway insertion followed by nasotracheal intubation, or non-head-

---

Table 27-3   Etiologies of aquatic cervical spine injuries*

- Head-first shallow-water dives
  Swimming pools
  Other shallow-water areas
- Head-first dives into submerged or surface objects
  Underwater rock ledges
  Underwater or surface swimmers
- Head-first beach hits by bodysurfers
- Head and/or neck trauma from boats, surfboards, etc.
- Foul play and suicide attempts

* Circumstances surrounding aquatic cervical spine injuries in the near-drowning necessitate ED personnel taking extreme care of the patient's neck when evaluating and treating the victim. High-risk cases are identified in this table. Their cervical spine status may not be known prior to arrival at the ED.

tilting tracheostomy are preferable ways of establishing adequate oxygenation of the near-drowning victim with an aquatic cervical spine injury.

APPROACH TO MANAGEMENT OF NEAR-DROWNING

For all near-drownings it is advocated that a sample of the responsible immersion fluid be safely collected in a sterile container for *chemical analysis* and *bacterial culture*. Chemical analysis of the fluid for electrolytes can assist in the evaluation of the pathophysiology for the individual near-drowner and can serve as a guide to IV fluid administration. In addition, certain liquid media contain substances that are direct pulmonary toxins when inhaled, such as *chlorine* in chlorinated swimming pools and the *hydrocarbons* in vats of paint, tanks of kerosene, or oil slicks near boat-launching ramps,

This fluid sample should also be submitted to the hospital laboratory for bacterial culture. It has been documented that the microorganisms in the fluid inhaled into the lungs contribute to the *pneumonia* sometimes affecting the near-drowner. Numerous bacteria have been cultured from seawater, marine organisms, and marine wounds, including staphylococci, streptococci, *Aerobacter, Escherichia coli, Proteus, Klebsiella,* and many species of *Pseudomonas.* Bacterial culture of the near-drowning immersion fluid can provide a 24- to 72-hour advance notice on bacteria that will be contributing to the pneumonia.

Samples for BGA must be drawn on all near-drowners. Serial analyses have been invaluable in the evaluation and management of the near-drowning victim, since hypoxemia and acidemia (particularly lactic acidemia) result from prolonged *asphyxiating immersion* or *submersion.* If hypoxemia is severe, myocardial cells can develop hypoxia and acidosis, and cardiac arrhythmias may ensue. No matter what the chemical composition of the near-drowning fluid medium is, any subsequent development of severe acute myocardial hypoxia and myocardial acidosis may lead to ventricular fibrillation or cardiac electrical asystole. (See Table 27-2.)

NONSYMPTOMATIC NEAR-DROWNING VICTIM

Some near-drowners appear well shortly after the near-drowning event and are brought to the ED for evaluation. This evaluation is to consist of:

1. Arterial blood-gas determination, with patient breathing room air

2. Chest x-ray (PA and lateral)

3. Thorough auscultation of the lungs

Derangement of one or more of the above is sufficient grounds for admission to the hospital, particularly if the PaO_2 is less than 80, the pH is less than 7.35, roentgenographic pulmonary infiltrates and/or edema are present, or auscultation reveals rales, rhonchi, or wheezes. If the above evaluatory triad is entirely normal, the emergency team may elect to discharge the otherwise well patient from the ED, excepting those inhaling the following fluids in any amounts:

• Chlorine or chlorinated liquids

• Hydrocarbons

• Hydrocarbon-contaminated liquids

• Sewage or other heavily bacterially contaminated fluids

• Other fluids containing direct pulmonary toxins

• Hypotonic or freshwater liquids

The effects of freshwater fluids, pulmonary-toxin-containing fluids, and bacterially contaminated fluids are *delayed* in causing pulmonary pathology in the apparently well near-drowner, and so the victim should be observed for several hours in the ED. At the end of the observation period, the near-drowner should be either discharged or admitted on the basis of a final *repeat arterial blood-gas determination (on room air), chest x-ray* (PA and lateral), and *thorough chest auscultation.* All near-drowning discharges from the ED should be reevaluated the next day for possible pulmonary complications. In endemic areas, near-drowning discharges should be reevaluated in 5 to 14 days for primary amebic meningoencephalitis and leptospirosis meningoencephalitis.

SYMPTOMATIC NEAR-DROWNING VICTIM

Symptomatic near-drowning victims present with a variety of signs, symptoms, pathophysiological aberrations, and physiological compensating mechanisms. These are often superimposed on preexisting medical problems. All diagnostic results must be considered in the context of the near-drowning event and the variables in near-drowning (Tables 27-1 and 27-2). The emergency medical care of the symptomatic near-drowner is to be individualized and determined by the initial *comprehensive* assessment (see Table 27-4), followed by careful observation of therapeutic effects and further diagnostic evaluations. The emergency team's therapeutic management of the near-drowning victim may include a number of the following modalities:

- Provide initial basic life support CPR, as indicated

- Provide advanced cardiac life support (ACLS), as indicated

- Ensure adequate patient oxygenation

- Provide thorough airway suctioning

- Use serial arterial blood-gas determinations to guide oxygen administration and sodium bicarbonate administration (after ACLS empirical bicarbonate administration)

- Provide continuous ECG monitoring, treat arrhythmias

- Minimize aspiration of vomitus (by employing thorough airway

---

Table 27-4	Assessment of the symptomatic near-drowning victim*

- Evaluation for airway integrity; breathing rate/rhythm; pulmonary auscultation
- Evaluation for carotid pulse, heart tones, and blood pressure
- 12-lead ECG and subsequent ECG monitoring
- Serial arterial blood-gas determinations
- Chest x-ray (PA and lateral—sometimes an AP expiration film)
- Serum electrolyte determinations (sodium, potassium, chloride, bicarbonate, calcium, magnesium)
- Blood glucose, lactate, and pyruvate
- Serum osmolality determinations
- Plasma-free hemoglobin determinations
- Complete blood counts with serial hematocrits
- Blood urea nitrogen determinations
- Urinalyses
- Urinary electrolyte and osmolality determinations
- Urine output monitoring
- Coagulation profile determinations, including fibrin-split products

* Preliminary *comprehensive* assessment of the symptomatic near-drowning victim includes the diagnostic modalities listed.

suctioning, nasogastric tube placement, gastric emptying, esophageal obturator airway placement, and/or endotracheal tube placement)

- Start or continue IV fluid administration
Freshwater sources: Use dextrose 5% in water at a keep-vein-open (KVO) infusion rate for medication administration until fluid overload status is known
Seawater sources: Use dextrose 5% in N saline (normal saline can be used in hyperglycemics); lactated Ringer's solution can be used if no clinical or electrolyte contraindications exist

- Treat anaphylaxis, if present

- Neutralize clinically significant aquatic organism toxins or overdose drugs (see Chap. 28)

- Control hemorrhage if significant bleeding is occurring

- Treat convulsions with anticonvulsants

- Obtain venous blood samples to submit to laboratory

- Insert CVP line or Swan-Ganz catheter for initial measurements and subsequent guide to IV fluid infusion rates

- Provide active rewarming for hypothermic immersion

- Obtain chest x-rays (cervical-spine and skull series if a cervical-spine injury is suspected)

- Immobilize cervical-spine fractures, if present, with sandbags, Crutchfield tongs, or Gardner tongs (and obtain neurosurgery consultation)

- Insert foley catheter for significant near-drowning

- Provide tube thoracostomy via large-bore intercostal needle or chest tube (a Heimlich valve is helpful) for tension pneumothorax

- Provide fiber-optic bronchoscopy for diagnostic evaluation, pulmonary lavage (to remove debris), and neutralization of gastric acids, as indicated

- Apply incremental oxygenating positive end-expiratory pressure (PEEP) as continuous positive pressure ventilation (CPPV) for near-drowner arterial hypoxemia that is unresponsive to traditional respiratory (ventilator) management

- Provide appropriate steroid therapy for cerebral hypoxia (apparently steroids are of little benefit in gastric HCl aspiration and some freshwater near-drownings)

- Provide broad-spectrum antibiotics for significant intrapulmonary aspiration, unless infectious disease consultant advises otherwise on the basis of bacterial composition of the near-drowning immersion fluid

- Provide definitive wound repair and more permanent fracture immobilization

- Submit urine specimens to laboratory for studies outlined previously, as determined by patient's condition

- IV salt-poor albumin administration for seawater near-drowners has benefited some

Resuscitation of near-drowners in recent years has improved as a result of experimental research, clinical research, and applications of research to patient care. Patients have survived total near-drowning submersion for 10 minutes (1964), 17 minutes (1964), 22 minutes (1963), 30 minutes (1974; 30 minutes immersion, minutes of total submersion unknown), and 40 minutes (1974). The latter two cases were both 5-year-olds immersed in hypothermia-causing ice-cold freshwater (that apparently evoked the diving reflex) and were neurologically normal upon examination 3 months and 13 months, respectively, after resuscitation. Basic and clinical research should provide the ED with solutions for the hypoxic brain damage, acute renal tubular necrosis, pulmonary parenchymal damage, lung infections seen in near-drowners and the nonresuscitable drowners.

BIBLIOGRAPHY

Chapman, R. L., et al., "The Ineffectiveness of Steroid Therapy in Treating Aspiration of Hydrochloric Acid," *Archives of Surgery,* vol. 108, 1974, pp. 858–861.

Chun, B., Okihiro, M. N., and Hale, R. W., "Analysis of Drowning Incidents on Oahu, 1960–1970," *Hawaii Medical Journal,* vol. 32, 1973, pp. 92–95.

Dietz, P. E., and Baker, S. P., "Drowning—Epidemiology and Prevention," *American Journal of Public Health,* vol. 64, 1974, pp. 303–312.

Donns, J. B., et al., "An Evaluation of Steroid Therapy in Aspiration Pneumonitis," *Anesthesiology,* vol. 40, 1974, pp. 129–135.

Fuller, R. H., "Drowning and the Postimmersion Syndrome—A Clinicopathologic Study," *Military Medicine,* vol. 128, 1963, pp. 22–36.

Modell, J. H., *The Pathophysiology and Treatment of Drowning and Near-Drowning,* Charles C Thomas, Springfield, Ill., 1971.

————, et al., "Effects of Ventilatory Patterns on Arterial Oxygenation after Near-Drowning in Sea Water," *Anesthesiology,* vol. 40, 1974, pp. 376–384.

Rivers, J. F., Orr, G., and Lee, H. A., "Drowning: Its Clinical Sequelae and Management," *British Medical Journal,* vol. 2, 1970, pp. 157–161.

Rosenthal, S. L., Zuger, J. H., and Apollo, E., "Respiratory Colonization with *Pseudomonas putrefaciens* after Near-Drowning in Salt Water," *American Journal of Clinical Pathology,* vol. 64, 1975, pp. 382–384.

Ruiz, B. C., et al., "Effect of Ventilatory Patterns on Arterial Oxygenation after Near-Drowning with Fresh Water," *Anesthesia and Analgesia,* vol. 52, 1973, pp. 570–576.

CHAPTER 28
DANGEROUS AQUATIC ORGANISMS
J. K. SIMS, M.D.

ACUTE medical and surgical emergencies may develop in human beings afflicted with injury or illness upon contact with organisms normally inhabiting aquatic environments. This chapter discusses these afflictions and ways to treat them. Afflictions may be categorized according to the following divisions:

1. Trauma, hemorrhage, and/or hemorrhagic shock

2. Envenomization: sting, spine, fang

3. Allergic reactions, acute dermatitis, anaphylaxis, infection, chronic dermatitis

4. Electric shock

Simplified treatment tables for worldwide use and for specific geographical areas have been devised for aquatic organism afflictions. *Each ED should formulate a list of the specific dangerous aquatic organisms indigenous to the area from which the facility's patient population is drawn and keep specific treatment modalities updated.* To do this the ED nurse should (a) read the worldwide marine organism geographical distributions found in Dr. Bruce Halstead's *Poisonous and Venomous Marine Animals of the World,* (b) consult reliable local experts on aquatic organism afflictions, or (c) telephone an "Aquadoc."[1]

TRAUMA, HEMORRHAGE, AND/OR HEMORRHAGIC SHOCK

Many aquatic organisms may grossly traumatize man. Examples include *sharks, sea urchins, stingrays, cone shells,* and *corals.* Identification of the offending organism is essential because of the venomous nature of some traumatogenic species. Determination of *wound* type, severity, and extent, and the responsible offending aquatic organism facilitates wound management (see Table 28-1).

Major pitfalls in the management of aquatic organism traumatic

Table 28-1	Management of aquatic trauma and hemorrhage
	• Support and correct any impairment of cardiopulmonary function
	• Control bleeding, replacing clinically significant blood or fluid loss
	• Treat for shock (according to type of shock)
	• Rule out fang and spine puncture envenomization early (treat immediately if present)
	• X-ray shark bite and stingray spine wounds (for retained teeth and spines, respectively) using soft-tissue x-ray technique
	• Evaluate and correct orthopedic and neurovascular derangements
	• Thoroughly irrigate all surface wounds with 0.9% NaCl solution, debride nonviable tissues, and *remove all foreign bodies:* 3% hydrogen peroxide irrigation provides mechanical cleansing, and scrub-brushing may provide effective wound cleansing Iodophors (e.g., Povidone-Iodine) cause less pain but provide *less* skin disinfection than iodine solutions (e.g., 1% iodine in 70% alcohol) Hexachlorophenes have limited bactericidal activity
	• Close wounds *primarily* and skin graft *early* as needed
	• Provide appropriate antitetanus, antirabies, anti–gas gangrene prophylaxis
	• Follow patient very closely for infection (some authorities recommend prophylactic antibiotics for marine wounds)

afflictions to man include: (a) failure to determine the full extent of the trauma, (b) failure to recognize fang or spine envenomizations, (c) failure to obtain adequate patient follow-up for early intervention into infection, (d) failure to adequately cleanse wounds of foreign material.

ENVENOMIZATION

STING NEMATOCYSTIC

Certain aquatic organisms, predominantly marine, have a microscopic stinging apparatus called an *envenomizing nematocyst* which can inject human beings with a multicomponent *venom*. These organisms include: *sea anemones;* elk horn coral; the *Portuguese man-of-war* (not a true jellyfish); many species of true *jellyfish,* stinging *fire coral* (not a true coral); dermatitis-producing *stinging seaweeds* (not true seaweed), and microscopic nematocystic branched organisms (e.g., *Lyptocarpus pennarius* and *Sarsia tubulosa*). Nematocyst venoms from several types of coelenterates include histamine, serotonin, and several allergenic polypeptide or proteinaceous components. This explains the allergic histamine-overdose and anaphylactic responses that the vast majority of envenomized patients demonstrate, excluding those symptoms of an Australian seawasp affliction. Sting (nematocystic) envenomizations may be managed by one or more modalities listed in Tables 28-2 and 28-3.

SPINE PUNCTURE

Another group of aquatic organisms, predominantly marine, bears a grossly visible *spine* that possesses an associated venom apparatus and venom. A traumatic puncture wound or laceration is thereby produced that is infiltrated with the species-specific *toxin,* resulting in severe *pain.* Spine puncture envenomizing organisms include some sea urchins, stingrays (and some manta rays), some *starfish* such as the Acanthaster *crown-of-thorns,* some *sharks* (e.g., the dogfish shark *Squalus acanthias*), *stonefish, scorpion fish, catfish,* aquatic *worms, weever fish,* certain surgeonfish (or tangs), and *cone shells.*

A number of toxins from the above organisms appear to be *heat labile* (i.e., inactivated by heat). Immersion of the wound site in hot water or application of hot compresses is the primary treatment modality. The hot-water therapy should be applied carefully

Table 28-2	Management of anaphylactic nematocystic envenomization

- Evaluate for anaphylaxis and treat appropriately if present. *Comprehensive anaphylaxis management requires:*
- Support of cardiocirculorespiratory function
- Administration of 100% oxygen to respiratory system
- Epinephrine administration subcutaneously, IV, or both
- IV fluid replacement of clinically significant extravasated fluid and electrolytes (particularly in hypotension)
- Vasopressor therapy for hypotension unresponsive to both epinephrine and IV fluid therapy
- Antihistamine administration: IV, IM, and/or po
- Removal of any remaining offending antigens (e.g., tentacles)
- Appropriate steroid administration, antitetanus therapy
- Cardiac monitoring and appropriate antiarrhythmic therapy
- Administration of antivenin (antitoxin), if available
- *Serial laboratory studies,* including electrolyte, hematological, clotting, immune, liver, renal, CNS/CSF, endocrine, arterial blood gases, skeletal muscle, and cardiac enzyme profiles, as necessary
- *Clinical follow-up for* delayed hypersensitivity, dermonecrosis, infection, gastric hyperacidity (and ulceration), renal failure, bleeding diathesis, CNS decompensation, convulsions, coma, tetanus, cardiac arrhythmias, pulmonary edema, laryngospasm, laryngeal edema, myocardial infarction, and heart blocks

For the highly lethal *Australian seawasp-type jellyfish* use:
- Immediate appropriate tourniquet application (*to confine toxin locally*)
- Administration of species-specific seawasp antivenin (from Commonwealth Serum Laboratories of Melbourne, Australia, or nearby aquarium may stock)
- Cardiac monitoring and/or cardiopulmonary support
- Analgesia, even IV opiates, for pain relief
- Ophthalmology consultation for eye injuries
- Antitetanus prophylaxis
- Close follow-up of integumentary injuries for infection, intervention, and skin-graft potential

to avert scalding the puncture site. Spine puncture envenomizations may be managed using the modalities in Table 28-4.

FANG ENVENOMIZATION

Fang envenomizations are the most serious injuries inflicted upon man by aquatic organisms. These envenomizations may be inflicted by *sea snakes* such as *Pelamis platurus,* freshwater snakes such as the cottonmouth water moccasin (*Agkistrodon piscivorus*), the blue-banded octopus (*Hapalochlaena maculosa*, not possessing true fangs but instead having salivary gland ducts conveying toxin to crushing jaws), and terrestrial venomous snakes that swim, such as the Eastern diamondback rattlesnake (*Crotalus adamanteus*).

The initial sensation of pain and the wound produced is variable. Trauma may range from a small laceration (characteristic for the octopus) to one, two, or more fang marks appearing to be puncture wounds or dots (1 to 20 dots). Treatment modalities for fang envenomizations are listed in Table 28-5.

Table 28-3   **Management of nonanaphylactic sting envenomizations**

- Nonanaphylactic envenomizations require observation and stabilization

- Remove offending nematocysts (e.g., tentacles) by the alcohol-powder-scrape-base method, using all steps:
  Coat tentacles and wound with hydrocarbon solution (e.g., methyl alcohol, ethyl ether, acetone, rubbing alcohol, or oils; (DO NOT USE FRESH OR DISTILLED WATER), then
  Coat wound site with a drying agent (e.g., flour, glove talc, baking soda, diver's talc, or Adolf's Unseasoned Meat Tenderizer*; (*Do not use sand, particularly wet sand*), then
  Remove inactivated tentacles with rubber gloves or a forceps, and carefully scrape off paste from above with a blade (*Do not use a scrub brush*)
  Coat wound with a dilute basic (alkalotic) solution to neutralize the acidic toxin (e.g., ammonia, supersaturated baking soda, or sodium bicarbonate)
  After effecting neutralization, irrigate wound with 0.9% NaCl solution and repeat sequence if pain recurs

- Give analgesia (even opiates) for pain

- Use IV calcium for skeletal muscle spasms

- Give antihistamines (preferably hydroxyzine)

- Give antitetanus prophylaxis

- Give analgesic cortisone preparations p.o., as skin aerosol, or as topical creme

- Obtain follow-up for sting site infection intervention

* Do not use Adolf's Meat Tenderizer on those allergic to papaya; papase or papain is a digestive enzyme for proteins.

Table 28-4   Management of spine puncture envenomizations

- Provide respiratory support as necessary

- Perform ECG and cardiac monitoring

- Provide appropriate antiarrhythmic and antipulmonary edema therapy (particularly for stingray afflictions)

- Differentiate spine puncture wounds from fang marks by examination and history

- Immerse puncture site in hot water for 15 to 90 minutes (with hot water replenishment) without scalding the patient ($MgSO_4$ or NaCl addition to solution is optional)

- Give IV *and* IM pentazocine or opiate analgesia; local anesthesia is sometimes helpful

- For stonefish, use the antivenin (contact Commonwealth Serum Laboratories, Melbourne, Australia, or nearby aquarium for stock)
  Some find a 0.1 to 0.5 cc local injection of 5% $KMnO_4$ helpful for *stonefish* stings if antivenin is unavailable. Others find a 0.5 to 1 cc local injection of emetine hydrochloride (1 grain/cc mixture) effective for stonefish stings

- Tourniquet use is advocated for stonefish stings but not for stingray stings; incision and suction are controversial

- Cryotherapy appears to worsen the pain (particularly in stingray afflictions)

- Vinegar soaking is sometimes helpful for sea urchin stings; pain of these stings may respond to phenylbutazone or thioridazine

- Sea worm bristles are easily removed with adhesive tape

- Give antitetanus prophylaxis

- Use of neostigmine/physostigmine is controversial

- Provide IM and po antihistamines if needed

- Administer appropriate steroids; provide take-home oral analgesics

- Treat traumatic spine puncture wounds appropriately (Table 28-1)

- Hospitalize patients with punctures of the peritoneal and thoracic cavities for surgical exploration

- Remove calcified spines (may sometimes be detected by soft-tissue x-ray)

- Obtain follow-up for infection

- Give IV calcium for skeletal muscular spasm and anticonvulsants for seizures

Table 28-5	Management of fang envenomizations

- Support cardiocirculorespiratory function and control shock
- Respiratory support with tracheal intubation, tracheostomy, and respirator may be required
- Apply venoconstrictive tourniquet to confine venom
- Local incision and suction of wound (not with mouth) is of value immediately for North American pit vipers, of little value for elapids and sea snakes, and contraindicated for some African snakes; *do not apply ice*
- Administer species-specific antivenin (contact Commonwealth Serum Laboratories of Melbourne, Australia, for sea snake antivenins and nearby poison control centers for others); watch for antivenin anaphylaxis or hypersensitivity
- Wipe venom off skin and clean wound
- Administer IV fluids, as appropriate
- Opiate administration is contraindicated
- Provide antitetanus prophylaxis
- Discourage exertion and movement
- Administer steroids
- Epinephrine administration may be required
- Consider early digitalization, as indicated
- Hemodialysis may be required for renal tubular necrosis
- Observe for at least 24 hours (i.e., *admit patient*)
- Consider atropine for bradycardia
- *Safely* obtain offending organism for positive identification
- Avoid fasciotomy if possible
- Obtain ECG, CBC, urinalysis, BUN, sedimentation rate, platelets, and electrolytes; watch for rapid electrolyte changes

ALLERGIC REACTIONS, ACUTE DERMATITIS, ANAPHYLAXIS, INFECTION, AND CHRONIC DERMATITIS

Many allergic reactions, acute dermatitis situations, and anaphylaxis circumstances occur from nematocystic sting envenomizations, fang venoms, and therapeutic antivenins.

A number of allergic and acute dermatitic reactions are labeled "swimmers itch" and actually may be caused by *nematocystic stinging organisms, sponges, algae, parasites, bristleworms,* and *bacteria* (e.g., *Escherichia coli, Pseudomonas*). Sponges (methdilazine hydrochloride is helpful as an antipruritic in sponge poisoning), algae, and bristleworm injuries may be treated according to the protocols listed in Table 28-2. Treatment of parasites and bacteria varies according to the organism diagnosed. The use of a Wood's lamp, Gram's stain, and/or cultures facilitate in making the diagnosis. Allergic reactions and nonparasitic, nonbacterial reactions should be managed as in Table 28-2 and 28-3.

Infection and acute and chronic *dermatitis* may result from retained foreign bodies (in aquatic-associated open wounds) or from aquatic bacteria. Probably no absolutely sterile aquatic environments exist year-round (unless processed by man). Many bacteria have been cultured from seawater (staphyloccus, streptococcus, *E. coli, Proteus, Aerobacter,* and *Pseudomonas*) and from freshwater sources including swimming pools. These bacteria may cause clinical problems. For example, *malignant otitis* caused by swimming pool *Pseudomonas* is an ENT emergency. *Mycobacterium marinum (Mycobacterium balnei)* is an important microorganism to consider when marine aquarium workers or hobbyists present with skin infections.

Thorough wound cleansing and debridement, removal of all foreign bodies, wound culture, close follow-up for infection intervention, and antitetanus prophylaxis are necessary in aquatic wound management. Diagnosis of a chronic dermatitis may require a skin biopsy. Antibiotic therapy should be directed according to the report of microorganisms cultured.

ELECTRIC SHOCK

Aquatic organisms that deliver an electric shock to human beings include the *electric catfish, electric eel, electric ray,* and *star-gazer fish*. Recovery has been described as uneventful despite severe jolts; treatment is symptomatic.

REFERENCES

1. "An Aquadoc for All Regions," *Emergency Medicine,* vol. 7, June 1975, pp. 194–200.

BIBLIOGRAPHY

Arena, J. M., *Poisoning,* Charles C Thomas, Springfield, Ill., 1974, pp. 532–541.

Campbell, C. H., "The Effects of Snake Venoms and Their Neurotoxins on the Nervous System of Man and Animals," in Hornabrook, R. W., *Topics on Tropical Neurology,* Davis Company, Philadelphia, 1975, pp. 259–293.

Halstead, B. W., *Poisonous and Venomous Marine Animals of the World,* U.S. Government Printing Office, Washington, D.C., vol. I (1965), vol. II (1967), vol. III (1970).

Humm, H. J., and Lane, C. E. (eds.), *Bioactive Compounds from the Sea,* Marine Science Series, vol. I, Marcel Dekker, Inc., New York, 1974.

Johnston, D. G., and Fung, J., "Bacterial Flora of Wild and Captive Porpoises: An Inquiry into Health Hazards to Man," *Journal of Occupational Medicine,* vol. 11, 1969, pp. 267–277.

Orris, W. L., "Aquatic Medical Emergencies," in Sproul, C. W., and Mullanney, P. J., *Emergency Care,* Mosby, St. Louis, 1974, pp. 212–223.

Russell, F. E., "Venomous Animal Injuries," *Current Problems in Pediatrics,* vol. 3, 1973, pp. 1–47.

Sims, J. K., "Venomous Sea Creatures." *Conference Report of the First International Water Safety Conference,* Kamuela, Hawaii, July 18–21, 1975, pp. 51–71.

Southcott, R. V., "The Neurologic Effects of Noxious Marine Creatures," in Hornabrook, R. W., *Topics on Tropical Neurology,* Davis, Philadelphia, 1975, pp. 165–258.

Strauss, M. B., and Orris, W. L., "Injuries to Divers by Marine Animals: A Simplified Approach to Recognition and Management," *Military Medicine,* vol. 139, 1974, pp. 129–130.

CHAPTER 29
EMERGENCY CARE OF DIVING ACCIDENTS

GERALEE BUMBAUGH, R.N.

IMAGINE yourself in charge of a small rural emergency facility in the Midwest. While on duty, a 26-year-old man arrives complaining of a gradual onset of increasing pain in the right elbow. He denies any trauma and appears to be in considerable amount of discomfort. The emergency physician finds the physical examination essentially negative except for pain in the right elbow. Baffled by the case, you return to the patient for a reevaluation. The patient then states he is a student at the nearby university and has just returned from a three-month vacation in the South Pacific. He expresses disappointment with the fact that he cannot continue his newly learned sport, scuba diving. "It's so much fun," he states. "I did as much diving as I could yesterday at all kinds of depths." With this history of "diving too long and too deep," this individual is a good candidate for a diving disease. The *bends, or decompression sickness,* is an important consideration.

DECOMPRESSION SICKNESS

Decompression sickness is a diving condition associated with scuba diving and military deep sea diving. Very simply, it occurs when the diver stays underwater for too long a period of time and goes to depths beyond the safe recommended limits (see Table 29-1).

The role of the ED nurse in the treatment of the patient with decompression sickness is fourfold. First of all, the nurse must be aware that such diving problems exist and that these problems can arise in almost any area in the world with today's jet age. Symptoms may present themselves anywhere from minutes to 48 hours after a dive.

PHYSIOLOGY

Secondly, it is important for the emergency nurse to understand the physiology behind the bends. When a diver goes underwater, his or her body undergoes changes due to the increase in the surrounding external environmental pressure. (Water is heavier than air and thus exerts more pressure). While the diver is underwater, he or she is breathing air (20 percent oxygen and 80 percent nitrogen) in a compressed form in tanks. When the body is exposed to this increase in pressure, considerable amounts of nitrogen gas go into solution. It is this *nitrogen* that causes the prob-

Table 29-1	Summary of the U.S. Navy's recommended diving limits. *(Adapted from U.S. Navy Diving Manual, vol. I, Navships, 0994-001-9010, U.S. Government Printing Office, Washington, September 1973.)*	
	Depth, feet	Decompression limit, minutes
	10	None
	20	None
	35	310
	50	100
	60	60
	100	25
	150	5
	190	5

Easy base line to remember: A diver can stay underwater at a depth of *60 ft* for only *60 minutes* to be in the "safe zone" and avoid the bends

lems associated with the bends. The nitrogen in the compressed air crosses the lung membrane by diffusion and is transported to the tissues. As the partial pressure of the nitrogen increases, the blood becomes saturated with this gas. As long as the body is maintained at an increased external pressure, the nitrogen is absorbed by the tissues and remains in solution. When the diver begins to surface and external pressure is reduced, the dissolved liquid nitrogen in the blood and tissues changes back into the gaseous state. It is then excreted from the body via the lungs. This takes time, however, and if the diver surfaces too quickly and the pressure decreases too rapidly, the unloading process of this nitrogen falls seriously behind. Gas bubbles appear in the bloodstream and tissues, and the diver may develop the bends.

SYMPTOMS

Thirdly, the nurse should be aware of the symptoms manifested by the patient with the bends. The most common symptom is *pain,* which is usually confined to a particular area, depending on where the nitrogen bubbles lodge. Most often the *joints* are affected, with the *legs* being the most common site. However, this pain can and does occur anywhere. It may appear at any time from minutes to 48 hours after the dive. Frequently, a diver may experience only mild symptoms such as rash, itching, and fatigue due to the excess of nitrogen in body tissues. These symptoms usually do not require medical treatment and subside as nitrogen levels in the blood return to normal.

More serious manifestations of the bends result from nitrogen bubbles developing in the *lungs, brain,* or *spinal cord.* Again, severity depends on the size of the bubbles and their placement in the body. The patient may present with such symptoms as dizziness, numbness, loss of vision, paralysis, loss of consciousness, convulsions, and cardiovascular collapse. Remember, however, that the most common complaint is *pain in the joints.*

TREATMENT

Finally, the emergency nurse must be aware of the methods of treating the bends. *Symptomatic treatment* and *recompression* are the only treatments. Recompression simply means submerging the patient under pressure to the point where the nitrogen gas converts back to the liquid state, thus relieving the pain. The pressure is then gradually released, allowing the body to eliminate the excess gas via the lungs.

Recompression can be done by two methods. The preferred and safer method uses a *dry recompression chamber*. This chamber is a large cylinder equipped with a stretcher, emergency equipment, and space for one attendant. The chamber is pressurized and can return patients to a painless state. The other method, which is inadequate and dangerous, is frequently instituted by other divers treating their friends and consists of taking the victim back under *actual water pressure*. Needless to say, this method is very hazardous and should be avoided at all costs.

To review, the nurse's responsibility is primarily symptomatic treatment and immediate transfer to the nearest recompression chamber staffed with adequately trained medical personnel. The preferred position is left lateral Trendelenburg; administration of 100 percent O_2 at 6 to 10 liters per mask should be instituted.

With prompt treatment of decompression sickness, the prognosis is good. However, almost every untreated case results in some degree of permanent injury. The severity of the injury depends on the specific location of damage. Bends is rarely fatal but frequently causes numbness, weakness, paralysis, or permanent crippling. This sickness need never happen. It can be prevented by proper training of divers, common sense, and strict adherence to the diving tables.

AIR EMBOLUS

Air embolus is another condition associated with divers, but it is less likely to be seen in the ED. Its symptoms occur rapidly and are usually fatal if not treated within minutes. The history of this diving disease is more dramatic and often requires immediate resuscitation at the scene.

PHYSIOLOGY

The physiology of air embolus can be explained by *Boyle's law,* which states that the volume of a gas increases as the external pressure decreases. A diver takes a normal breath underwater and, forgetting to exhale, begins to surface. The normal lung volume increases as the external pressure decreases. This may progress to the point that alveoli rupture, sending air emboli into circulation, affecting the brain, heart, and lungs.

SYMPTOMS AND TREATMENT

Unconsciousness is usually the first symptom, and unconsciousness underwater is sure death without immediate resuscitation. Many of today's drownings associated with scuba diving are caused by air emboli but are rarely diagnosed until autopsy. The treatment for air embolus, as with decompression sickness, is *immediate recompression* in a dry chamber with trained personnel.

In summary, the emergency nurse must:

1. Be aware that diving accidents occur and can present in any ED, no matter the locale.

2. Understand the basic physiology of diving diseases.

3. Get an accurate history.

4. Recognize some of the common symptoms.

5. Know the location of the nearest recompression chamber and the procedure for emergency transfer. It is important to note here that since these are conditions relating to external body pressures, victims must *not* be transported by air unless a very low flying aircraft is available, i.e., helicopter.

BIBLIOGRAPHY

Dueker, C. W., *Medical Aspects of Sport Diving,* Barnes, New York, 1970.

Hart, G., "Treatment of Decompression Illness and Air Embolism with Hyperbaric Oxygen," *Aerospace Medicine,* October 1974, pp. 1190–1193.

Strauss, R., and Prockop, L., "Decompression Sickness among Scuba Divers," *JAMA,* vol. 223, no. 6, Feb. 5, 1973, pp. 637–648.

U.S. Navy Diving Manual, vol. I, Navships 0094-001-9010, U.S. Government Printing Office, Washington, September 1973.

CHAPTER 30
EMERGENCY OCULAR CARE
PERCIVAL H. Y. CHEE, M.D., F.A.C.S.

THE part of the eye that most concerns a nurse in an emergency care situation is the *external eye*, and it is necessary that he or she be aware of its normal appearance (see Fig. 30-1). Near the medial canthus on the upper and lower lids are the *puncta*. These are connected to the canaliculi which enter the *lacrimal sac*, the normal drainage site for tears. The *sclera* is the most obvious part of the eye and is normally white. Blood vessels are in the conjunctiva which overlies the sclera. The *cornea* is crystal clear and should have no haziness or opacities. The limbus is the demarcation line between the sclera and the cornea. The *iris* is the colored portion of the eye and forms the posterior border of the anterior chamber which is filled with *aqueous humor,* a clear fluid. The *pupil,* which is normally round, is the space formed by the iris. If there is any distortion, a pathologic entity should be considered. The *lens* is behind the iris. The *conjunctiva,* which ends at the limbus and covers the entire sclera, forms a cul-de-sac in the upper and lower portions of the eye. The conjunctiva on the globe itself is called the *bulbar conjunctiva;* as it is reflected onto the eyelids, it becomes the *palpebral conjunctiva.* The conjunctiva is normally clear with few vessels.

Figure 30-1 Anatomy of the normal eye.

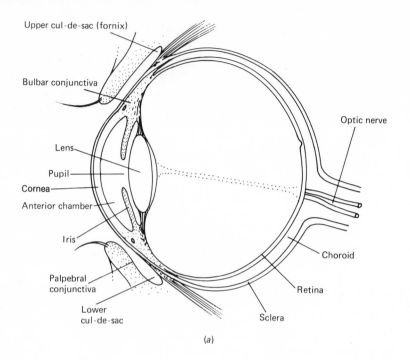

Upper cul-de-sac (fornix)

Bulbar conjunctiva

Optic nerve

Lens

Pupil

Cornea

Anterior chamber

Iris

Palpebral conjunctiva

Lower cul-de-sac

Choroid

Retina

Sclera

(a)

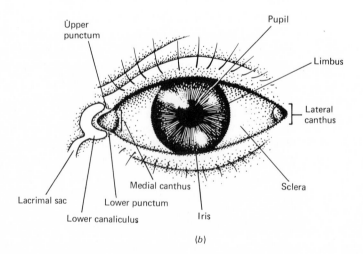

Upper punctum

Pupil

Limbus

Lateral canthus

Lacrimal sac

Lower punctum

Lower canaliculus

Medial canthus

Iris

Sclera

(b)

BASIC EQUIPMENT

The equipment described in this section is basically for a nurse to use under the direction of a physician. A *Snellen chart* and/or a *near-vision card* should be available in the ED. A *Finoff head hand light* should also be available. In addition, some method of double-everting the eyelids, such as a *Desmarres retractor,* is necessary. A *lid speculum* for opening the eyes during irrigation or foreign body removal is helpful.

Medications that may be of help in the ED are:

1. A topical *ocular anesthetic,* such as proparacaine

2. Some medication for *dilating the eyes,* such as tropicamide 1%

3. Some *miotic,* such as pilocarpine 1, 2, 3, or 4%

4. Some method of *determining the pH,* such as litmus paper

5. *Fluorescein strips,* individually packaged

6. *Antibiotic eye drops* and ointment

INITIAL EMERGENCY CARE AND OBSERVATIONS

After a patient is logged into the ED, the nurse should obtain a *brief ophthalmic history* including the chief complaint, how long the problem was present, and a brief medical history such as whether the patient is a diabetic or hypertensive. If the patient is a woman, determine whether she is using hormonal therapy for any reason. This information and remarks on observation of specific abnormal conditions should be relayed to the ophthalmologist. The exception to this process is in *chemical injuries,* when irrigation *must* be carried out as the initial step. This is explained in greater detail in a subsequent section.

Visual acuity should be assessed using a Snellen chart at 20 feet. If the chart cannot be placed at 20 feet, adjustments in recording of the vision may be made. For example, if the chart is placed at 10 feet and the patient can read the 20/20 line of the chart, then the vision is recorded as 10/20, the distance being the numerator. If no Snellen chart is available, a near card may be used to obtain some measure of vision. If no other means of vision testing is available, newsprint, which is roughly equal to 20/50, may be used. The best obtainable vision of both eyes, not just the impaired one, is recorded. If the patient wears glasses, this fact should be noted and glasses should be worn in vision testing. The right eye is tested with the left eye covered; then the left eye is tested with the right eye covered. If the patient cannot see the 20/400 E on a Snellen chart, some measure of visual function must still be recorded, such as FC 8' (finger counting at 8 feet), HM 3' (hand movements at 3 feet), or LP (light perception).

COMMON OCULAR EMERGENCIES

CHEMICAL TRAUMA

Any patient with a history of chemical agents entering the globe must be *treated promptly,* prior to taking history, obtaining the name and address, or any other step. The affected eye must be *immediately irrigated.* Irrigation, if no other method is available, can be done with a gentle flow of water from an open tap. A gentle flow of *saline* or water *through a tube* is the superior method.

If pH paper is not available for a more accurate measure, irrigation must be carried out *for at least 30 minutes.* If available, the pH of the secretions of the eye should be checked as soon as possible. To check normal pH, place a piece of litmus paper in a normal conjunctiva and compare the two. If the paper reveals that the chemical entering the eye was acid, irrigation should be carried out until the paper returns to a normal pH and then may be stopped. If the original chemical was alkaline, irrigation must continue until a few minutes after a check of the pH of the cul-de-sacs indicates a normal state. Then the cul-de-sacs must be checked again about 5 to 10 minutes after irrigation was stopped to see if the pH is still normal since alkaline chemicals tend to continue to act. One must be sure to pull the lids away from the globe to irrigate the cul-de-sacs copiously. In chemical injury cases, a lid speculum, which allows maximum exposure of the cul-de-sacs, should be used whenever possible.

Tear gas and *Mace injuries* should be treated as chemical injuries, unless there is penetration of the cornea from the force of the Mace hitting the globe.

BLUNT OCULAR TRAUMA

Blunt ocular trauma may be due to the face striking the dashboard in an auto accident or could be due to objects acting as missiles into the *eye* or orbit, such as baseballs, tennis balls, or champagne corks. If there is a history of such an occurrence, one must be careful not to place any *undue pressure* on the eye that sustained any trauma until ascertaining that there was no entrance into the eye or no rupture of any part of the eye. If at all possible, a *visual acuity* must be obtained. A swollen eye may be opened by placing gentle pressure only on the *bony orbits* and lifting the lid. Generally speaking, all blunt ocular trauma should be examined by a physician as soon as possible because of the possible severe complications. The *possible complications* of blunt ocular trauma are:

1. *Decreased Visual Acuity Secondary to a Hyphema.* If the pupil cannot be seen, then there is a possibility that the hyphema is total so as to give an eight-ball hemorrhage. If a hyphema in the anterior chamber is suspected, both eyes should be loosely patched to decrease ocular movement due to refixation on objects. The patient should be allowed to sit up while waiting to be examined by an ophthalmologist so that blood will settle in the lower portion of the anterior chamber.

2. *Choroidal, Scleral, or Corneal Rupture.* There is always the possibility of a choroidal, scleral, or corneal rupture. If there is a choroidal rupture, an ophthalmoscopic examination must be performed. A scleral rupture may also be hidden. However, an *iris prolapse,* because of a rupture at the limbus, can be seen as a small knuckle of pigmented material under the conjunctiva. The pupil will be displaced in such a case. A *retinal detachment* or *vitreous hemorrhage* may also occur due to this type of trauma.

3. *Blowout Fracture.* If there is severe blunt trauma, a blowout fracture must be considered, even in the absence of any double vision, since there cannot be double vision if one eye does not see clearly. A blowout fracture may be diagnosed by *x-rays* of the *orbit.* If there is *lid emphysema,* a fracture is present until proved otherwise. This symptom occurs when the patient attempts to blow the nose and the lid fills with air.

4. *Dislocated Lens:* A dislocated lens can be diagnosed only with a slit lamp.

SHARP OCULAR TRAUMA

If there is a history of a sharp penetrating injury, *no pressure* should be placed on the eye. Though a penetrating injury may appear to be very minimal, severe visual loss could result from it, and any pressure on the eye could further compound the injury by causing loss of its intraocular contents. In the case of any sharp ocular trauma, it is imperative that an ophthalmologist be contacted to examine the eye to rule out any severe problems. The nurse must examine the pupil carefully to make sure that it is *round, regular,* and *reactive.* If there is a history of metal striking metal or hammering of any type with the feeling of something hitting the eye, it is imperative that an intraocular foreign body be considered. X-rays to rule out an intraocular foreign body are necessary.

Small foreign bodies are commonly found on the globe of the eye; these can be washed out with gentle irrigation. If the foreign body is adherent, removal with gentle movement of a cotton-tipped applicator may be attempted. If it cannot be removed, a physician should be called immediately. If there is a sensation of a foreign body in the eye but no foreign body can be seen on the cornea, then the *tarsal conjunctiva* should be checked by everting the upper lid. This can be done by pulling the eyelid down at the lash line and then everting the lid backward on the edge of the tarsal plate. If a foreign body is present, it should be gently wiped off by a cotton-tipped applicator, preferably after topical anesthesia has been administered per order of a physician. Commonly, after removal of a tarsal foreign body, the patient may still complain of a foreign-body sensation. This is because of *abrasions of the cornea.* If on fluorescein staining abrasions are noted, treatment involves an antibiotic drop and tight patching.

OTHER EXTERNAL EYE TRAUMA

An *avulsion* of the *nasolacrimal system* requires surgical repair under the operating microscope. It should be noted that even what appears to be a minor laceration of the medial portion of the eyelid must be examined for a laceration of the nasolacrimal system. Frequently, a laceration that appears minor is actually very deep, and because of good apposition of tissue, appears to be less severe than would be found under a thorough examination.

A common cause of trauma to the eyes is the *over-wearing of hard contact lenses.* The patient will present to the ED with a swollen, painful eye or eyes. By staining the cornea with fluorescein, one can see a diffuse stain over the entire central cornea. The pain normally begins 4 to 6 hours after removal of the contact lens. The same symptoms with a similar stain can be seen after overexposure to an ultraviolet sun lamp or exposure to a welder's arc. The treatment is the same, namely, *analgesia* and *proper patching* of the *eye*.

Another common problem regarding contact lenses is the *loss* of a *hard contact lens in the upper cul-de-sac*. If this happens, removal is facilitated by double eversion of the eyelid. This can be done by placing a Desmarres retractor just above the tarsal plate and everting the upper tarsus onto the retractor blade, then swinging the retractor up to double evert the lid, opening the cul-de-sac so that the entire upper fornix can be seen.

NONTRAUMATIC EMERGENCIES

Noninjury emergencies fall basically into four groups. These groups are broad classifications, and a patient may have symptoms which overlap. The groups are: (1) *a painful eye;* (2) *a red eye;* (3) *swollen eyes;* and (4) *loss of vision.* A definitive report of the patient's condition with the four classifications in mind provides the opthalmologist with valuable information when requesting initial orders by phone. An overview of the nontraumatic emergencies is provided.

PAINFUL EYES

Two common causes of a painful *eye* are a *foreign body* and a *comeal abrasion.* Fluorescein staining helps to determine the specific cause. A foreign body should be looked for if an abrasion is seen. Other causes for pain are *acute glaucoma* or *acute iritis; conjunctivitis* may cause some pain to certain individuals.

RED EYES

The red eye may be due to *acute conjunctivitis, iritis, glaucoma,* or a *comeal problem* (see Table 30-1). Conjunctivitis can be either allergic, chemical, viral, or bacterial. In any case, it is not visually threatening except for the possible rare *gonorrheal conjunctivitis,* which is extremely purulent. A *comeal infection* must be seen by an ophthalmologist immediately because of the possibility of perforation. *Acute glaucoma is a true emergency,* and an ophthalmologist must be called immediately as this is vision-threatening. The treatment for acute glaucoma begins with pilocarpine drops, *every few minutes* in an attempt to break the attack.

Table 30-1   Common Causes of Red Eye

	Acute conjunctivitis	Acute iritis	Acute glaucoma	Corneal infection or trauma
1. Vision	Normal	Slightly blurred	Marked blur	Blurred
2. Discharge	Moderate to copious	None	None	Watery and/or purulent
3. Pain	Nonburning	Moderate	Severe	Some irritation to very painful
4. Cornea	Clear	Clear	Hazy	Abrasion on fluorescein Ulcer may be present
5. Pupil	Normal	Small	Semi-dilated	Normal
6. Light response of pupil	Normal	Poor	Poor to none	Normal
7. Ocular pressure	Normal	Normal	Elevated	Normal

SWOLLEN EYES

A swollen eye in a child can be serious because of the possibility of *bacterial sinusitis* and *cellulitis*. It can also be due to *conjunctivitis* or *acute dacryocystitis* secondary to a nasolacrimal block. If there are signs of sepsis, then sinusitis must be considered strongly; antibiotics are the treatment of choice along with medications to open the sinus passage. If the eye is swollen and the patient is a known *diabetic* who appears to be somnolent, one must consider a *fungal infection*. A physician should be contacted immediately since this can be life-threatening.

LOSS OF VISION

In loss of vision, an ophthalmologist must be called to determine the cause. Intermittent loss of vision may be due to the entity known as *ophthalmic migraine*. This is seen commonly in women and may be aggravated by birth control pills. However, intermittent loss of vision is also due to *transient ischemic attacks,* which is a prestroke sign.

Sudden painless loss of vision can be due to *vascular accidents:* a retinal artery occlusion, a venous occlusion, or a vitreous hemorrhage in the eye. *Hypertensives* and *diabetics* tend to have these problems. If the patient is seen immediately after loss of vision occurred, a retinal artery occlusion may be helped by *ocular massage* in an attempt to push a thrombus into a distal arteriole. A vitreous hemorrhage may herald a *retinal detachment.* It is imperative that this patient be bilaterally patched and placed at bed rest with the head elevated in order for the blood to settle so that a retinal tear may be diagnosed, if it is present. Other possibilities of visual loss are an optic neuritis, retrobulbar neuritis, and retinal detachment.

BIBLIOGRAPHY

Anderson, R., "Ocular Emergencies," in Sproul, C., and Mullanney, P., *Emergency Care: Assessment and Intervention,* Mosby, St. Louis, 1974.

Coe, R., "Emergency Eye Care," in Stephenson, H. E., *Immediate Care of the Acutely Ill and Injured,* Mosby, St. Louis, 1974, pp. 130–136.

McGavic, J. S., "First Aid in Eye Injuries," *Medical Clinics of North America,* vol. 40, 1956, pp. 1595–1608.

Mayer, Leo, "Emergency Care of the Eye," *Postgraduate Medicine,* vol. 29, 1961, pp. 199–208.

Vail, O., "Emergency Treatment of Eye Injuries," *Postgraduate Medicine,* vol. 35, 1964, pp. 150–154.

Vaughan, D., Cook, R., and Asbury, T., *General Ophthalmology,* Lange, Los Altos, Calif., 1975.

CHAPTER 31
EAR, NOSE, AND THROAT PROBLEMS
GENE W. DOO, M.D.

THE ED staff is a highly trained group of professionals who are specialists in all facets of emergency care. Ironically, however, the ED has too often become an outpatient department in which the entire spectrum of problems in a given specialty may be seen. It is the purpose of this chapter to cover the management of the acute as well as some of the more common ear, nose, and throat problems that may be encountered.

EAR

ACUTE EXTERNAL OTITIS

Acute external otitis or "swimmers ear" is one of the most common ear infections seen. The etiology is usually the use of a Q-tip cotton swab, bobby pin, or other object to clean the ear. The pain is constant and often worse when chewing or eating. The canal often is swollen shut, red, weeping, and very tender to the touch. Treatment is the application of antibiotic ear drops, analgesics, and perhaps systemic antibiotics. Often a cotton wick needs to be inserted past the swollen tissues to allow the drops to get into the ear canal. To prevent external otitis, remember the saying, "Nothing in your ear smaller than your elbow."

ACUTE MASTOIDITIS

Acute mastoiditis is uncommon but may present with the same physical findings of a swollen, very tender ear. All the soft tissues may be edematous, and the ear may be pushed forward if the infection has ruptured through the *mastoid cortex.* There is usually a history of a preceding upper respiratory tract infection. Mastoid x-rays are important. Unlike acute external otitis, there is usually a fever and more systemic signs and symptoms. Hospitalization, intravenous antibiotics, and possibly a simple mastoidectomy or incision and drainage are the steps to be followed.

ACUTE VIRAL LABYRINTHITIS

This disease is usually associated with vertigo, nausea, vomiting, and nystagmus. A prior history of an upper respiratory tract infection is often present. One must rule out more serious problems such as stroke and brainstem lesions. Hospitalization and further evaluation are necessary.

AEROTITIS

Aerotitis, or *barotitis media,* is commonly seen with a history of a recent plane trip or diving with a cold. Hearing loss, otalgia, tinnitus, or vertigo may be present. There may also be a retracted eardrum with yellow serous fluid, an air fluid level, or blood behind the eardrum. Analgesics, decongestants, and antibiotics are prescribed. Myringotomy may be needed.

SUDDEN DEAFNESS

Sudden deafness may accompany an ear infection, a cold, diving, or other situations in which middle and inner ear pressures are affected. Viral infections, vascular problems, and idiopathic conditions may also occur. Tinnitus and vertigo may be present when other physical findings are absent. Hospitalization to treat the suspected cause is indicated.

In the case of sudden deafness due to scuba diving, decompression is indicated. With changes in middle or inner ear pressure, the round window membrane may be ruptured or the stapes bone dislocated. In this case, emergency exploration has been suggested.

TRAUMATIC EAR INJURIES

Traumatic injuries to the ear are common. A perforated or ruptured eardrum may be caused by a blow to the ear, explosion, foreign bodies, or a sudden change in air pressure. Bleeding from the ear, hearing loss, vertigo, and pain are commonly present. Systemic antibiotics are recommended. The ear must not be syringed or cleaned, and the clot should be left in place. At times, an otologist may evert the edges of the perforation to provide faster healing. These perforations usually heal spontaneously. A *myringoplasty* can later be performed if healing is not complete.

A *basilar skull fracture* can affect the temporal bone. Deafness, vertigo, cerebrospinal otorrhea, or facial paralysis may occur. Treatment of the head injury is primary. Systemic antibiotics for at least 2 weeks may be needed if cerebrospinal fluid otorrhea is present. Further evaluation and treatment of the hearing loss may later be needed. Facial paralysis often requires further exploration.

FOREIGN BODIES—EAR

Foreign bodies in the ear usually occur in children. Insects can be first killed with a few drops of *alcohol* and removed with irrigation. Round objects are especially difficult to remove. A soft 10- or 12-gauge French red rubber catheter with the tip cut squarely off can be inserted with suction in an attempt to remove the smooth object. It is imperative to immobilize the child before any attempt at removal is made. Resistant objects often require a short general anesthetic for removal.

NOSE

Infections of the nose may be serious since a danger triangle encompasses the area between the eyes to the angles of the mouth. In this region, the veins are valveless and flow occurs in both directions. Retrograde flow may proceed from the angular veins on each side of the nose to the ophthalmic veins and then intracranially to the cavernous sinus (see Fig. 31-1). This sinus is located on the sides of the body of the sphenoid bone and is heavily

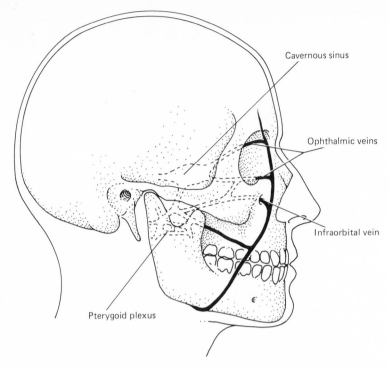

Cavernous sinus

Ophthalmic veins

Infraorbital vein

Pterygoid plexus

Figure 31-1 Chief connections of the anterior facial vein to the cavernous sinus.
(Taken from Hollinshed, W., Anatomy for Surgeons: The Head and Neck, vol. I, Hoeber-Harper, New York, 1960.)

trabeculated. Blood flow is, therefore, very slow, increasing the likelihood of *thrombosis* due to infection. Septic thrombi may then spread intracranially.

VESTIBULITIS

Vestibulitis is an infection occurring just inside the nose. Commonly, it is due to plucking of a nasal hair, irritation from rubbing, or nasal picking. Warm compresses and head elevation are indicated, and further nasal irritation should be avoided. Since *furuncles* and other infections of the nose and face are usually caused by staphylococcal penicillinase-producing microorganisms, antibiotics effective against this bacterial strain should be prescribed. Close observation is imperative. All nasal and facial infections should be treated aggressively and followed closely.

FACIAL AND NASAL FRACTURES

Facial fractures are commonly seen in the ED, since these are usually associated with high-speed auto accidents. More serious cervical, cerebral, and systemic injuries must be ruled out and treated first. Establishing an *airway* and controlling *hemorrhage* into the airway are primary. Although the facial trauma may appear to be a simple one, cervical spine x-rays are necessary. The facial fractures can be later evaluated and treated.

A simple nasal fracture may be anesthetized and reduced in the ED. Usually, though, one waits until the swelling has decreased, and the patient is sent home with compresses and analgesics. Again, x-rays are important to obtain because of the frequent medicolegal problems.

SEPTAL HEMATOMA

Often associated with a simple nasal fracture is a *septal hematoma* in which blood collects between the nasal septum and the overlying mucoperichondrium. *Septal abscess* may quickly follow, and subsequent *cavernous sinus thrombosis* and its complications occur. A septal hematoma is incised and drained immediately, as is the septal abscess. The organism is usually staphylococcus, and appropriate antibiotics are used.

NASAL HEMORRHAGE

To successfully treat nosebleeds, *good suction* and *visualization* are important. A powerful aspirator and a 10- or 12-gauge Fraquier suction tip are useful. An electric headlight is simple to use and is needed for illumination. Emergency departments should be equipped with nasal hemorrhage trays with the necessary equipment.

To control bleeding, *topical epinephrine* 1:1000 may be sparingly used on cotton pledgets. Cocaine solution 4 or 10% is a good topical anesthetic and has the added advantage of being a vasoconstrictor. Pontocaine 2 or 4% is an *effective* anesthetic but more toxic as it does not vasoconstrict and thus is more rapidly absorbed into circulation.

The emergency nurse must be aware that local anesthetics are often *toxic*. The toxic dose of cocaine is 100 mg. This amounts to 1 cc of 10% cocaine or 10 to 12 sprays from a Devilbiss atomizer. Pontocaine or tetracaine is toxic at 60 mg or 1½ cc. Xylocaine is safer, and approximately 300 to 500 mg is the toxic level.

Most nosebleeds are fortunately *anterior* and quite easy to stop. Following anesthesia, anterior nosebleeds are treated with packing or cautery. Once hemostasis is achieved, the patient can be discharged with instructions for bed rest. Tranquilizers should be provided, and the patient must be advised to see his physician in 1 to 2 days. If bleeding reoccurs, the patient should return to the ED, and hospitalization may be required.

Posterior nosebleeds are more serious and require posterior packing. Various types of posterior packing are used. A 14-gauge French foley catheter with a 30-cc bag is inserted into the bleeding side. When it is seen in the pharynx, the balloon is inflated with about 10 cc air or saline and the catheter is pulled forward lodging into posterior choanae. Anterior packing with ½-inch Vaseline gauze impregnated with antibiotic ointment is then packed against the balloon. Anteriorly, it is fixed against the nares with an umbilical clamp. Narcotics are needed as well as intravenous fluids and hospitalization.

NASAL FOREIGN BODIES

Removal of a nasal foreign body in a child is often felt to be an innocuous procedure. Problems arise when the foreign body is pushed into the nasopharynx and the child inhales, causing a subsequent laryngeal obstruction. To avoid this, the child should be immobilized with a papoose board and the head hung over the edge of the examining table. A mouth gag, tongue depressor and palate retractor, and long forceps should be on hand in the event the object passes into the pharynx.

THROAT

Oral pharyngeal infections are serious since airway obstruction may occur.

PERITONSILLAR ABSCESS

Peritonsillar abscess, or *quinsy,* usually follows a bout of tonsillitis and is commonly unilateral. It pushes the involved tonsil and uvula to the opposite side. Pain, salivation, elevated temperature, and a "hot potato voice" are present. Systemic antibiotics, bed rest, analgesics, fluids, and saline gargles are adequate for the early phlegmonous stage. However, persistent or increased swelling requires incision and drainage. *Tonsillectomy* is indicated not less than 1 month after the acute stage has subsided.

PARAPHARYNGEAL ABSCESS

These abscesses occur when the peritonsillar abscess spreads through the superior constrictor muscle into the *pharyngomaxillary* or *lateral pharyngeal space.* The carotid vessels, internal jugular veins, and important nerves are in this space, as is a potential connection to the *superior mediastinum.* With infection, neck swelling and *trismus* are present. The patient cannot open his mouth widely because of the spasm of the internal pterygoid and masseter muscles. Speech is difficult because of the limited ability of mandibular movement. Intravenous antibiotics are required, and incision and drainage are necessary if *fluctuation* exists.

RETROPHARYNGEAL ABSCESS

Retropharyngeal abscess is most commonly seen in infants under 2 years of age. Older children may lacerate the *posterior pharynx* with a foreign body, e.g., a Popsicle stick. The posterior pharynx bulges forward, and pyrexia and toxemia are present. Incision and drainage in infants are done with great care and preferably in the OR. There is the possibility of cardiac arrest with sudden pressure release and increased pharyngeal vagal tone.

LUDWIG'S ANGINA

Infection of the *sublingual* and *submental space,* or Ludwig's angina, is serious. The muscles under the tongue are attached to the hyoid bone and resist the swelling inferiorly. Consequently, the tongue is pushed up and backward, and sudden airway obstruction is imminent. Antibiotics, wide external incision, and drainage with possible tracheostomy are indicated. A nasal tracheal tube behind the tongue could be lifesaving in an acute obstruction with this entity.

FOREIGN BODIES: ESOPHAGEAL, BRONCHIAL, AND LARYNGEAL

Laryngeal foreign bodies require instant *tracheotomy* or *laryngoscopy* and *removal.* The problem is more commonly seen in restaurants where a piece of food, commonly meat, is inhaled.

Reports of life-saving tracheostomies done in restaurants are commonly seen in the newspapers.

Esophageal and *bronchial* foreign bodies create no emergency as long as the child does not cough up the object and then inhale it, obstructing the larynx or trachea. The child should be carried by an adult and calmed while preparation for endoscopic removal is underway in the operating suite.

CROUP

Laryngotracheobronchitis or croup is usually of viral etiology in young children. Inspiratory stridor and a barking cough are symptomatic, with subglottic edema present on the lateral x-ray of the soft tissues of the neck. Usually having the parent hold the child while in the ED provides a calming effect, making evaluation for treatment easier. If the child is admitted, careful monitoring of vital signs and placing the child in a croup tent are helpful. Nasotracheal intubation or tracheostomy is seldom required.

ACUTE EPIGLOTTIS

Acute epiglottis is a serious and rapidly progressing infection which may quickly compromise the airway. Hemophilus influenza is felt to be the etiologic agent. *Inspiratory stridor* may be present, with airway obstruction occurring suddenly. Again, keeping the child calm with a familiar person is important. Depression of the tongue reveals a swollen or cherry-red epiglottis. A lateral soft tissue x-ray of the neck reveals a swollen epiglottis; *nasotracheal intubation* or *tracheostomy* is required.

Acute epiglottitis in an *adult* is easily misdiagnosed. Little, if any, inspiratory stridor is present. Usually, the patient presents with an *inordinate amount* of *pain* in the throat. Routine oropharyngeal examination with the tongue blade reveals a mild erythema of the pharynx. Unfortunately, the larynx is rarely examined by mirror laryngoscopy. Many adult patients have come back to the ED several times complaining of *severe pain* in the throat. Often the last visit brings them in completely obstructed. Again, one must suspect this entity in an adult who presents with pain in the throat out of proportion to the physical findings. Hospitalization and establishing a safe airway are imperative.

LARYNGEAL TRAUMA

Trauma to the larynx is more commonly seen with the advent of safety seat belts. A sudden collision or stop throws the patient's head forward, striking the windshield. The neck and larynx are thrust forward against the dashboard. Pain, dysphagia, dysphonia or aphonia, and hoarseness are common presenting symptoms. Increasing airway obstruction may be present requiring that an immediate airway be established. Laryngeal trauma is often missed in the multiple-injury patient. Therefore the staff must be cognizant of this possibility as a seemingly stable patient may suddenly obstruct as the laryngeal edema increases.

BIBLIOGRAPHY

DeWeese, David D., and Saunders, William H., *Textbook of Otolaryngology*, 4th ed., Mosby, St. Louis, 1973.

Freeman, G., "Ear, Nose and Throat Emergencies," in Sproul, C., and Mullanney, P., *Emergency Care: Assessment and Intervention*, Mosby, St. Louis, 1974, pp. 257–269.

Hollinshead, W. Henry, *Anatomy for Surgeons:* vol. 1, *The Head and Neck*, 2d ed., Hoeber-Harper, New York, 1968.

Maloney, W. H., *Otolaryngology*, Harper & Row, Hagerstown, Md., 1971.

CHAPTER 32
RESPIRATORY DISTRESS IN CHILDREN

MARLENE MONIZ, R.N.

RESPIRATORY distress in children can be categorized into three major types: the obstructive type, the restrictive type, and pure hypoventilation.

OBSTRUCTIVE TYPE

Obstruction of the airway is evident by decreased peak flow rates when simple spirometry is done.* The obstruction may be high in the airway, causing croupy or brassy coughing, retractions of the chest wall, wheezing stridor, and decreased breath sounds. If the obstruction is lower in the airway, all the above symptoms may be evident with the exception of the croupy cough.[1] The obstruction

* Simple spirometry and peak expiratory flow rates are tests done to determine pulmonary functions. Simple spirometry measures *vital capacity,* the volume of air maximally exhaled from the lungs following maximal inspiration. Peak expiratory flow rate is the measurement of the *highest voluntary velocity* of air exhaled after maximal inspiration.

can be caused by airway edema, foreign body, tumor, infection, or congenital anomalies.

RESTRICTIVE TYPE

With the restrictive type of respiratory distress, vital capacity is decreased. The breath sounds are decreased and subcostal retractions, tachypnea, and nasal flaring may be evident.[1] A restrictive pattern may be seen in children with penumonia, chest muscle paralysis, or tight, binding chest dressings.

PURE HYPOVENTILATION

This type of respiratory distress is evidenced by cyanosis, headache, decreased breath sounds, an elevated $PaCO_2$ and a decreased PaO_2. Anesthesia and drug overdose are possible causes of pure hypoventilation.

CAUSES OF RESPIRATORY DISTRESS AND TREATMENT

ACUTE EPIGLOTTITIS

The acute obstructive *supraglottic laryngitis,* or acute epiglottitis, is probably one of the most common respiratory emergencies seen in 3- to 6-year-old children.[2] This is due to *Hemophylus,* type B, and has a dangerously rapid course of approximately 2 hours. The child appears shocky and toxic with respiratory difficulty. The child sits up in bed, breathes slowly and deeply, and has saliva pooling in the mouth due to difficulty in swallowing.[2] The swollen cherry-red epiglottis present in the posterior pharynx can completely block the airway. *The doctor must be aware that forceful depression of the tongue to visualize the area may completely occlude the airway.* It is imperative that a *lateral neck x-ray* be taken to confirm epiglottitis.

Time is of the essence in the treatment of acute epiglottitis. In the early clinical phase, *intubation* or *tracheotomy* must be performed. Once the endotracheal, nasotracheal, or tracheotomy tube is passed, the airway obstruction is relieved, danger has passed, and the child breathes easier. The tube usually is needed for 3 to 5 days until the edema is resolved and x-ray reports show no swelling in the supraglottic area.

CROUP

Acute subglottic edema, croup, or acute *laryngotracheobronchitis* is the most common type of obstruction occurring among 6-month to 3-year-old children.[2] This illness is usually caused by a virus but has a less rapid and dangerous course than acute epiglottitis. It is characterized by inflammation of the larynx and tracheobronchial tree directly below the vocal cords. The child usually has inspiratory stridor and a croupy, hoarse cough, often suggestive of a "sea-lion" or "brassy" bark.[2] The child tends to lie down and breathes rapidly.

Croup can be treated medically, but surgical intervention is sometimes needed. Medical management consists of *moist air* to reduce swelling of the airway lumen. This mist can be given in the home by steam vaporizers or by running hot water in a small, enclosed room, thus providing an area of high humidity and mist similar to a croup tent. *Hydration* is needed to both loosen thick tenacious mucus and decrease body fever. If oral fluids cannot be tolerated, intravenous fluids must be given. Antibiotics or sulfonamides may be prescribed by the physician to prevent secondary infections. Racemic epinephrine 2.25 percent in 1:8 dilution may be aerosolized per IPPB with low pressures or mask to promote bronchodilatation, thus relieving the edema and swelling.[3] This treatment may need to be repeated within the next 2 hours before effective results are noted.

Surgical management is indicated when there is diminished airway entry. Circumoral cyanosis, increased use of accessory chest and costal muscles, and an increase in pulse and respiration rates may also be noted. If a tracheotomy tube placement is needed, time is of the essence. If at all possible, the tube should be inserted in the OR where proper ventilation and sterility can be maintained. The tracheotomy tube need be in place only until the edema has diminished and airway patency is adequate.

ASTHMA

The asthmatic child in varying degrees of respiratory distress is frequently encountered in the ED. Asthma may be of two types: the *intrinsic* type due to the reaction of the respiratory tract to an infection, and the *extrinsic* type due to the sensitization of a person to an allergen, usually dust or food.[4] Children may possess the allergic type of asthma after the first 3 months of life, and this may be associated with skin eczemas and wheezing.

Environmental factors (i.e., pollen, fumes, or smoke) affect the asthmatic's airways causing edema, increased secretions, and bronchial constriction. The edema usually develops rapidly, and the child experiences sudden shortness of breath and a feeling of suffocation. In the ED, the child is often sitting up, leaning forward, and showing great use of accessory chest and abdominal muscles.

The child is usually intent on breathing, devoting all the energy to this task. He or she is usually quite apprehensive and should be watched carefully for signs of increased hypoxia. An atmosphere of calm reassurance is very desirable. *Wheezing* is usually quite pronounced and heard all over the room. This wheezing is actually a result of the *ball-valve* effect of the bronchi (see Fig. 32-1). Coughing is often present. The cough is dry and tight, becoming more marked and productive of thick, white or yellow frothy mucus as the edema subsides. The child may vomit and show signs of relief as the thick mucus is expelled from the airway.

In the treatment of asthma, laboratory reports may be helpful. Unless infection is present, the complete blood count is normal with a possible *elevated eosinophil level.* Sputum culture may show bacterial invasion if there is an infection. The chest x-rays are

Figure 32-1 Bronchi with mucus plug. On inspiration, the bronchi lengthens and becomes larger in diameter, thus permitting air to pass the obstruction fairly easily. On exhalation, the bronchi shortens and diminishes in diameter, causing increased difficulty with exhalation, and the characteristic wheeze is produced.

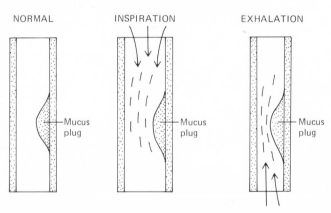

usually hyperinflated but may be normal. X-rays may also be done to rule out pneumonia or pneumothorax. Function testing shows a markedly *decreased peak flow rate,* thus confirming obstruction in the airways.

Treatment consists of the administration of subcutaneous aqueous epinephrine 1:1000 in divided doses, 15 to 20 minutes apart, as prescribed by the physician. Usually this will not exceed three successive injections. A longer-acting brand of epinephrine may be used for prolonged relief upon discharge from the ED. Side effects of epinephrine are tachycardia, headache, nausea, and hypertension, and so the child must be observed very closely when this bronchodilator is given.

Bronchodilatation can also be attained with *isoproterenol* 1:200 diluted 1:8 or 1:10 with normal saline and given per IPPB or mask aerosol to reduce spasm, open airways, decrease the work of breathing, and provide needed oxygen.* Pulse and blood pressure must be carefully monitored as this medication also produces tachycardia, cardiac arrhythmias, hypotension, and headaches.

The need for *fluids,* either orally or intravenously, cannot be overemphasized. Dehydration occurs readily as the work of breathing is increased and secretions become increasingly viscid and difficult to expectorate.

If the above modes of treatment are unsuccessful in controlling the wheezing, *aminophylline* administered intravenously over 20 to 30 minutes may be given. If the child is not relieved within 20 to 30 minutes, hospitalization is recommended, along with expectorants, continuous intravenous fluids, and cortisone, if needed. Aminophylline IV every 6 to 8 hours alternating with a bronchodilator per aerosol mask or IPPB every 6 to 8 hours, followed by chest physiotherapy to loosen and move secretions, has proved quite effective.

OTHER CAUSES OF PEDIATRIC RESPIRATORY DISTRESS

Other illnesses can contribute to respiratory distress in children and cannot be overlooked. Severe diarrhea and vomiting definitely alter blood electrolytes and gases, which in turn, affect respiratory

---

* Inflation pressures for children should range from 8 to 16 cmH$_2$O for IPPB. If mask aerosol is given, instruct the child to inhale deeply with mouth open for better penetration of particles down the tracheobronchial tree.

rates and patterns. Abdominal distention pushes the soft tissues against the diaphragm, causing shallow, rapid breathing. If this type of breathing continues for extended periods of time, the child becomes fatigued, and *acidosis* develops. Many ingested medications or household products cause hypoventilation or hyperventilation in children, depending upon the effects on the central nervous system. If the ingested liquid is not caustic to the airway, the child should be encouraged to vomit. Foreign objects and toys can be lodged in the airway; if so, they must be removed carefully following direct visualization by laryngoscope or bronchoscope.

DANGER SIGNS

The danger signs every emergency nurse must watch for are:

1. Marked decrease in inspiratory breath sounds and no wheezing. Although the absence of wheezing should indicate improvement, if it is accompanied by decreased breath sounds, the child may be more obstructed.

2. Increase in use of accessory muscles, thus increasing the work of breathing and leading to fatigue.

3. Decrease in level of consciousness.

4. Increase in cyanosis despite the administration of 40 percent oxygen per mask.

5. $PaCO_2$ of 55 mmHg or over in arterial blood sample.

6. PaO_2 of 65 mmHg or under in arterial blood sample.

These signs denote respiratory failure, and intensive, monitored care is needed immediately.

REFERENCES

1. "Airway Obstruction," unpublished article, Tulane University and Hospital, New Orleans, 1970–1971.

2. Fearon, B., "Acute Obstructed Laryngitis in Infants and Children," *Hospital Medicine*, December 1968, pp. 51–67.

3. Adar, J., Ring, W., Jordan, W., and Elwyn, R., "Ten-Year Experience with IPPB in the Treatment of Acute Laryngotracheobronchitis," *Anesthesia and Analgesia,* vol. 50, no. 5, July–August 1971, pp. 649–653.

4. "Respiratory Allergies," in *Introduction to Respiratory Diseases,* Chap. 3, American Lung Association, 1975.

BIBLIOGRAPHY

Arit, M. L., Doeshuk, C., and Stern, R., *Pediatric Respiratory Therapy,* Year Book, Chicago, 1974.

Nelson, W., Vaghan, V., and McKay, R., *Textbook of Pediatrics,* Saunders, Philadelphia, 1969.

Reeves, K., "Acute Epiglottitis—Pediatric Emergency," *American Journal of Nursing,* vol. 71, no. 8, August 1971, pp. 1539–1541.

Richards, L., and Siegel, G., *Pediatric Clinics of North America,* vol. 16, no. 1, February 1969.

CHAPTER 33
CHILD ABUSE
GWENDOLYN R. COSTELLO, R.N., M.P.H.

THE nurse in the ED plays a vital role in the identification of *child abuse* and *neglect.* Many victims of the *battered-child syndrome,* if not seen initially by a private physician, are brought to the ED for treatment. Certain studies have shown that 10 percent of all injuries seen in the ED in children under 6 years of age were the result of child abuse.[1] For the safety of the child, it is critical that the correct diagnosis be made at this time. Much skill is required at this case-finding stage to properly set the stage for effective, humane, positive intervention. In assisting the physician, child, and family, the nurses need a working knowledge of the dynamics of child abuse, the criteria for assessing child abuse, and their responsibility to the child and family.

DYNAMICS OF CHILD ABUSE

Child abuse is a broad area and needs defining if the nurse is to understand how to function in respect to this field. Looking at the problem in three major categories makes the definition of child abuse clearer.

The first category of child abuse is *inflicted injury;* this includes the battered-child syndrome. Burns, fractures, internal injuries, and poisoning are some examples. *Sexual molestation* is the second category and includes incest, rape, and fondling. The third area is *environmental neglect* which includes the psychosocial failure-to-thrive infant and the child suffering from lack of supervision or medical care.

In discussing the dynamics of child abuse, authorities in this field have put forth useful information gathered from research and clinical experiences. Some significant factors that increase the risk of child abuse in a family as presented in the literature are discussed briefly here. The reader is encouraged to review the work of Steele and Pollack.[2]

In their study, Steele and Pollack found that abusing parents had emotional problems that were serious enough to warrant therapeutic intervention. The issue causing these parents to be seen by psychiatrists was the dysfunction occurring in parent-child interaction in the form of child abuse or neglect. In exploring the dynamics of parent-child interaction, some significant findings were revealed that may be used as "red flags" or signals that this family is in need of assistance. One very significant finding was that these parents expect a great deal from their children. These *unrealistic expectations* usually are centered around the growth and developmental milestones of the normal child, for example, a suitable age to begin toilet training. The study also found a *sense* of *righteousness*. These parents had been raised in a manner similar to the one in which they were raising their children; they had been expected to perform well, to gratify parental needs very early in life, and then had been criticized, punished, and frequently abused for failure to do so. In addition, the parents were frequently difficult to relate to. Their *self-image* was *poor,* so they withdrew from contact, thus reducing the chances for criticism. An understanding, noncritical nurse in the ED at the time of crisis intervention is vital.

The quality of neglect has been incorporated in the broad area of child abuse. To truly understand the dynamics of child abuse, it is important to remember that although the mother may have given the child much attention, the attention may have been given in a negative manner that could lead to emotional abuse or in a perfunctory manner that could lead to emotional neglect.

In detecting possible child-abuse victims, socioeconomic status is often considered. Although families in the lower socioeconomic class are reported as child abusers or neglecters more frequently than middle or upper socioeconomic classes, there are no data to support the theory that it therefore occurs more frequently in the former. Families in the middle or upper socioeconomic classes have more alternative ways to handle family stress situations and therefore may not be reported to official agencies.

EMERGENCY NURSING INTERVENTION

The nurse's skill in developing a high level of suspicion for abuse and neglect is an important part of the case-finding procedure. But this is only the beginning. The nurse must also comprehensively and precisely record all observations. This enables the individual responsible for coordinating services to this family to assess the risk to the child. Once a family is determined to be in need of protective services, a *multidisciplinary effort* should be employed.

Recent literature has provided a much-needed data base for case-finding, diagnosis, treatment, follow-up, and prevention of child abuse and neglect. Helfer, Kempe, and their contributors have spearheaded research and program development that has increased understanding of this multidisciplinary problem.[3] Some of their findings which are listed below provide helpful diagnostic data.

In initial contacts with the parents, frequently the history given as to the cause of the injury does not appear compatible with the type or extent of injury. With more questioning, other versions of the cause of injury may be given. This lack of candor as to the true etiology of the injury is seen as an important clue to establishing the diagnosis of child abuse. As long as denial of the true situation persists, the child is at risk. This is not to say that the professionals involved in caring for the child and its family are on a "who-done-it" mission, but merely that the dynamics operating within the family need to be altered to provide a safe environment for the child.

The emergency nurse may also see the mother who repeatedly brings in her infant for minor problems. Actually, this mother may be trying to draw attention to the fact that all is not well between her and the baby. An alert, compassionate nurse should be aware of the underlying problem that is really being presented. The nurse should then take the time to attempt to elicit information regarding what the mother sees as the real difficulty. It is desirable that some form of follow-up services be initiated at this time.

The emergency intervention needed for the dead infant or child that is brought into the ED must also be discussed. Although nothing can be done for the victim, it is important to remember that if child abuse or neglect played a part in the death of the patient, consideration must be given to preventive aspects if there are other children in the family, or if there is the possibility that more children could be born by the couple. Careful and thorough diagnostic evaluations must be done to rule out child abuse or neglect. Factual historical data, in addition to skilled observation, must be made at this time. *Documentation* of all the information gathered is essential. *Protective services* must be considered as part of the therapeutic program that should be initiated in the ED.

CHILD ABUSE LEGISLATION

Many nurses express concern over the possible legal reprecussions that may develop if a child abuse case is reported. In reality, in many states, legal difficulties may develop if the case is *not* reported. There now exists both federal and state legislation to help meet the needs of the abused child. However, there is variance from state to state in regard to a commonality of certain basic elements in the laws. Therefore, it is imperative that a nurse be familiar not only with legislation on a federal level, but also with the law governing child abuse and neglect in the state where the nurse is practicing.[4]

Much has been written in the field of child abuse and neglect. Research endeavors are being expanded; demonstration centers have been funded to develop and evaluate specifically what kind of interventions are successful and therefore necessary to combat this serious medicosocial problem. This chapter is intended to alert and provoke nurses into assessing their own emergency situations and developing multidisciplinary solutions to meet the needs of these unfortunate families.

REFERENCES

1. Holter, J. C., and Friedman, S. B., "Child Abuse: Early Care Finding in the Emergency Department," *Pediatrics,* vol. 42, no. 1, July 1968.

2. Steele, B. F., and Pollack, C. B., "A Psychiatric Study of Parents Who Abuse Infants and Small Children," in Helfer, R. E., and Kempe, C. H. (eds.), *The Battered Child,* University of Chicago Press, 1968.

3. Helfer, R. E., and Kempe, C. H., (eds.), *The Battered Child,* University of Chicago Press, 1968.

4. Public Law S1191 93rd Congress.

BIBLIOGRAPHY

Chamberlain, R., "The Nurse and the Abusive Parent," *Nursing '74,* October 1974, pp. 73–75.

Gil, D. G., "Unraveling Child Abuse," *American Journal of Orthopsychiatry,* vol. 45, no. 3, April 1975, pp. 346–356.

Gregg, G., "Infant Trauma," *American Family Physician,* vol. 3, no. 5, May 1971, pp. 101–105.

Kempe, C. H., and Helfer, R. E., *Helping the Battered Child and His Family,* Lippincott, Philadelphia, 1972.

Newberger, E., *"Child Abuse,"* in Feinbloom, R., et al., *Child Health Encyclopedia,* Delacorte Press/Seymour Lawrence, 1975.

Reece, R. M., "Child Abuse," in Baumslag, N., *Family Care,* Williams & Wilkins, Baltimore, 1973.

The Lippincott Manual of Nursing Practice, "The Battered Child (Child Abuse)," Lippincott, Philadelphia, 1974.

CHAPTER 34
GYNECOLOGIC EMERGENCIES
LAURENCE A. REICH, M.D.

E MERGENCY care, by its very nature, is surrounded by crisis. Health care personnel who deliver emergency services and the consumers who seek those services can do much through educational processes to diminish this orientation and maximize one which is more satisfactory. While it is the intention of this chapter to provide the reader with a brief, workable system to process and use information pertaining to emergencies in obstetrics and gynecology, the reader should notice that, when possible, appropriate suggestions are offered to reduce the need for such emergencies.

It is not within the scope of this chapter to provide a complete guide to obstetrics and gynecologic emergencies. Those of a more serious consequence will be presented and the reader will find a reference list at the conclusion of the chapter for more detailed and comprehensive information. It will be the format of this chapter to offer information based upon symptom presentation rather than disease models. The two most common obstetrical or gyne-cological presenting symptoms are *pelvic pain* and *vaginal bleeding,* and often they coexist. Pregnant patients with these complaints should receive immediate attention and/or referral.

HISTORICAL DATA COLLECTION

Prior to diagnosis and treatment, a brief problem *history* is essential. It is extremely useful to have the patient describe the *presenting problem* or complaint in the most specific terms possible. Vague descriptions often lead the interviewer on circuitous, repetitive routes, if not astray. Attention is directed toward those questions which pertain to the social and physiologic events associated with the reproductive system.

Useful information includes: (1) the first day of the last normal menstrual period; (2) a menstrual calendar or menstrual history; (3) pain or bleeding associated with sexual intercourse; (4) previous pregnancies and their associated complications; (5) the history of a current pregnancy including its management and complications thus far; (6) any history of pelvic infection or associated venereal diseases; and (7) any previous or current treatment for obstetrical or gynecologic problems.

Should the nurse notice uncomfortable or awkward feelings pertaining to questions related to sexual behavior, helpful suggestions include sharing these feelings with the patient (i.e. "If you're embarrassed about the question I'm asking, I hope the feeling soon passes," or "The information I want to obtain may require some awkward discussion for both of us, so let's handle any uneasiness that occurs together"). Role playing in front of a mirror or with other professionals is extremely useful and often assists in allaying anxiety.

BLEEDING AND PAIN ASSOCIATED WITH PREGNANCY

It is crucial that the nurse become aware that most obstetrical-gynecological patients are young and healthy rather than medically debilitated. Thus, in both the pregnant and nonpregnant patient, symptoms associated with bleeding may *initially* seem vague and nonthreatening. Since physiologic reserves are usually quite adequate, one may be lulled into a sense of false security and institute prolonged observation, only to find a later catastrophic deterioration. *Do not* be fooled by the fact that the individual looks healthy, has normal vital signs and laboratory data, and is without pallor and associated dizziness or syncope. By the time signs of shock have become manifest, vital time has been lost and physiologic reserves have been severely depleted.

Bleeding in the pregnant individual can occur as an episode of scant vaginal spotting or as a massive hemorrhagic event. The amount of bleeding is not an adequate index of pathologic involvement. The most frequent causes of bleeding in the first half of pregnancy include *abortion* and *ectopic pregnancy*. *Placenta previa* and *abruptio placenta* are events most often implicated in bleeding during the latter half of gestation. Intact or completely separated placentas do not bleed—it is the partially separated placenta which results in bleeding.

Labial, vaginal, or cervical involvement is ruled out by direct inspection. Assisting the patient in developing skills toward relaxation during pelvic examinations is of immeasurable importance. Most individuals tense their pelvic, thigh, and abdominal muscles during this examination. *Muscle relaxation* can be a learned skill, and nurses who have knowledge of these techniques are of great value to their patients.[1,2]

BLEEDING AND PAIN IN EARLY PREGNANCY

Often these symptoms occur prior to a definitive diagnosis or even a suspicion of pregnancy. The patient may or may not know the dates of her last period. In fact, her last menstrual flow may have been related to withdrawal bleeding associated with oral contraceptives which she has discontinued without medical advice.

ABORTION

Bleeding or *spotting* associated with cramping of varied intensity, following one or more missed menses, can raise suspicions of a *threatened abortion*. If tissue has been passed, the diagnosis is confirmed, and the patient may require a uterine aspiration or suction curettage. Occasionally the entire products of conception are passed in toto, and no surgical intervention is necessary. If the pregnancy is still viable, most patients are sent home and await abating or increasing symptoms. While a variety of hormonal preparations have been utilized in the past, none have proved effective. The current concerns over drug usage during pregnancy warrant *extreme caution* regarding the use of *chemical compounds* in these situations. Rarely is hospitalization necessary unless curettage is to be performed under general anesthesia. Emotional support is of great value and should be dispensed liberally. The patient should be asked to save any tissue that is passed at home.

ECTOPIC PREGNANCY

A *missed period* and accompanying *abdominal pain* especially of an increasing nature, with or without associated signs of shock, nausea, or vomiting, should serve as an early warning sign of possible *ectopic pregnancy*. Pain may be unilateral and directed toward either adnexal region. This event can be associated with drastic sequela and demands immediate attention regardless of the degree of presenting symptoms. Bleeding is usually minimal, and difficulty may be encountered in establishing a diagnosis. Ectopic pregnancy must be differentiated from appendicitis, enteritis, ruptured ovarian cyst, and a pelvic infectious process. While the history of a missed menstrual period is quite helpful, this particular sign may also exist in the presence of functional ovarian cysts and in individuals with an irregular menstrual history. Pelvic examination is usually helpful; however, occasionally it will not be conclusive. If the ectopic pregnancy is leaking or has ruptured, a *culdocentesis* may aid in establishing the diagnosis.

If an ectopic gestation is suspected, the patient should be hospitalized, kept at bedrest, NPO, and an infusion of 5% D and L/R started. Serial hemoglobins and hematocrits may provide useful information, and should be typed and cross matched. If the signs and symptoms are minimal and little change in the status occurs over the next several hours, occasionally an *endometrial aspiration* and *frozen section* of the extracted tissue can aid in establishing a diagnosis.

A much less common cause of bleeding in early pregnancy is a *hydatidiform mole,* and the interested student is referred to an appropriate gynecologic text for information on this subject.

BLEEDING AND PAIN IN LATE PREGNANCY

The diagnosis of pregnancy is almost always assured by the symptoms presenting during this stage of gestation. However, rare occurrences of astonished women in early labor have been documented. Pain, cramping, and spotting may be associated with premature labor in the second half of pregnancy. Depending upon gestational viability and other variables such as the presence or absence of ruptured membranes, attempts are usually made to delay labor. Abdominal pain can also result from various events not involving pregnancy, such as a ruptured ovarian cyst, appendicitis, cholelithiasis, and even pancreatitis. The point to be made is that although one first rules out events related to the gestational process, an astute attendant does not overlook other causes of pain simply because the patient is pregnant. Most emergency services transfer patients presenting with pain or bleeding in late pregnancy to obstetrical units where careful fetal and maternal monitoring can more easily be performed.

PLACENTA PREVIA AND ABRUPTION

Placenta previa and abruptio placenta are two possible causes of bleeding in late pregnancy. *Placenta previa* is defined as a placenta which has separated from the uterine wall; *abruption* is defined as a placenta which is encroaching upon or covering the internal cervical os. Most textbooks classically differentiate bleeding associated with placenta previa from that accompanying abruption by the description of *abdominal pain*. While abdominal pain usually accompanies *abruption,* this is not always the rule, and further examination is necessary. Vaginal and pelvic examinations are always deferred in patients presenting with bleeding in the second half of pregnancy until obstetrical expertise is available. However, abdominal examination for the presence of uterine activity and a fetal heart tone is certainly indicated and advisable.

Should previa, abruption, or premature labor be suspected, initial laboratory work and intravenous solutions should be ordered. If the patient appears to be in distress, a *lateral recumbant* position is preferable since the supine position allows the heavy uterus to partially occlude venous return by compressing the vena cava.

Should a pregnant patient present with either a *prolapsed cord* or prolapsed *fetal extremity,* the most advantageous immediate treatment consists of placing the patient in the *knee-chest position* and rapidly transporting her to the labor and delivery suite. While waiting for an elevator, an intravenous infusion can be started.

Intrapartum and immediate postpartum hemorrhage is not a subject for this chapter, since it is usually handled in the labor-delivery room complex. Delayed postpartum bleeding can occur after the patient is sent home from the obstetrical unit and is usually associated with subinvolution of the placental site or retained placental fragments. Laboratory work to assess blood loss and intravenous support are usually ordered while awaiting specific obstetrical management.

HYPERTENSIVE CRISIS AND AMNIOTIC EMBOLUS

Two rare and acute obstetric emergencies, which present with a broad range of symptoms, are mentioned only as an introduction to the reader. The *hypertensive crisis,* peculiar to pregnancy, known as the *preeclampsia-eclampsia syndrome* may present with a variety of clinical manifestations, which may include elevated blood pressure, proteinuria, generalized edema, hyperreflexia, and oliguria. The presenting signs and symptoms can be as overt as noted in classic textbook descriptions or ambiguously couched in vague, almost nondescript complaints. Because of the catastrophic nature of the progressive form of this disease and the ability to forestall its associated crises if discovered early, it is far better to err on the cautious side of observational admission when in doubt. Individuals thought to be involved in the process of a hypertensive crisis in pregnancy should receive immediate evaluation by a trained attendant. It is imperative that the patient be made as comfortable as possible within a *quiet environment* so that a *seizure* is not precipitated.

Amniotic fluid embolus is a dreaded and rare sequela to several obstetrical situations, including the dead-baby syndrome, intrauterine sepsis, a tumultuous home delivery, and the disseminated intravascular coagulation syndrome. This accident is *usually fatal* before it is ever diagnosed.

BLEEDING AND PAIN NOT ASSOCIATED WITH PREGNANCY

Symptoms suggestive of the acute gynecologic abdomen either present as a definitive gynecologic emergency or are referred to a gynecologic service when a specific diagnosis is not immediately entertained by the medical or surgical specialties.

Because of the possibility of a concealed hemorrhage, any *pain* associated with a *missed menses* should arouse the suspicion of *ectopic pregnancy.* Since a pregnancy test is conclusive only when the pregnancy contains viable trophoblastic tissue, this procedure may not afford diagnostic help. Often a leaking or ruptured functional ovarian cyst or hormone-dependent ovarian tumor can produce symptoms confusingly similar to an ectopic pregnancy. A *detailed* and *accurate history* often makes the difference in correct diagnoses. Should any tumor or cyst leak (usually bleeding) or rupture, valuable evidence may be obtained by a *culdocentesis*. Blood work to assess hemorrhagic conditions and intravenous infusion should be started prior to such a procedure.

PELVIC INFLAMMATORY DISEASE

Pelvic inflammatory disease, bilateral salpingitis, or torsion of an ovarian cyst or pedicle may present as acute abdominal pain. Infection and inflammatory processes when caused by gonorrhea or secondary bacterial invasion during the menstrual flow usually present symptomatically, shortly after the menses has ended. The pain is usually low in the abdomen and bilateral in nature. Often an adequate pelvic examination is difficult to perform. Pelvic laparotomy is rarely indicated unless a toboovarian abscess has ruptured or is leaking. Treatment usually consists of *admission* and *intravenous antimicrobial chemotherapy*. Appropriate laboratory data, including hemoglobin, hematocrit, BUN, creatinine, ESR, and bacterial cultures, are essential in following these individuals, until an informative pelvic examination can reveal the extent of pelvic organ debilitation. It is the bias of this author *not* to treat salpingitis on an *outpatient* basis with *intramuscular antibiotics*.

DYSFUNCTIONAL UTERINE BLEEDING

Dysfunctional uterine bleeding is usually related to some derangement in the *hypothalmic-pituitary-ovarian axis* and is often associated with the phenomenon of *anovulation*. Investigation of inter- and intramenstrual bleeding that is heavier or longer than the usual cyclic event is mandatory. Functionally, this type of bleeding may occur at the waxing or waning of the reproductive years (i.e., menarche and menopause).

Dysfunctional uterine bleeding associated with *oral contraceptives* can also occur. This bleeding especially happens when the pills are stopped and then started again without reference to the cyclic shedding of the endometrial lining.

For the individual with dysfunctional bleeding, controlling the symptoms on an emergency basis may necessitate the use of estrogenic compounds and rarely a curettage. Labial, vaginal, and cervical inspection is mandatory, since often small tissue tears occur leaving arterial "pumpers" in the vaginal barrel, which are compressed during speculum examination. Unless massive hemorrhage has occurred, outpatient management is most often adequate. Emergency nurses must also provide adequate patient teaching and emotional support since these women are often quite apprehensive, especially those in their perimenopausal years.

SEXUAL ABUSE

No discussion of gynecologic emergencies can be undertaken, regardless of its brevity, without the inclusion of approaches to the management of *sexual assault*. Sexual problem-solving as a sub-specialty has arrived in many areas of the United States. However, most of the recent treatises on sexual abuse have come out of the wide variety of women's caucases. While sexual abuse or assault has often been substituted for the term "rape," the concept is at best poorly defined. Most health care personnel have abrogated their responsibility to the awesome legal system in the sense that legal definitions, opinions, and jurisprudence often set the pace and tone for patient policy rather than the health and well-being of the individual. Sexual abuse includes assault, both upon men and on women, and need not apply to only forced genital intercourse. Definitions are archaic, and many health professionals might do well to examine their own biases and prejudices before pinning "labels" on individuals. Contrary to popular medical and legal opinions, the patient presenting with a complaint of having been sexually assaulted *need not* be subjected to pelvic examination unless the physical assault has been severe enough to cause external or internal bleeding or trauma. Should the patient be desirous of pressing legal charges through an attorney or the police, an examination is legally mandatory.

It is this author's expressed bias that individuals who are abused sexually be afforded measures to *prevent venereal disease* and *pregnancy*. Many centers are now using *menstrual aspiration* if an expected menses is delayed rather than the "morning after pill" at the time of the assault.

Emergency personnel have learned to deal effectively with the physical aspects of sexual abuse. The emotional needs of the sexually abused patient are often more difficult to handle in the emergency setting. One possible solution to this problem is the use of an *advocate system* which could bridge the gap between the medical and legal communities. Ideally, an advocate could examine, treat, take depositions, and perhaps even testify for the assaulted individual. This system would be particularly helpful if the abused person is a young and frightened child.

No matter what system is used, emergency personnel must become more sensitive to the emotional needs of this type of patient. Before searching for acid-phosphatase preparations and worrying about legal matters, emergency personnel must first concern themselves with the *person* who has been abused. A calm, empathic approach can do much to lessen the emotional trauma associated with sexual abuse.

EMERGENCY DELIVERIES

As policemen and taxi drivers are only too well aware, not every birth occurs in a planned, placid fashion attended by a physician. Deliveries in the ED may not be frequent, but the basic skills needed to manage them should be part of the ED nurse's knowledge. The ED nurse is often not provided with educational opportunities to learn how to manage deliveries. Confidence and proficiency in handling these cases can be obtained only by study and practice. Emergency deliveries are no different from cardiopulmonary resuscitations, cardiac arrests, or fractured bones in this respect. Annual or semiannual courses mandated by hospital regulations are the basic means of providing the necessary skills. Close cooperation between delivery room and ED staffs is desirable. Labor and delivery nurses can easily inform the ED of the procedures practiced by their particular services. Excellent information on labor, delivery, and complications is readily available in standard reference texts. Equipment requirements and procedural instruction lists can be drawn up with the help of the medical staff.

REFERENCES

1. Reich, L. A., and Pion, R. J., *Sex in Pregnancy: Audiocassette,* Enabling Systems, Inc., Honolulu, 1975.

2. ———, *Learning about Your Pelvic Exam: Audiocassette,* Enabling Systems, Inc., Honolulu, 1976.

BIBLIOGRAPHY

Barnes, A., *The Social Responsibility of Gynecology and Obstetrics,* Johns Hopkins, Baltimore, 1965.

Greenhill, L., and Friedman, F., *Obstetrics,* Saunders, Philadelphia, 1974.

Hellman, M., and Pritchard, R., *William's Obstetrics,* 14th ed., Appleton-Century-Crofts, New York, 1971.

Kistner, R. W., *Gynecology,* 2d ed., Year Book, Chicago, 1971.

CHAPTER 35
PSYCHIATRIC EMERGENCIES
CHRISTINE N. LANGWORTHY, A.C.S.W.

PSYCHIATRIC emergencies comprise a good part of most emergency department's daily census and are often some of the most troublesome cases for the emergency staff to handle. In this chapter the focus is on attitudinal as well as management problems from the point of view of a psychiatric social worker. In addition, information regarding the psychiatric patient's psychological makeup is presented which may help in understanding the dynamics of this patient as well as suggesting alternative management approaches.

CLASSIFICATION OF PSYCHIATRIC EMERGENCIES

Psychiatric emergencies can be classified into several main categories. These are psychosis, acute anxiety attacks, family crises, suicide attempts and depression, psychophysiologic disorders, acute and chronic alcoholism, and drug abuse. In addition to these more neatly defined problem areas, there are those people who wander into the ED asking to be treated whose problems do not

fit into any of the above psychiatric categories. People with dis-
position problems, such as not having a place to live, and people
with character or personality disorders, such as hostile, dependent,
or manipulative patients, are included in this category. Patients
with a personality disorder do not necessarily have specific psychiatric problems, but are particularly difficult to deal with because
of their overt maladjusted behavior. These patients are often the
most troublesome because their behavior provokes feelings which
may be difficult to handle and can interfere with patient care. The
care and management of these patients as well as problems in
dealing with the more specific categories of psychiatric patients are
discussed.

THE PSYCHOTIC PATIENT

Perhaps one of the most disturbing types of patients to find in an
ED is the fearful, psychotic person, such as a patient with the diagnosis of *acute paranoid schizophrenia*. This patient can be extremely frightening since by definition he or she is out of contact
with reality. The person is experiencing a *thought disorder* which
includes delusions and/or hallucinations that others are at fault and
are out to do harm. Consequently, the ED staff becomes the target
of this person's aggression, as would anyone else who gets in the
way.

In dealing with this grossly psychotic patient, one thing that is
helpful to remember is that the person is acting out of fear more
than anything else, even though the psychotic behavior might also
be frightening to the staff. In this patient's delusional frame of reference everyone is to be suspected. As a result, the need to protect self by striking out verbally or physically becomes overwhelming.

Because the *reality* of this person is so greatly *distorted* (as it is
with other types of acutely psychotic patients), he or she cannot
usually respond to demands or explanations regarding this behavior and the present situation. What the person can respond to is
nonverbal cues and communication at a feeling level. This includes
direct eye contact, slow movements, directness, and reassurance.
Ideally, this patient should be promptly placed in a room, alone,
and an attempt made to minimize confusion and contacts with
people. One person at a time should speak "to," not "about," the
patient. Often the manner and *attitude of the staff* member, rather
than the specific care (other than the administration of medica-

tion), have the greatest effect in calming this patient. Finally, it is important to acknowledge one's fear if it is there and act upon it. The acutely paranoid patient often does strike out and should not be approached lightheartedly.

THE HOSTILE, BELLIGERENT PATIENT

An equally difficult patient to handle in an emergency setting is the hostile, belligerent patient. This is often a person with a *character disorder,* or one who is drunk or hysterical, rather than a person who is out of contact with reality. The former type of patient is aware of what he or she is doing at some level of consciousness and is using various symptoms to manipulate. In psychodynamic terms, this patient is often asking to be "kicked" (*negatively reinforced*) because this is the only response from other people that is comfortable and consistent with this person's own negative identity. Thus a self-fulfilling cycle is perpetuated. In order to accomplish it, this patient is often very good at attacking the weak points in the target's personality, and a power struggle results. The issue then becomes "who's right" or "who will win," rather than what the problem is and what can be done to help it.

Since the patient, knowingly or not, sets up this pattern and it is so easy to fall into, what is an alternative response? First of all, it is important to try to *hear the message* that the patient does need help of some sort and what is specifically requested. It is helpful to remember that underneath the brazen exterior is often a very helpless, inadequate, and lonely person who has a limited repertoire of skills to satisfy wants and needs.

Secondly, after pinpointing the request, it becomes necessary to differentiate between what can and cannot be done to resolve the problem and to determine what part of the problem is the patient's responsibility. This is the point at which frustration, anger, and guilt can appear if limits are not set. However, it is usually the staff member, rather than the patient, who is left feeling inadequate. This kind of patient usually does not know how to cooperate very well, and certainly prefers manipulation to taking partial responsibility for the resolution of a problem.

Thirdly, if after the ED staff have done their part in meeting the request for help and the patient is still acting out or will not cooperate, the person may have to be asked to leave. At this point it is important to be *firm* but not totally rejecting; that is, be specific about which behaviors are unacceptable rather than convey the message that the person as a whole is unacceptable. This information could be of help if the patient is interested in formulating a more positive approach to people.

THE ACUTELY ANXIOUS PATIENT

Another category of patient often seen in the ED is the acutely anxious person. This person can be responding to a real crisis, such as a death or injury of a loved one, or a crisis which has been exaggerated or is unidentified. With this patient also it is important to have a minimal number of people around as confusion often aggravates the situation. This person is often but not always willing to talk, but needs help in focusing feelings as well as getting in perspective the facts of the situation. Anxiety is often a mask for other emotions, primarily *anger* and *sadness,* and the patient may require more time than the ED staff can give if this problem is to be resolved in any way other than by medication. However, often reassurance of what the problem is and where the patient can go for help can alleviate many of the symptoms.

THE DEPRESSED PATIENT

The depressed person or the person who makes a *suicide attempt* is another very common category of psychiatric patient seen in the ED. This category also includes the patient who has *overdosed,* which is the most common method of attempting suicide. The overdosed patient is perhaps the most provocative in terms of stirring up feelings in staff members. Feelings of anger and disgust or sadness are most commonly felt. There are several reasons why these feelings are aroused.

First of all, this patient makes it very plain that he or she cannot handle problems and expects someone else to do something about it. This *helplessness and dependency* can be quite irritating to emergency staff who are generally an independent, rather resourceful, group of people.

Secondly, there is certainly an element of *frustration* in treating a patient who deliberately attempts self-injury, especially if the patient is a repeater and the emergency staff has worked previously to save this person's life. There is both a feeling of helplessness in doing such fruitless work and a fear of being manipulated by someone who repeatedly comes into the ED because of attempted self-destruction.

Thirdly, many times there is identification with a staff member's own feelings of sadness and depression which makes it difficult to view the patient's plight objectively.

In relating to this patient, it can be very detrimental to give an uncaring, overcritical response, as the patient is asking for something which cannot be gotten by more appropriate means at this time. A suicide attempt or gesture is a desperate and/or immature way of getting a need met, and it is easy to respond in a parental, overcritical, or overnurturant way. What the patient needs is *adult-to-adult communication,* i.e., concern and interest with the message that it is up to the patient to cooperate and take responsibility. Sharing feelings with this patient, even anger, can be helpful if a *positive, caring relationship* which can tolerate constructive criticism and expression of negative affect has been established.

THE PSYCHOPHYSIOLOGICALLY ILL PATIENT

Also a common problem to the emergency staff is the psychophysiologically ill patient. In this category are people with reports of backaches, headaches, fainting spells, and other neurologically related problems for which no organic basis can be found. This type of patient usually reports vague symptoms of chronic problems, generally focused around *anxiety* or *tension* but not always precipitated by a crisis. The most prominent personality characteristic of these patients is *extreme dependency.*

A question that is often brought up in regard to treatment of these patients is whether it is more helpful to the patient and to the staff to reassure him or her that the problem is understood, or whether it is better to confront the person with the fact that the illness is emotionally based. First of all, the latter may not always be true; secondly, defenses are rigid and unyielding when they are linked to somatic complaints, and no matter what explanations are given, this patient is unlikely to change. While insight helps very little with this patient, providing *alternative environmental structures* and *supports* does help, and this type of planning can cut down on the frequency of visits to the ED. This patient can also respond to *limit-setting,* after a relationship is established, specifying which kinds of problems are appropriate for an ED and which problems require on-going outpatient care.

THE ALCOHOLIC PATIENT

The alcoholic patient technically is a psychiatric problem, but in reality presents a dichotomous picture. This patient often gets informal support and acceptance from the emergency staff, but can also get the lowest priority in terms of time and attention to medical and emotional problems. The alcoholic differs from other psychiatric patients in that alcoholism is usually more socially acceptable and is a problem which is easier for most people to identify with. Also, there is more community support for the alcoholic in terms of rehabilitation programs than there is for the psychiatric patient. Although this patient is on the whole easier to manage than most psychiatric patients, the alcoholic does present some particular problems because of an apparent lack of self-control. However, it is important to remember that in most instances the alcoholic can hear, can understand, and can control. This patient also requires supportive but firm messages of what is and is not acceptable behavior and what are the ED's limits on the help it can offer.

BIBLIOGRAPHY

Beck, A., Kovacs, M., and Weissman, A., "Hopelessness and Suicidal Behavior: An Overview," *JAMA,* vol. 234, no. 11, Dec. 15, 1975, pp. 1146–1149.

Bellak, L., "The Role and Nature of Emergency Psychotherapy," *American Journal of Public Health,* vol. 58, February 1968, pp. 344–347.

———, Prola, M., Meyer, E. J., and Zankerman, M., "Psychiatry in the Medical-Surgical Emergency Clinic," *Archives of General Psychiatry,* vol. 10, 1964, p. 267.

Berliner, B. S., "Nursing a Patient in Crisis," *American Journal of Nursing,* vol. 70, October 1970, pp. 2154–2157.

Bridges, P. K., *Psychiatric Emergencies, Diagnosis and Management,* Charles C Thomas, Springfield, Ill., 1971.

Errera, P., Wyshak, G., and Jarecki, H., "Psychiatric Care in a General Hospital Emergency Room," *Archives of General Psychiatry,* vol. 9, 1963, p. 105.

Farnsworth, D. L., "Medical Perspectives on Alcoholism and Around-the-Clock Psychiatric Services," *American Journal of Psychiatry,* vol. 124, June 1968, pp. 1659–1663.

Feldman, F., "The Tripartite Session: A New Approach in Psychiatric Social Work Consultation," *Psychiatric Quarterly,* vol. 42, 1968, pp. 48–61.

Frazier, S. H., "Comprehensive Management of Psychiatric Emergencies," *Psychosomatics,* vol. 9, January–February 1968, pp. 7–11.

Hankoff, L., Mischorr, M., Tomlinson, K., and Joyce, S., "A Program of Crisis Intervention in the Emergency Medical Setting," *American Journal of Psychiatry,* vol. 131, no. 1, January 1974, pp. 47–50.

Hollis, Florence, *Casework, a Psychosocial Therapy,* Random House, New York, 1964.

Lion, J. R., Bach-y-Rita, G., and Ervin, F. R., "Violent Patients in the Emergency Room," *American Journal of Psychiatry,* vol. 125, June 1969, pp. 1706–1711.

Milgram, B., "Psychiatric Emergencies," *Emergency Medicine,* February 1973, pp. 174–181.

CHAPTER 36
THE ALCOHOLIC AND DRUG ABUSER IN THE EMERGENCY DEPARTMENT

PAMELA K. BURKHALTER, R.N., M.S.N., MA.

ALCOHOLICS and drug abusers are frequent visitors to the ED. They seek, either voluntarily or involuntarily, such ED services as treatment for trauma, illness, overdose, or detoxification. Often these patients are perceived by the staff to be difficult, unpredictable, aggressive, resistant, and passive, or in general as presenting management problems. This chapter is, therefore, written to provide information on some of the factors that underlie the behavior of alcoholics and drug abusers in the ED.

PSYCHOSOCIAL COMPONENTS OF ALCOHOLISM

Alcoholism usually begins with moderate drinking which can eventually progress to chronic, excessive drinking. The progressive illness develops over time in *three* phases.

PHASE ONE

At first, the person consumes alcoholic beverages to achieve relief from, or avoid, psychological or physical stressors. Although not an alcoholic at this time, the person may begin to (consciously or unconsciously) associate alcohol intake with relief (see Fig. 36-1).

Figure 36-1

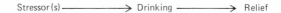

Stressor(s) ──────────> Drinking ──────────> Relief

PHASE TWO

With continuation of the pattern, the person starts to psychologically depend on alcohol in order to avoid stressors. *Dependence* here refers to reliance on the chemical, alcohol, which masks or rearranges an unpleasant reality. Because alcohol succeeds, at least partially, in distorting the person's perception of an unrewarding and/or harsh world, its continued intake becomes reinforcing (see Fig. 36-2).

Figure 36-2

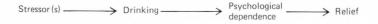

Stressor(s) ─────> Drinking ─────> Psychological dependence ─────> Relief

PHASE THREE

As this self-reinforcing pattern continues, *tissue tolerance* develops in which more alcohol is required by the cells to bring about the desired distortion. Additional behavioral tendencies become prominent in this phase:

1. *Loss of control.* The person seems unable to break the cycle of repeated alcohol intake. It must be noted, however, that recent research indicates that alcoholics do have the ability to control alcohol intake under certain circumstances.

2. *Craving.* The heightened need to drink excessively results from both psychological dependence and tissue tolerance. The term *craving* does not imply wild-eyed, bizarre behavior! Rather, it implies a persistent biological and psychological need to continue to drink.

3. *Amnesias* (blackouts). These memory losses may occur before, during, or after a drinking episode. Frequently they are a source of great concern to the alcoholic and his or her significant others and, as such, may be a source of motivation to seek treatment.

4. *Withdrawal syndrome.* When alcohol intake is decreased or stopped, the alcoholic begins to experience a variety of physical and psychological symptoms. (This syndrome is discussed below.)

Of these behaviors, the loss of control is considered the key factor indicating the specific presence of *alcoholism*. Thus, a vicious cycle evolves (see Fig. 36-3). The relief the alcoholic now experiences is shaky and tends to reinforce the need to increase drinking.

PERSONALITY CHARACTERISTICS OF ALCOHOLICS

A single "alcoholic personality," per se, does not exist. What does exist are several personality traits that many alcoholics may exhibit to some degree at some time during the drinking career.

Many alcoholics experience major conflict over the need to feel *independent* and the need to be *dependent.* Usually dependency, in many forms, predominates. This conflict may act as a prime stressor leading to continued drinking while leaving the conflict unresolved.

As alcoholics drink, they are able to experience and project varying levels of *omnipotence,* or powerfulness and control. By sobering up, their perceptions of reality clear, and these feelings of power are erased. Frequently, alcoholics then tend to experience feelings of worthlessness and loss of self-esteem.

Because alcoholics often experience conflict between independence and dependence, they may be very *angry* and *frustrated* people. The anger tends to be used as the rationale for inappropriate social and interpersonal behavior; i.e., "How can it be my

Figure 36-3

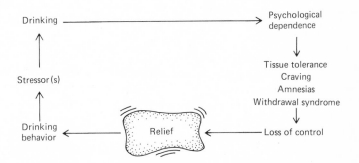

fault? I was drunk." Low frustration tolerance also seems to be quite common with the alcoholic.

Alcoholics generally employ *defense mechanisms* as a means of coping with unrelieved stress and anxiety. Of the many defense mechanisms used by most people, the alcoholic seems to rely on denial, rationalization, and projection.

DENIAL   As perhaps the best known of the alcoholic's defense mechanism repertoire, denial serves several purposes. It prevents acknowledgement of the seriousness and potential threat to the alcoholic that his or her behavior presents. It allows a person to remain unlabeled as a deviant, i.e., an alcoholic. It implies an ability to be independent of the chemical, alcohol. Denail of dependence, of a drinking "problem," and most of all, of loss of self-control, is a significant behavior pattern of the alcoholic person.

RATIONALIZATION AND PROJECTION   Hand in hand with denial are the behaviors associated with excuse-finding for alcoholic behavior (rationalization) and placing blame or responsibility on others for the alcoholic's behavior (projection). By seeking to absolve themselves of responsibility for their behavior, alcoholics try to convince themselves that "everything is all right."

Another significant personality characteristic possessed by many alcoholics is *depression* that may (1) motivate the person to start heavy alcohol consumption, (2) lead to continued drinking, or (3) be the result of uncontrolled drinking. To date, depression (primary or secondary) has not been identified as a direct causative factor in the development of alcoholism.

The behavior patterns presented here are found in many alcoholics. It must be remembered, however, that *many* alcoholics do not display all these behaviors, or, if they do, the behaviors are in modified form. In general, the nurse should avoid making broad general statements about the behavior or personality of alcoholics. Such labeling, which often can be derogatory, serves only to perpetuate stereotypes and impede therapeutic nurse-patient relationships.

ALCOHOL WITHDRAWAL SYNDROME

Because alcohol acts as a *depressant* to the CNS, a *reflex hyperactivity* results when alcohol intake is decreased or stopped. The visible symptoms manifested by the person make up the withdrawal syndrome that can be broken down into *three* stages.

TREMULOUS STAGE Onset for this stage may vary considerably from as soon as 3 to 6, 12, 24, 36 hours or longer after the last drink. Common symptoms include tremors, anxiety, flushing, anorexia, nausea, vomiting, tachycardia, depression, insomnia, bloodshot eyes, and general agitation. These symptoms can usually be alleviated with intake of alcohol or administration of sedatives that mimic the action of alcohol on the CNS.

ACUTE HALLUCINOSIS STAGE The major characteristic of this stage is the appearance of hallucinations that may be visual, auditory, or tactile. This break with reality tends to be frightening to the person, especially when the hallucinations are threatening. Psychomotor agitation continues in this stage. It should be noted that appearance of hallucinations indicates the imminence of *delirium tremens.*

DELIRIUM TREMENS STAGE Onset for this most serious of the withdrawal stages may range from 24 to 72 hours or longer. The extremely *high mortality* rate, 5 to 30 percent, is attributed to hyperthermia, peripheral vascular collapse, head trauma, or infection.[1] In addition to extreme agitation, psychomotor hyperactivity, and hallucinations, delusions appear that are seldom related to the hallucinations. Symptoms of this stage may include tachycardia, diaphoresis, tachypnea, elevated blood pressure, fever, and convulsive activity—grand mal or petit mal. Frequently the person is terrified and combative in response to threatening delusions and hallucinations. The person should also be carefully evaluated for presence of head trauma, infections, or other injuries and illnesses that might add to, or be responsible for, the severe symptoms.

With careful, knowledgeable assessment and planned intervention, the life-threatening delirium tremens stage can be prevented. The goal of intervention is to duplicate the action of alcohol on the CNS, thereby preventing uncontrolled withdrawal. The person can then be gradually withdrawn from alcohol and, one hopes, avoid the life-threatening aspects of advanced withdrawal.

NURSING INTERVENTION WITH THE ALCOHOLIC

The ED nurse has an invaluable role to play in the prevention of serious withdrawal symptoms as well as in the initial care of the acutely withdrawing person brought to the ED, as the following list of functions shows.

1. Thorough *assessment* of the patient's physical and psychological status is imperative on admission. This should include observation of orientation to time, place, and reality as well as careful assessment of neurological, muscular, skeletal, and other body system intactness and responsivity.

2. *Knowledge* of accepted *chemical agents* useful in alleviating and reducing the symptoms of uncontrolled withdrawal is also important, for example, Valium, Librium, Sparine, chlorpromazine, paraldehyde, meprobamate, diphenylhydantoin, and many others. The chemicals prescribed by the physician will vary as to specific drug, route of administration, dosage, and frequency. The nurse, however, can suggest the consideration of chemical intervention as assessment is begun.

3. Provide a physically *safe environment* for the severely agitated person. Equipment dangling overhead must be removed or secured to prevent head or body injury. Cords and bed controls (if present) should also be removed. Dimmed room lighting, or a consistent source of dim light in the alcoholic's room or cubicle, is frequently helpful in reducing sources of stimulation.

4. Prevent *excessive* tactile, auditory, or visual *stimulation,* i.e., people and noise. Decreased stimulation helps to calm the hallucinating and delusional person.

5. Recognize that the alcoholic is *ill* in the truest sense of the term; he or she is not able to control withdrawal behavior without assistance or support.

In addition to these suggested areas of consideration, the ED nurse needs to evaluate his or her own *attitudes* toward the alcoholic. Very judgmental, negative, and condemning attitudes may block the nurse's ability to evaluate objectively the needs of the person who is acutely withdrawing.

PSYCHOSOCIAL COMPONENTS OF DRUG ABUSE

With all the emphasis placed on the "drug revolution" of the sixties, remarkably little consistent information has been generated regarding the "whys" and "whos" of illicit drug use. (On the other hand, much is known about "what" drug abuse is and the forms it takes.) For each study that purports to have identified a personality profile of the drug abuser, another study can be found to refute it. This is especially true for the tremendous volume of research conducted into the effects of marijuana. Thus, to attempt to identify specific traits or behavior patterns of the potential drug abuser here would be difficult at best. The emphasis in this section, then, is on describing behaviors often found in certain drug abuser populations that frequent EDs.

The paradigm presented above describing the development of alcoholism over three phases also applies to many forms of drug abuse, especially narcotic and barbiturate-sedative abusers. People who abuse hallucinogens and stimulants frequently do not experience physical dependence and a concomitant physical withdrawal syndrome. Psychological dependence, however, does contribute to continued drug ingestion, experimentation, and/or combining of drugs. The underlying motivation for some drug abusers is a desire to experience mind expansion or cosmic awareness, or to adventure into "inner space."

DRUG ABUSE AND PERSONALITY

Personality characteristics of drug abusers consist of all the characteristics of nonabusers. It is simply not possible to describe the personality profile of the barbiturate or amphetamine abuser, for example, since abusers come from all socioeconomic backgrounds, age groups, and ethnocultural heritages. In addition, the trend recently has been one of *multiple* drug abuse, indicating that abuse of a single category of drug is much less common than previously believed. In spite of this inability to make conclusive statements about personality traits of drug abusers, limited descriptions of recurring idiosyncracies of personality have been identified.

HALLUCINOGEN ABUSERS   Traits descriptive of the abuser of hallucinogens (LSD, mescaline, marijuana, etc.) include hostility, high anxiety, dependence, impulsiveness, irresponsibility, nonperformance, and pleasure-seeking. Intellectually, psychedelic abusers have been variously characterized as underachievers, above average academically, or as indistinguishable from nonusers. Others state that the personality of the psychedelic abuser can range from total normality to acute psychosis.

AMPHETAMINE ABUSERS   The so-called "speed freak" personality may consist of varying degrees of disillusionment, rebellion, anxiety, tension, alienation, escape from sexuality, or curiosity and hedonism. In addition, significant levels of depression have been found in amphetamine abusers as evidenced by acute sadness, agitation, and psychomotor dulling. A general dissatisfaction with life has also been identified in some amphetamine abusers.

BARBITURATE ABUSERS   Persons who excessively use barbiturates and sedative-hypnotics may be depressed or anxious, or they may use the drugs to offset the "up" associated with "speed." As with the other types of drugs, the "barb" abuser may be seeking an avenue to express rebellion, dissatisfaction with life, frustration, anger, or a deep-seated desire to hurt significant others.

Once a person has developed a drug-abusing behavior pattern, several other personality traits may appear. Common among these traits is a degree of deceptiveness and denial very similar to that found in the alcoholic. In order to continue to blot out, distort, or rearrange reality, drug abusers must explain the behavior to themselves. They may do so by use of defense mechanisms such as rationalization, projection, denial, and repression. For the adolescent drug abuser who has not yet developed mature coping behaviors, the recourse to defensive maneuvers forms a consistent pattern.

It should be carefully noted, however, that *depending on which drug is abused,* and the prevailing societal attitudes toward the drug, the drug abuser may not be labeled as deviant in any way. This contradiction has become most obvious in reference to use of marijuana, which appears to have acquired a degree of societal sanction in many parts of the United States.

NARCOTIC ABUSERS   More commonly, the person who abuses narcotic drugs is referred to as an *addict.* Although the physical and psychological dependence may be just as great with the barbiturate abuser, the *addict* label has acquired a distinctly negative, fear-tinged connotation. Largely this is due to the criminalization of the narcotic abuser as he or she seeks to support a dependence that is totally rejected by society.

The stereotype of the drug addict as a "sex fiend" or "dope fiend" has served to preserve some basic misconceptions among the public. The narcotic addict's sex drive is dulled or repressed as drug-seeking and drug-using behavior becomes the major occupation. Thus, fear of sexual aggression from the heroin addict, for instance, seems to be somewhat unjustified. Apprehension regarding criminal behavior of addicts is, to an extent, realistic. The addict must obtain an expensive illegal drug supply for which financial resources are necessary. Theft, assault, and prostitution often serve as the means to obtain such financing.

To achieve and maintain the narcotic addict life-style, the abuser develops certain well-known personality characteristics. Addicts have been described as cunning, devious, perverted, amoral, unfeeling, and, above all, manipulative. They are skilled at "conning" others and playing interpersonal games to achieve their ends. These very well-developed and frequently reinforced behaviors are quite adaptive to the addict's life but act as almost impenetrable barriers in many treatment situations including the ED.

The narcotic addict, when in contact with treatment facilities, may present a recalcitrant, helpless picture to the nurse. Genuineness of this behavior, unfortunately, is often lacking. The addict needs health care services for illness, infection, trauma, or overdose. Once the immediate crisis is over, however, the addict may seem totally ungrateful and unappreciative of the assistance received. For the nurse, this is a "hard pill to swallow." As one way to partially cope with the frustration experienced when caring for the addict, the nurse can remember that (1) paradoxical behavior is often a part of the drug abuser's personality, (2) the behavior represents a defensive coping style, and (3) this behavior is appropriate to the addict's life-style to which he or she generally returns after discharge.

Alcoholics and drug abusers possess the same characteristics as nonabusers of chemical substances. Differences become clear, however, in the *degree* of expression and dependence on various behaviors. The psychological and/or physical dependence characteristic of the excessive user of chemicals also fosters excess in use of defense mechanisms and other coping behaviors.

Nursing has much to offer these patients in terms of physical care as well as initial psychological intervention. A first step in being able to develop nursing approaches applicable to these patient populations is a basic understanding of the patient's personality dynamics. To this end, the information discussed in this chapter has been presented.

Table 36-1 A drug abuse reference chart for the ED.

Drug of abuse	Street names	Route of administration
Stimulants		
1. Amphetamines	Uppers, pep pills, wakeups, A, cranks, chalk, ups, lid poppers, sparkle plenties,	By mouth in pill or capsule form. Intravenous after liquefying, i.e., "shooting up." User may experience a "flash" or "rush"—a rapid, euphoric, intense feeling of well-being, a jolt of energy.
Benzedrine (amphetamine sulfate)	Greenies, footballs, bennies, cartwheels, roses, hearts, peaches	
Methedrine (methamphetamine)	Speed, meth, crystal	
Dexedrine (dextroamphetamine sulfate)	Dexies, Christmas trees, hearts, oranges	
2. Cocaine	C, majo, happy dust, coke, snow, dust, bernies, flake, stardust, gold dust, incentive, sniff	Sniffing ("snorting"). Injecting. "Speedball": Combination of cocaine and heroine or morphine sniffed or taken intravenously.
Sedatives		
1. Alcohol: Beverage alcohol, e.g., wine, whiskey, gin, beer	Booze, hooch, sauce, suds	By mouth straight or mixed.
2. Barbiturates	Downers, sleepers, barbs, candy, cap, goofers	By mouth in pill or capsule form.
Sodium amytal	Blue angels, blue devils, blue birds, blue heavens	
Tuinal (amobarbital sodium or secobarbital sodium)	Tooies, Christmas trees, rainbows, double trouble	
Luminal (phenobarbital)	Phennies, pink lady	
Nembutal (pentobarbital sodium)	Yellow jackets, goof balls, dolls, nimbies	
Seconal (secobarbital sodium)	Red devils, seggy, red birds, seccy, reds	

Drug of abuse	Street names	Route of administration
3. Methaqualone (Quaalude) (nonbarbiturate sedative)	Sopors, luding, soapers, the live drug, mandrakes, heroin for lovers, wallbangers	By mouth in pill or capsule form.
Hallucinogens 1. Marijuana	Mary Jane, hash, stuff, hay, joints, reefers, pot, grass, dope, hemp, tea, love weed, roach, weed, doobie, gold, number	Smoked in cigarette form. Eaten alone or with food.
2. LSD (lysergic acid diethylamide tartrate)	Acid, the hawk, blue acid, sugar cubes, royal blue, pearly gates, heavenly blue, instant zen, 25, trip	By mouth usually. In food soaked with the drug. "Freaked out": a bad drug experience. Also in pill, liquid, or capsule form.
3. Psilocybin	Magic mushroom, sacred mushroom	Mushrooms by mouth, or in pill, capsule, or liquid form.
4. Dimethoxamphetamine	STP (serenity-tranquility-peace), syndicate acid, DOM	By mouth in pill or capsule form.
5. Mescaline (peyote)	Mesc, cactus, big chief, half moon, the button tops, a moon, P, mescal beans, tops, the bad seed, mescal button	By mouth, subcutaneous, intramuscularly.
6. Dimethyltryptamine	DMT, forty-five minute psychosis, businessman's special	Parsley, tobacco, or marijuana are soaked with the drug which is then smoked. May be injected.
7. Phencyclidine	Angel dust, peace pill, hog, PCP, synthetic marijuana	Capsules by mouth, or the powder is sprinkled on parsley, marijuana, or tobacco and smoked.

Table 36-1 (continued)

Drug of abuse	Street names	Route of administration
Narcotics		
1. Morphine and heroin	Heroin: Junk, shit, snow, horse, stuff, dope, hard stuff, boy, skag, joy powder, smack, H, crap, harry, brother, caballo Morphine: Morf, monkey, Miss Emma, morphie, M, dreamer, unkie, white stuff, hocus	Subcutaneous: "Chippying," "skin pop-ping," "joy popping." Intravenous: "Mainlining." Injecting paraphernalia called "works," "artillery," "biz."
2. Codeine	Schoolboy, junk	By mouth in pill or liquid elixir form.
3. Hydromorphone (Dilaudid)	D, lords	Injectable.
4. Meperidine (Demerol, Dolantal, isonipecaine, pethidine)		By mouth or injectable.
5. Methadone (Adanon, Amidon, Dolophine)	Dolls, dollies, 10-8-20	By mouth or injectable.
Volatile substances	Gasoline, glues, paint, nail polish, lighter fluid, cleaning fluids, and other flammable liquids	Vapors are sniffed; plastic bags may be used to concentrate vapors, then bag contents are inhaled.

REFERENCES

1. Anderson, Richard H., and Weisman, Maxwell N., *The Alcoholic in the Emergency Room,* The National Council on Alcoholism, New York, June 1972, p. 3.

BIBLIOGRAPHY

Ashley, Richard, *Heroin: The Myths and the Facts,* St. Martin's, New York, 1972.

Blane, Howard T., *The Personality of the Alcoholic,* Harper & Row, New York, 1968.

Block, Marvin, *Alcohol and Alcoholism: Drinking and Dependence,* Wadsworth, Belmont, Calif., 1970.

Burkhalter, Pamela K., *Nursing Care of the Alcoholic and Drug Abuser,* McGraw-Hill, New York, 1975.

Catanzaro, Ronald J. (ed.), *Alcoholism: The Total Treatment Approach,* Charles C Thomas, Springfield, Ill., 1968.

Cortina, Frank M., *Face to Face,* Columbia University Press, New York, 1972.

Crowley, Thomas J., The Reinforcers for Drug Abuse: Why People Take Drugs," *Comprehensive Psychiatry,* vol. 13, January 1972, pp. 51–62.

Hayman, Max, *Alcoholism: Mechanism and Management,* Charles C Thomas, Springfield, Ill., 1966.

Keup, Wolfram (ed.), *Drug Abuse: Current Concepts and Research,* Charles C Thomas, Springfield, Ill., 1972.

Kissin, Benjamin, and Gross, Milton M., "Drug Therapy in Alcoholism," *Current Psychiatric Therapies,* vol. 10, 1970, pp. 135–144.

Knott, David H., and Beard, James D., "Acute Withdrawal from Alcohol," *Emergency Medicine,* May 1969, pp. 38–41.

Louria, Donald B., *Overcoming Drugs,* McGraw-Hill, New York, 1971.

McNichol, Ronald W., *The Treatment of Delirium Tremens and Related States,* Charles C Thomas, Springfield, Ill., 1970.

Weil, Andrew, *The Natural Mind,* Houghton Mifflin, Boston, 1972.

INDEX